The Mindful Health Care Professional

A PATH TO PROVIDER WELLNESS AND PATIENT-CENTERED CARE

Dr. Carmelina D'Arro

ELSEVIER

Elsevier
3251 Riverport Lane
St. Louis, Missouri 63043

Senior Content Strategist: Lauren Boyle
Senior Content Development Specialist: Vaishali Singh
Publishing Services Manager: Deepthi Unni
Senior Project Manager: Kamatchi Madhavan
Design Direction: Renee Duenow

Printed in India

Last digit is the print number: 9 8 7 6 5 4 3 2 1

Working together
to grow libraries in
developing countries

www.elsevier.com • www.bookaid.org

for
all people who entrust a health care professional with their well-being

for
all those who dedicate themselves
to the well-being of others

May they all find healing
in the bonds forged
through Presence.

PREFACE

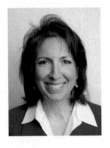

*Don't turn your head. Keep look-
ing at the bandaged place. That's
where the Light enters you.*
Rumi[1]

One could say I started writing this
book over 50 years ago. I am pres-
ently 55 years old. No, I was not
writing in the crib (if so, writing
would be much easier for me!), but the experiences that
shaped me as a health care professional started from the
very beginning of my life. Each moment of trauma, each
moment of shame, each moment of abandonment—each
moment of wounding—called for healing and attuned me
to the wounds of others.

My personal journey harkens back to the Greek myth
of Chiron, the archetypal wounded healer. The deep
wound of this centaur-like creature forces him to con-
front his own pain and suffering, and, by doing so, he
learns to cope with suffering and heal himself. As a result, he develops a profound sense of empathy, enabling
him to heal others. My own wounds reflect a family
history of pain resulting from war, poverty, and abuse.
This legacy manifested for many years as low self-
esteem, perfectionism, and workaholism despite achieving outward success in more than one profession, first as
a concert pianist and then as a dentist. Anxiety and
depression knocked at my door regularly, never bad
enough to cancel patient appointments, but bad enough
to make life miserable at times. In retrospect, I can see
clearly that it is *because* of my struggles, not in spite of
them, that I am able to embrace the suffering of others
in a way that heals.

How did I cope with suffering, find healing, and by
doing so, learn to help others heal? The simple act of
paying attention to the present moment experience, no
matter how uncomfortable, and allowing it space and
kindness—in a nutshell, mindfulness. So many times, I
was plagued by negative thoughts about myself: "I'm
lazy, I'm stupid, I'm going to fail," or, "I am a bad dentist." With practice over time, steadiness emerges that
can withstand the buffeting blows of self-criticism. With
practice, kind presence emerges followed by understanding and peace. With practice, this presence seeps
into encounters with others, especially with those who
suffer.

This book contains the fruits of my journey as a
wounded healer. Out of a deep desire to understand and
relieve my own suffering and that of others, a collection
of resources has arisen, which has enriched my work as
a dentist and the work of other health care professionals
I have taught, as I hope it will yours, too.

As I tune into my experience in this moment, I notice
the impulse to edit some more and a worry that I must
capture my thoughts the "right" way, to inspire you to
read on. Along with that, I notice a tightness in my
chest. I breathe with this worry, this impulse, this tightness, invite them in and allow them all space. Now, I
have a fluttering in the heart with a sense of excitement
at the possibility that, in experiencing this book, a seed
of change may take root in you so that you may heal
yourself and those in your care.

REFERENCES

1. Rumi J, Barks C. *Delicious Laughter: Rambunctious Teaching Stories From the Mathanawi of Jelaluddin Rumi.*
Athens: Maypop; 1990.

Dr. Carmelina D'Arro

ACKNOWLEDGMENTS

I thank the many mindfulness teachers—in retreats, lectures, practice groups, and books—who taught me how to stay steady in the storms of life and to find real happiness and peace. This includes a special psychotherapist, Dr. Jean Hauser, who introduced me to mindfulness meditation many years ago. I believe she saved me from becoming another grim statistic and launched me on a mission to share mindfulness with others.

I thank the many trailblazers for mindfulness in health care who have inspired me and served as mentors, including Patricia Dobkin, Nareg Apelian, John Lovas, Diane Riebel, Debbie Holexa, Ron Epstein, and Michael Baime. I thank my teachers at UConn Dental School, who modeled competence, commitment, and compassion, as well as my residency director, Mark Schmidt, who had much more confidence in me than I did in myself. I thank my speech coach Dilip Abayasakara who helped me grow as a speaker and who introduced me to the magic of mind-mapping for writing and speaking. Thank you to my DESEAA Toastmasters club for lending me your ears and support as I practiced sharing the concepts in this book.

I thank the many patients who have entrusted me with their health and their stories, many of which are shared here. I thank the librarians at Christiana Care for helping me gather the references needed to do this research. Thank you to the administrators at Christiana Care Health Center, McGill University Faculty of Dentistry, and Delaware Technical Community College for the privilege of teaching this material, as it gave me the chance to understand and develop more fully the models and concepts presented here. I thank Caitlyn McDonough for her administrative support early on and Jon Nelson for bringing the tree model to life with his graphics artistry.

I am grateful to all the reviewers for their feedback and encouragement, including Patricia Dobkin, Nareg Apelian, Connie Cicorelli, Mikaela Frazier, Kwan Ngai, Jessica Muller, Kevin Toussaint, Max Baer, Martha Barry, Cherie Rebar, and Brittany Sykes, especially those whose words are featured throughout these pages—they didn't realize at the time that their spontaneous personal notes and insights entered on the margins would become the voices of HCPs for this book (with their permission)! Thank you, Dustin Samples, for your editorial work and helping me reach the submissions finish line. Thank you, Jocelyn Dumas, at Elsevier who was a champion for this project early on; she understood my passion and sense of urgency for this project.

I thank my parents for providing me with the education they could only dream of for themselves and for the financial support that allowed me the space to do this work. I thank my closest friends who provide ballast and joy every day. Thank you to Pendle Hill in Wallingford, Pennsylvania; Centre Monthly Meeting in Centreville, Delaware; and Holly Haven in Rehoboth Beach, Delaware for providing me a writing sanctuary over the past few years. Speaking of sanctuary... Thank you to Charlie whose patience, confidence, empathy, intelligent sounding board, and domestic support provide stability and sustenance to keep going every day.

Dr. Carmelina D'Arro

CONTENTS

VIDEO CONTENTS

Not all health care encounters are created equal. Consider the following: many encounters involve a consultation; others involve a procedure with sedation or general anesthesia. Finally, there are the many encounters involving technical procedures without sedation—with a fully conscious patient. Such medical and dental procedures, be they diagnostic or therapeutic, often induce pain or evoke anxiety. The doctors, nurses, and allied health professionals who provide these procedures have the unique calling to simultaneously manage not only the *human body* and all of its technical complexity but also the *human being* attached to that complex anatomic structure. Despite this unique calling, the education and training of many health care professionals (HCPs) still resemble that of a skilled technician.

It is important to clarify the distinction between curing and healing. The focus of *curing* is to remove the objective signs and symptoms of disease, and this is the focus of most health care. On the other hand, *healing*, while it may also include curing, focuses on the subjective experience of the patient by inquiring, "What is this person's experience of their condition? Of this procedure? Of their life?" Healing aims to alleviate suffering and to avoid creating more suffering whenever possible. Attempts to cure without healing can create harm, like when a dentist coerces a patient to endure a painful tooth extraction (as we will see in the opening story of Sally in Chapter 1) and, by doing so, creates trauma. Conversely, healing can occur in the absence of a cure, as when a nurse practitioner stops to truly listen to a woman's story of lost pregnancies in the aftermath of yet another.

People seek health care not to get procedures and tests done but to heal some form of suffering, and Chapter 1 offers evidence of this universal expectation. In the words of the beloved physician and medical ethicist Eric Cassells:

The relief of suffering, it would appear, is considered one of the primary ends of medicine by patients and layperson, but not by the medical profession... Patients and their friends and families do not make a distinction between physical and nonphysical sources of suffering in the same way that doctors do.[1]

It is time for all HCPs, especially procedure-oriented ones, to embrace a larger role than just an educated technician—more than just a body mechanic. We are called to be healers. Research shows that this is what patients want, and the qualities and relational skills of a healer are the very criteria that patients use to evaluate competence.[2] Further, the lack of these qualities and skills is what leads patients to sue.[3]

Are the qualities and skills of a healer learnable? Research has shown that, indeed, they are[4]; therefore, they should be fundamental to the education and ongoing development of all HCPs. This book intends to light a path to the following end: embracing the role of the HCP as a healer for the benefit of both the patient and the provider. It represents the fruits of 25 years of clinical experience and inquiry about patient preferences. It represents more than 10 years as a dental educator and mindfulness teacher and 30 years of meditation practice. The intended audience of this book is any HCP, especially any doctor, nurse, or allied health professional who is procedure-oriented, at any stage, including learners, seasoned practitioners, and educators.

What are the qualities and skills of a healer? Research shows patients, especially when they are hurting or afraid, want their HCP to be calm, attentive, and empathetic. In Chapter 2, you will find time-tested, evidence-based practices that cultivate these very qualities. Next, how does an HCP connect with a patient in a way that conveys safety, care, and respect? Chapter 3 unveils the 6 essential communication skills. Whereas previous communication models focused entirely on the *consultation*, this book provides a model for communication before, during, and after *procedures* (including procedures in which patients can't talk!). In Chapter 4, we will apply the mind-training practices and communication skills covered in Chapters 2 and 3 to common clinical challenges, such as delivering bad news and requests for unethical care. Finally, Chapter 5—my favorite chapter—reveals a multitude of simple, efficient, non-pharmacologic interventions that allow procedures like injections and radiographs to flow more easily for the patient and the provider, too.

Being a healer requires, first and foremost, caring for oneself. So many external forces, like pandemics and administrative demands, are challenges to the sanity and wellness of HCPs all over the world. In addition, like myself, many HCPs are wounded healers with historical scars of their own to reckon with. This book provides core practices for attuning the mind and heart in a way that reduces stress and enhances the HCPs own emotional, mental, and physical well-being. When HCPs are well and resilient, they are more present and empathetic to the person in their care.

Lastly, while caring for ourselves enables us to care for others, the converse is also true: caring for others is ultimately a way to care for ourselves. In the words of Erich Fromm, "But in giving he cannot help bringing something to life in the other person, *and this which is brought to life reflects back to him*" (emphasis added).[5] This message is echoed in the prayer of Saint Francis of Assisi: "It is in giving that we receive." May this book help all HCPs receive the many gifts that come from serving others fully.

REFERENCES

1. Cassell EJ. The nature of suffering and the goals of medicine. *N Eng J Med.* 1982;306(11):639–645.
2. Riley JL 3rd, Gordan VV, Rindal DB; Dental Practice-Based Research Network Collaborative Group. Components of patient satisfaction with a dental restorative visit: results from the Dental Practice-Based Research Network. *J Am Dent Assoc.* 2012;143:1002–1010.
3. Zoppi K, Epstein RM. Is communication a skill? Communication behaviors and being in relation. *Fam Med.* 2002;34:319–324.
4. Riess H, Kelley JM, Bailey RW, et al. Empathy training for resident physicians: a randomized controlled trial of a neuroscience-informed curriculum. *J Gen Intern Med.* 2012;27:1280–1286.
5. Fromm E. *The Art of Loving.* New York: Perennial Library, 1989.

What is Your Job?

Stabbing, throbbing toothache in the middle of the night, again. Sally had been having pain for months in her lower left back tooth. She couldn't afford treatment and dreaded having dental work done ever since her traumatic dental experience as a child. So, she medicated herself for months and went to the ED once, too. Finally, she couldn't take it anymore.

The dental clinic nearby was swamped on the day she had her appointment. The receptionist told Sally to sign in on the sheet and thrust a stack of forms in front of her. After a long wait, she heard, "Smith!" as the assistant summoned her out of the waiting room. She shuddered and silently shuffled behind the assistant down a long hall to the treatment room.

"I'm going to take an x-ray of your tooth," announced the assistant as she raised Sally's chair into position. Sally's heart pounded, and she felt suffocated. She wanted to escape but knew that if she didn't take care of the problem, she would end up in the ED again. She writhed in pain as the assistant wrestled with the x-ray device. "Hold still," the assistant demanded. Finally, the assistant was done, but the worst was yet to come.

After a long wait, the dentist finally came in. He darted straight to the computer to see the radiograph. "That's got to come out. Get me some local," he said to the assistant and left the room. "Sign here," said the assistant as she thrust the consent form and pen in front of Sally. The dentist returned. "Your tooth has to be extracted. Any questions?" He

proceeded to recline the chair and commanded, "Open wide." She felt a sharp stabbing in the back of her mouth, and her whole body tensed up. She couldn't breathe at all. She felt pushing and pulling and terrible sharp pain. "Ow!" Sally cried. "You're okay," said the dentist as he continued to push and pull. She clutched the armrests and braced herself. Tears streamed down her cheeks. "You're OK. Stay open!" the dentist demanded. By the time Sally's tooth was out, she felt completely drained. The next time Sally went to the dentist was twenty years later.

Sadly, I have heard this story told many times in many variations throughout my career as a dentist. The common theme consists of pain that was ignored or minimized and boundaries that were violated. "I told them it hurt and they kept going." "I cried for help but they ignored me." Most of the time, the health care professional (HCP) delivered quality technical care. Most of the time, the patient was cured of their infection or disease. In Sally's case, the dentist applied scientific knowledge to accurately diagnose Sally's problem and devise a treatment plan. He extracted Sally's tooth well based on the current standard of care—no roots left behind. Yet, clearly, there was something missing in the interaction between this HCP and the patient. This story highlights that quality care is more than just excellent technical care.

What is your job as an HCP? Based on how we are trained, licensed, and compensated, the HCP's role is primarily mechanical, involving scientific knowledge and technical skill. Biochemistry, anatomy, physiology, pharmacology, clinical skills training: these are the typical core subjects of our education and credentialing—in summary, scientific knowledge and technical skills. After education and training, we are compensated by performing a procedure: specifically, one that matches a billable code. But, as the story of Sally illustrates, focusing only on scientific knowledge, technical skills, and billable codes can actually result in deeply wounding a patient.

Perhaps considering the role of the HCP from the patient's perspective will help elucidate why Sally's dental experience left her more wounded than healed, despite her technical procedure being well-done.

YOUR JOB FROM THE PATIENT'S PERSPECTIVE

You may have heard patients assert, "I have the best doctor!" or "She is the best dental hygienist." Even people who know nothing about medicine or dentistry are convinced they know the quality of care they receive. If their assessment is not based on technical skills, what are the patient's criteria when judging the quality of their care?

Video 1.1 captures the voice of a patient describing her doctor. Notice how much of her opinion is based on the doctor's technical skill and knowledge versus other factors.

Everything this patient describes involves her interactions with her doctor and the way he relates to her. Several studies on dental patient satisfaction suggest that her sentiments are representative of most patients. A large-scale study on patient preferences by Riley et al. gathered information from 197 dental practices and almost 6000 patient satisfaction surveys, revealing that "a patient's judgment of dentists' skills and quality of care are based on *personal interactions with the dentist, the level of comfort, and post-treatment sensitivity*" (emphasis added).[1] The same researchers cite many studies showing that "patients evaluate the quality of their care according to a range of criteria, particularly their dentist's interpersonal communication." Further, "In terms of patients' own definition of quality of care, empathy emerges as a key factor."[2]

In addition to studies on patient satisfaction, malpractice trends further elucidate patients' definition of quality of care. The Harvard Medical Practice Study gathered data on 31,429 patients in 51 hospitals in NY State.[3] Out of this cohort, they found 280 adverse events. One would expect that most adverse events would result in a lawsuit, yet, out of the 280 adverse events, only 8 resulted in lawsuits. One would also expect that there would not be lawsuits filed by patients who had not experienced an adverse event. Yet, there were a total of 39 such lawsuits! So, the vast majority of the lawsuits (39 out of 47 total cases) were not the result of a technical problem with the care delivered.

What Makes Patients Sue?

Several studies have shown that problems with the technical quality of care do not usually lead patients to sue. "The number of lawsuits suffered by a physician is not related to the quality of medicine practiced."[3] In fact, one study reported, "No relationship was found between prior malpractice claims history and the technical quality of practice."[4] What, then, makes patients sue, if not a breach in the technical quality of care?

Research has found that most of the issues that lead patients to sue are related to the doctor–patient relationship. An article on communication skills from the *Journal of Dental Education* asserts unequivocally that "… *poor communication* is the most common cause of patient dissatisfaction" (emphasis added).[5] In medicine, "Breakdowns in communication between patients and physicians…are critical factors leading to malpractice litigation."[6] One particular aspect of communication that, when missing, triggers the most patient complaints is empathy, as we will discuss more later.

The quality of the doctor–patient relationship is especially important in the case of adverse events as it will determine the outcome. A study of malpractice cases in oral surgery practices concluded that "most of the lawsuits in oral surgery practice can be prevented… by dealing with the impact of the surgical error through good patient rapport and communication."[7] Similarly, several studies of physicians have confirmed that "Patients who suffered bad outcomes were less likely to sue if their physician's bedside manner was caring and compassionate."[3] The mounting evidence of the importance of good bedside manner prompted the American Medical Association to issue the following statement: "It is increasingly apparent that one of our best protections against a professional liability lawsuit is the creation of a good physician-patient relationship."[8]

While good bedside manner reduces the risk of lawsuits, this is not the main reason we are called to be caring and compassionate. "The originators of client-centered and patient-centered health care were well aware of the moral implications of their work, which was based on deep respect for patients as unique living beings, and the obligation to care for them on their terms."[9]

BENEFITS OF PATIENT-CENTERED CARE

Avoiding lawsuits is just one of many benefits of compassionate, patient-centered care, not only for the patient, but also for the HCP. To start, patient-centered care avoids harming patients in the way that Sally was harmed. Medical research found "empathetic communication skills are associated with increased patient satisfaction, improved adherence to therapy, decreased medical errors, fewer malpractice claims, better outcomes, decreased burnout and increased physician well-being."[10] A review study in dentistry cites a host of benefits associated with empathy: "negotiated treatment plans, treatment adherence, increased patient satisfaction, reduced dental anxiety."[11] Finally, a benefit that any HCP can appreciate is time savings; both active listening[12] and empathy[13] have been found to shorten the time of a patient encounter.

Considering these benefits, one would expect that bedside/chairside manner and relational skills would be a fundamental part of education and licensure requirements. Yet, "systematic development of [communication] skills in student practitioners tends to be limited and is often overshadowed by curricular time spent teaching technical skills rather than integrating behavioral and technical abilities."[14] Both medical and dental education cultures still give "privileged status to scientific knowledge," and "insufficient attention tends to be paid to reflection, values, and wisdom."[15]

What little is taught about relational skills and ethics is overridden by *the hidden curriculum*—"The values and behaviors that trainees learn by observing what actually takes place in hospitals and clinics rather than what is explicitly taught in their communication skills classes."[16] In the same way that a child adopts the values of parents and authority figures by modeling, trainees absorb the values of professional role models—a role model's way of relating to patients speaks much louder than what is taught in the classroom. The hidden curriculum in the health care professions conveys the value of detachment and casts patients as "victims of disease, objects for learning, subjects for research."[17]

Why aren't HCPs taught more about patient-centered care if it is so critical to quality care? Medical and dental education and training still reflects the legacy of a paternalistic model of care. In the days of paternalism, the doctor would dictate the treatment plan to patients, based on their own priorities. In the days of paternalism, patients assumed a "Whatever you say, doc" attitude and tolerated their treatment. Yet, patients are no longer satisfied with just being passive recipients of care. Researchers confirm, "Patients want to be involved and educated about treatment options and for health care professionals to listen, pay attention to their concerns, and treat them as individuals."[14] We have entered the age of evidence-based medicine and patient-centered care. Evidence-based medicine includes the triad of best external evidence, individual clinical expertise, and *patient values and expectations*.[18] Patient-centered care, according to the official statement from the Institute of Medicine (renamed the National Academy of Medicine) consists of "providing care that is respectful of and responsive to individual patient *preferences, needs, and values*, and ensuring that the patient values guide all clinical decisions."[19]

The path to patient-centered care has been hard to define: "Patient-centered care is integral to health care quality, yet little is known regarding how to achieve patient-centeredness in the hospital setting."[20] What is clear is that patient-centered care requires attention to the connection between the provider and the patient. "Relationship is itself an important therapeutic tool, one that often gets little formal acknowledgment."[21]

The HCP must uncover and respond to "individual patient preferences, needs, and values,"[19] before, during, and after treatment, especially during challenging technical procedures. But how exactly should they do this? Unfortunately, like good customer service, patient-centered care is more than a formulaic checklist of words or behaviors. A recent personal experience illustrates this point. After realizing I hadn't been receiving all of my phone messages, I called my cell phone company. The customer service representative responded with a robotic, "that sounds very frustrating, I'm sorry you are having this problem," followed by the classic line, "you are a valued customer, and we are committed to providing you excellent service." Even though the representative said the right words and resolved the issue, I felt patronized by their choreographed approach.

Caring for a patient in a way that honors their unique needs and values is truly an art form and a labor of love. At times, it can be as simple and as subtle as a pause or an understanding look. Discerning this requires being *present*. Imagine the words and actions of the HCP like the fruit of a tree. For a tree to bear fruit, it must be well-rooted. Likewise, for an HCP's words and actions to meet the patient's needs in the moment, the HCP must be rooted, grounded, present. What are the qualities of a patient-centered HCP, and, even more importantly, is it possible to cultivate these qualities? This is the subject of Chapter 2.

REFERENCES

1. Riley JL III, Gordan VV, Rindal DB; Dental Practice-Based Research Network Collaborative Group. Components of patient satisfaction with a dental restorative visit: results from the Dental Practice-Based Research Network. *J Am Dent Assoc.* 2012;143:1002–1010.
2. Mercer SW, Reynolds WJ. Empathy and quality of care. *Br J Gen Pract.* 2002;52:S9–S12.
3. Virshup BB, Oppenberg AA, Coleman MM. Strategic risk management: reducing malpractice claims through more effective patient-doctor communication. *Am J Med Qual.* 1999;14:153–159.
4. Entman SS, Glass CA, Hickson GB, et al. The relationship between malpractice claims history and subsequent obstetric care. *JAMA.* 1994;272:1588–1591.
5. Orsini CA, Jerez OM. Establishing a good dentist-patient relationship: skills defined from the dental faculty perspective. *J Dent Educ.* 2014;78:1405–1415.
6. Levinson W. Physician-patient communication. A key to malpractice prevention. *JAMA.* 1994;272:1619–1620.
7. Marei HF. Medical litigation in oral surgery practice: lessons learned from 20 lawsuits. *J Forensic Leg Med.* 2013;20:223–225.
8. Frankel RM. Emotion and the physician-patient relationship. *Motiv Emot.* 1995;19:163–173.
9. Epstein RM, Street RL Jr. The values and value of patient-centered care. *Ann Fam Med.* 2011;9:100–103.
10. Riess H, Kelley JM, Bailey RW, et al. Empathy training for resident physicians: a randomized controlled trial of a neuroscience-informed curriculum. *J Gen Intern Med.* 2012;27:1280–1286.
11. Jones LM, Huggins TJ. Empathy in the dentist-patient relationship: review and application. *N Z Dent J.* 2014;110:98–104.
12. Leebov W, Rotering C. *The Language of Caring Guide for Physicians: Communication Essentials for Patient-Centered Care.* 2nd ed. USA: Language of Caring, LLC; 2014.
13. Morse DS, Edwardsen EA, Gordon HS. Missed opportunities for interval empathy in lung cancer communication. *Arch Intern Med.* 2008;168:1853–1858.
14. Wener ME, Schönwetter DJ, Mazurat N. Developing new dental communication skills assessment tools by including patients and other stakeholders. *J Dent Educ.* 2011;75:1527–1541.
15. Lovas JG, Lovas DA, Lovas PM. Mindfulness and professionalism in dentistry. *J Dent Educ.* 2008;72: 998–1009.
16. Riess H. Can empathy be taught? *Medscape.* February 2013. Available at: https://www.medscape.com/viewarticle/778463. Accessed March 2019.
17. Hafferty FW, Franks R. The hidden curriculum, ethics teaching, and the structure of medical education. *Acad Med.* 1994;69:861–871.
18. Sackett DL. Evidence-based medicine. *Semin Perinatol.* 1997;21:3–5.
19. Institute of Medicine (US) Committee on Quality of Health Care in America. *Crossing the Quality Chasm: A New Health System for the 21st Century.* Washington, DC: National Academies Press (US); 2001.
20. Aboumatar HJ, Chang BH, Danaf JA, et al. Promising practices for achieving patient-centered hospital care: a national study of high-performing US hospitals. *Med Care.* 2015;53:758–767.
21. Barnett L, Chambers M. *Reiki: Energy Medicine.* Rochester: Healing Arts Press; 1996.

At the Roots: What We Are

The physician professional is defined not only by what he or she must know and do, but most importantly by a profound sense of what the physician must be.[1]

Dr. J Cohen

For a moment, think of a time when you were in pain or afraid and a medical or dental professional cared for you. Set aside what they *did* for you and recall what they were like—what were the *qualities* they embodied that made you feel safe, comfortable, cared for, understood? Most likely, they were not rushed or agitated but calm and confident. Most likely, they were not distracted but rather focused on you and your experience. Most likely, they were not judgmental but accepting and empathetic.

Now, you are the health care professional (HCP), and you are called to embody these same traits. But what if, like many other HCPs, you are not feeling calm but stressed or overwhelmed? What if you are feeling scattered, stuck on your phone, and struggling to focus?

What if, instead of empathetic, you feel judgmental or irritated?

NEUROPLASTICITY AND MINDFULNESS

One evening, an elderly Cherokee brave told his grandson about a battle that goes on inside people. He said "my son, the battle is between two 'wolves' inside us all. One is evil. It is anger, envy, jealousy, sorrow, regret, greed, arrogance, self-pity, guilt, resentment, inferiority, lies, false pride, superiority, and ego. The other is good. It is joy, peace love, hope serenity, humility, kindness, benevolence, empathy, generosity, truth, compassion and faith." The grandson thought about it for a minute and then asked his grandfather: "which wolf wins?..." The old Cherokee simply replied, "the one that you feed."[2]

Historically, people believed that the brain forms during a critical period in early life and then remains static. After that critical time, a person is either empathetic or not, calm or not, focused or not. Over the past few decades, research in neuroscience has debunked this theory and confirmed what the Cherokee chief taught his grandson; the human brain is, in fact, anatomically and functionally mutable throughout life, and its development depends on what we feed it. Mindfulness is a way of feeding the good wolf. Mindfulness meditation practices create observable changes in brain anatomy and function,[3,4] and these changes can help both HCPs and their patients.

Mindfulness is the English translation of the Pali word *sati*, which means *awareness of the present moment* as well as *remembering* (what is skillful and beneficial).[5] Jon Kabat-Zinn defines mindfulness as "the awareness that emerges through paying attention, on purpose, in the present moment, and non-judgmentally."[6] The definition of mindfulness involves two parts: the "what" and the "how," as captured by Bishop et al.:

The first component involves the self-regulation of attention so that it is maintained on immediate experience, thereby allowing for increased recognition of mental events in the present moment. The second component involves adopting a particular orientation toward one's experiences in the present moment, an orientation that is characterized by curiosity, openness, and acceptance.[7]

Mindfulness is a trait, and mindfulness practices are meditation techniques that cultivate the qualities characterizing mindfulness: equanimity, attentiveness, self-awareness, and empathy (EASE). There are two main types of mindfulness practice: *focusing practices* that typically feature the breath, body sensations, or sounds as the focal point of attention, and *mindful awareness*, which is characterized by attending to all of the different aspects in the triad of experience, including thoughts, emotions, and sensations as they arise. All practices are done with an intention of kindness, curiosity, and acceptance.

Where Does Mindfulness Come From?

Although they originated from ancient Buddhist traditions, mindfulness practices have been disseminated in recent years in a secular form by a wave of contemporary Western teachers, including Jon Kabat-Zinn, Sharon Salzberg, Jack Kornfield, Joseph Goldstein, and Tara Brach. Jon Kabat-Zinn is largely credited for introducing mindfulness into health care. In 1979, he began teaching a secularized and standardized 8-week curriculum at the University of Massachusetts called Mindfulness-Based Stress Reduction (MBSR). The genius of Jon Kabat-Zinn was the creation of a standardized, secularized curriculum, which has allowed scientists to investigate the effects of mindfulness practices on the mind and body. Many studies have compared subjects before and after the 8-week MBSR course and have measured significant differences in mental and physical health[8] and even brain anatomy and function.[3]

Mindfulness in Health Care

Mindfulness training is beneficial to the well-being of both HCPs and their patients. "Several studies have demonstrated reduced stress, increased coping, and improved empathy among HCPs after completing an MBSR program."[9] Clinicians who are mindful are noted to be more patient-centered and highly rated by patients.[10] "Mindful physicians can be easily identified by patients and colleagues—they are present, attentive, curious, and unhindered by preconceptions."[11] Benefits of mindfulness practice to nurses include: "avoid burnout by decreasing tension; improve focus in order to quickly identify problems and administer appropriate interventions; and remain attentive to help patients and family members stay informed and relaxed."[12]

A summary of the research on the impact of mindfulness training programs on premed, medical, and practicing doctors and other HCPs states: "In general, results

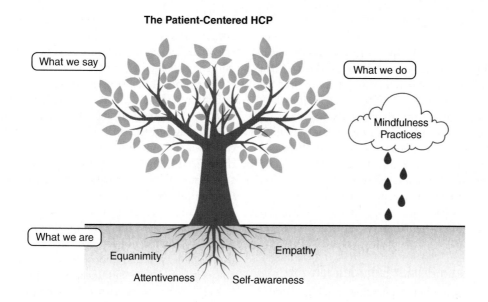

The Patient-Centered HCP

What we say

What we do

Mindfulness Practices

What we are

Equanimity

Empathy

Attentiveness

Self-awareness

Fig. 2.1 The Qualities of the Patient-Centered Provider. *HCP*, Health care professional.

indicate that such programmes are beneficial in terms of reducing negative emotions and stress, as well as enhancing mindfulness, empathy, and self-compassion."[13]

Because of its benefits to both HCPs and patients, mindfulness increasingly is being incorporated into medical and dental education to cultivate "healing presence"[14] as well as attentiveness and professionalism.[1] In fact, several medical schools have incorporated mindfulness training into their curricula.[13] Dr. John Lovas, a dentist and pioneer of mindfulness in health care writes, "Mindfulness training may be a practical way to help re-establish the ideal of wise health care professionals doing their best for patients and in the process deriving profound satisfaction as well as improved personal well-being and health."[1]

As an HCP, you have already demonstrated incredible strength and resilience. You have accomplished your level of knowledge and skills through discipline and hard work. You have faced the challenges of caring for patients and have found ways to endure. Now, you have the opportunity to learn mind training practices to develop additional qualities that will benefit you and your patients. These practices are simple to learn, free to practice, legal, and nonpharmacologic. The goal is not to fabricate anything but simply to water the seeds that already exist in you. Think of mindfulness practices as "feeding the good wolf" from the Cherokee story.

In the metaphor illustrated in Fig. 2.1, the roots of the tree represent the core qualities of the patient-centered HCP: EASE. The mindfulness practices cultivate these qualities and are represented by the water which nourishes the roots of the tree.

For each of these core qualities, supporting mindfulness practices will be provided. All of the formal mindfulness practices presented in this chapter come directly from the 8-week MBSR curriculum, an evidence-based curriculum taught worldwide. As a qualified MBSR teacher myself, I will be sharing the practices from this curriculum through text and accompanying videos. Through the videos and stories, I offer a model of a humanistic HCP, one who demonstrates commitment to the care of the whole person—not only the patient, but also themselves.

PRACTICING MINDFULNESS MEDITATION AND SUGGESTED PROGRAM

No reasonable person would exercise at the gym and then complain that they did not see an immediate improvement in their body. Similarly, the benefits of mindfulness practice are not often experienced while practicing; rather, they emerge slowly—sometimes when least expected. In other words, it takes some effort and patience. Consider formal mindfulness practice as "brain hygiene" or "mental flossing." Just as you brush and floss your teeth every day (hopefully!) to maintain oral health, it is recommended to set aside a few minutes to practice every day for your mental and physical health. If all you can manage is 2 minutes, this will still be beneficial. Evidence shows that frequency of practice is more important than length of time per session.[15,16]

Try to find a regular time that you reserve for practice instead of just waiting for an opportunity (which rarely comes since most of us are so good at filling our time with activity). I find that by practicing at the beginning of the day, I am more likely to practice, and the benefits seep into the day from the start. Others may find it easier to practice at the end of the day or at another time when there is no urgency to get anywhere.

Parasympathetic Primer Experiences

HCPs are known for being high-achieving, high-energy people, and this can make it very challenging, if not impossible, to try to meditate. Many HCPs are stuck in fight or flight reactivity, and this may explain the relative lack of traction of mindfulness practice among HCPs despite all of the benefits. Our "high-voltage" nature may reflect the types of personalities that are attracted to the profession, or it could be the result of the demands of the profession. Regardless, stress, anxiety, trauma, and traumatic stress are common among HCPs. *If you have a history of trauma, please see the Cautionary Note at the end of this chapter before starting mindfulness meditation.*

The "parasympathetic primer experiences" (PPEs) are intended to help "dial down" to a lower voltage by dissipating excess energy and inducing relaxation quickly. In doing so, these practices aim to soften the landing into what, for some, may be the unfamiliar terrain of stillness.

Tips on Dealing With Difficulties as You Practice

In the beginning, everyone who practices mindfulness meditation reports the same finding, "My mind is constantly wandering," and many immediately conclude, "I'm special, I can't do this." I can affirm that you are, indeed, special, but not for this reason! *Everyone's* mind wanders constantly, and, in fact, the human brain is hard-wired to do so to scan for potential threats to our safety and happiness. Scientists have even mapped out the neural network of the wandering mind and call it

the default mode network (DMN; more on this soon), but neuroscience is also showing how regular mindfulness practice over a short time can rewire the brain to be calmer, more focused, and more kind.

As you practice, if you find you are encountering difficulty, know that you can modify the instructions in a way that feels right to you. If the anchor of attention offered does not feel comfortable or stabilizing, you can choose a different one. The three recommended anchors include *the breath, body sensations,* and *sounds.* In addition, if the body position in the practice does not feel comfortable physically or psychologically, choose a position that feels right to you—*standing, sitting, walking,* or *lying down.* Finally, for most of the practices, you will be instructed to keep eyes closed. If that feels uncomfortable, you may choose to *open your eyes.* If difficulty persists despite modifications, you are encouraged to *simply listen to the words and the tone* of the guided practice for just a few moments and see what unfolds. Chances are that something will shift before long (it always does, eventually!) and you will have learned how to stay steady instead of reacting—a very important lesson for all of life.

Table 2.1 outlines the suggested program and includes hyperlinks to the videos of guided meditations included in the text, for your convenience. You do not need to follow the recordings every time you practice. After practicing a few times, if you prefer, you can try the practice silently on your own. However, many people find that each time they listen to the guidance, they notice something new or are reminded of an instruction they forgot. In addition, if you find you have a strong preference or aversion to any particular practice after giving it a fair trial, choose any practice that suits you in the moment. Although each practice is presented in association with one EASE quality, all practices cultivate all four qualities of EASE, so all are beneficial.

One final note: Many people find encouragement and strength by practicing with a group. HCPs who do not have a cohort to practice with might consider joining an MBSR class or a local practice group. Resources for more mindfulness information and training can be found in Appendix A.

Enjoy your mindfulness meditation journey!

Journaling

Each day you practice, you are encouraged to write your observations and reflections in a journal. A recommended

TABLE 2.1   Mind Training Program

Module	Theme	Parasympathetic Primer Experience (PPE)	Formal Practice	Informal Practice
1	Equanimity	Progressive muscle relaxation (PMR) 1. Introduction to PMR (see Video 2.1) 2. PMR practice (see Video 2.2)	Introduction to Body scan (see Video 2.3) Body scan seated (see Video 2.4) Body scan lying down (see Video 2.5)	Gratitude practice
2	Attentiveness	Mindful movement 1. Mindful standing movement (see Video 2.6) 2. Lying down movement (Audio 2.1) 3. Standing movement (Audio 2.2)	Awareness of breath (see Video 2.7) Walking meditation (see Video 2.8)	Mindfulness of daily activities: Washing hands (see Video 2.9)
3	Self-awareness	Diaphragmatic breathing (see Video 2.10)	Choice of anchors (see Video 2.11) Multiple anchors (see Video 2.12)	Three breaths (see Video 2.13) STOP (see Video 2.14)
4	Empathy and compassion	EFT tapping (see Video 2.16)	Compassion practice (see Video 2.15) Awareness of breath with emphasis on self-compassion (Instructions in the text)	Compassion practice at work (see Video 2.18) Compassion practice while driving (see Video 2.17)
5 (optional)	Integrating EASE	Any previous PPE	Recognize, allow, investigate, nurture (RAIN)	Any previous informal practice

TABLE 2.2   Recommended Journal Structure

Date	Practice/Duration	Emotions	Body Sensations	Believed Thoughts
Example: 1/1/23	Body scan/10 min	Impatience	Tightness in chest, forehead	• I can't do this (judgments) • Planning what will I have for dinner (leaning to the future) • I should have done that dental procedure differently (leaning to the past)

journal structure is provided in both Table 2.2 and in the appendices.

Note to educators: What distinguishes a skilled technician from an HCP? It is the quality of their presence—the healing qualities of EASE. Because these qualities are essential to becoming a resilient, compassionate, and ethical HCP, educating and training in these qualities is also essential—as essential as training surgeons in suturing techniques.

Some might consider cultivation of personal qualities not the domain of professional training. Yet, in a world that has become dominated by forces that are rapidly feeding "the bad wolf" and cultivating such qualities as anxiety, depression, and distractedness, HCPs must consciously, deliberately focus on feeding the good wolf.

Educators are encouraged to carve out time in class for mindfulness practice. This allows students who do not practice at home to at least experience the practices in class. Some possibilities for practice include starting a lecture with 2 minutes of meditation or starting clinic sessions with the sound of a bell that offers students a cue to take three conscious breaths.

Note that there are individuals whose vulnerabilities may be laid bare by mindfulness meditation in a way that could be destabilizing (see the **Cautionary Note** at the end of this chapter regarding trauma-sensitivity). Thus it is advisable to offer students the option to listen to the practices without actively engaging. This way, the practices will be available to the students later, when they are ready. Student-performance evaluations can be based on samples of journal entries, participation in group discussions, or recognition of key concepts of the meditation practices on a written examination.

THE FIRST "E" IN EASE: EQUANIMITY

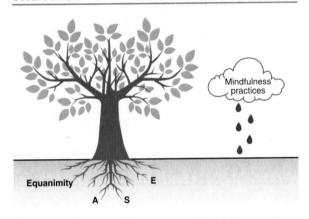

Eyes sparkling, the newly inducted president of the American Dental Student Association poses for a picture. This beautiful, young Korean-American is Jiwon Lee, a shining star in the dental class of 2014 at Columbia University. By the spring of her senior year, she had successfully passed her exam qualifying her for graduation.[17] On April 1, 2014, just weeks before graduation, she disappeared. Authorities searched for several weeks. Finally, her body was found in the Hudson River. Investigations revealed that she suffered from depression.[18]

Jiwon's tragic story resonates with my own struggles with depression early in my career. Harsh self-criticism continually overshadowed my sense of self-worth and confidence and sent me teetering over the valley of depression. It was as if a crowd of voices was following me, shouting indictments: "You're lazy, you're stupid, and

everyone is going to know!" I struggled to maintain a sense of balance, and equanimity was not a familiar place.

Equanimity is "remaining centered in the middle of whatever is happening" and the ability "to see without being caught by what we see."[19] This is not to be confused with "aequanimitas"—a detached, clinical stance toward patients—extolled by the father of modern medicine, William Osler, as avoiding becoming "emotionally affected by or involved in the suffering of patients"[20] (more on this in the discussion on empathy later in this chapter). Equanimity helps the HCP to deal with the stresses of personal life and patient care. It has also been shown to help leaders in health care:

> Equanimity allows the nurse leader to remain in control and assess situations clearly and accurately. It provides the nurse leader with the sense of self-confidence and the propensity to envision solutions with calmness and grace. It's with these thoughts that equanimity stands as first in the proposed sequential conceptual triad model of nurse leader resiliency.[21]

Finally, equanimity, or "a calm, competent image," has been found to be associated with patient satisfaction.[22]

Although Jiwon's story is extreme, it is not unusual among HCPs. Some researchers assert, "Individuals who pursue careers in health care professions may have higher pre-existing rates of depression and anxiety."[23] "As high as 72% and 67% of final year dental students have been reported to suffer from stress and pathological anxiety respectively."[24] Once their education and training are completed, HCPs continue to experience stress and mental health disorders; for example, researchers report, dentists are "prone to professional burnout, anxiety disorders and clinical depression."[25] Before the Covid-19 pandemic, "Numerous global studies involving nearly every medical and surgical specialty indicate that approximately 1 in every 3 physicians is experiencing burnout at any given time."[26] During the pandemic (between May and October of 2020) a survey of more than 20,000 HCPs in the United States revealed a burnout rate of 49%.[27] As for nurses, "Over the past decade, nurses have consistently reported the *highest levels of job stress* of all healthcare professionals" (emphasis added).[28]

Note: If you sense that you may be depressed, you are encouraged to take the Beck Depression Inventory (https://www.ismanet.org/doctoryourspirit/pdfs/Beck-Depression-Inventory-BDI.pdf). If test results indicate you are suffering from depression, please seek the support of a mental health professional as soon as possible. Because depression alters perception and judgment, it can result in self-destructive impulses and suicide.

What are the stressors for HCPs? You know them well because you face them every day! Factors both external (work related) and internal (originating from oneself) are plentiful, and each health care specialty and HCP have their own personal "favorites." Some external stressors include "time-related pressures, fearful patients, too much work, financial worries, problems with staff, equipment and material problems, poor working conditions."[29] For nurses and intensive care unit clinicians, *moral distress* arises "when clinicians are constrained from taking what they believe to be ethically appropriate actions or are forced to take actions they believe are ethically inappropriate," such as being unable to minimize suffering because of the risks of exacerbating a medical condition.[30] For dental professionals, "providing treatment to uncooperative patients" is "one of the most important work-related stressors."[31]

There are a few lesser-known external stressors that also deserve discussion—to shed light on them, to validate our experience of them, and to thereby gain some perspective and power over them. These include *sharing bad news, emotional labor*, and *information technology*.

Sharing bad news, such as poor prognosis or the need for extensive treatment, can arouse stressful feelings in the HCP. "Psychological experiments showed that the bearer of bad news often experiences strong emotions such as anxiety, a burden of responsibility for the news, and fear of negative evaluation."[32] My colleague, Jessie, a dental hygienist, describes her experience of informing a patient about their periodontal disease:

> I have been mostly successful as explaining what periodontal disease is comes easily to me. However, when the patient is angry, in a bad mood, or questions my knowledge, I become anxious.

Practical ways of sharing bad news skillfully are discussed in Chapter 4.

Emotional labor, a term coined by sociologist Arlie Hochschild, involves the work of "managing one's own emotions" including "evoking and suppressing feelings."[33] In health care, emotional labor is commonly associated with performing painful procedures.[34] Again, Jessie comments:

> I sometimes find myself failing to remove all the deposit (tartar) because a person is in pain. Even with topical and/or local [anesthesia], a patient can still be in pain. It's frustrating because I don't want to scar the patient. I only ever do what they allow me to do, and I always tell them to ask me to stop if I am hurting them too much. This leads to me feeling as if I am not doing a good job as a hygienist. I have to frequently remind myself that I can only do so much.

You might also experience emotional labor when a patient's expectations are unreasonable and you struggle to be pleasant as you smile through clenched teeth!

Information technology is a final external stressor that we should discuss here. Health care has become dominated by computers. It is mind-boggling to consider how much time and energy HCPs spend navigating computer systems. The sheer volume of data HCPs must track is ever-growing, resulting in what some call "click fatigue." Paul Coyne, RN, chief nursing informatics officer of one hospital describes a "cyclical paradox in health care":

> Healthcare leadership seeks metrics to determine how to best provide patient care, and turns to IT... IT seeks more data to feed algorithms and dashboards, and turns to frontline clinicians to input the data into the EHR. Frontline clinicians manually enter this data and turn to leadership and say they are burned out. And the cycle repeats.[35]

Computer systems frequently are not user friendly (not surprisingly, if they are designed by non-HCPs), and many times computer delays and malfunctions create barriers to basic functionality. I remember several occasions when I was trying to extract a patient's tooth and unable to view the digital radiographs (the only way to see most of the tooth!), leaving me to choose between waiting for professional computer help indefinitely in the middle of surgery or continuing to work blindly.

In addition to the many external stresses described earlier, internal sources of stress plague many HCPs. Researchers in dentistry report that the profession attracts "compulsive personalities who display unrealistic expectations and strive for unattainable standards of excellence."[25] Many HCPs are prone to perfectionism and fear that "if we don't judge ourselves harshly, then we'll become lazy, incompetent or unsuccessful."[36] This drive to perfection and the fear of failure compel many HCPs, including myself, to push excessively and to worry a lot. My dentist colleague and fellow meditator, Mikaela F, describes her experience:

My main problem is not while I see patients, it is when I get home! My brain goes a mile a minute thinking about things I worry I did not do well enough, crowns cemented that were not perfect, the possibility of lawsuits over my self-perceived insufficient dentistry—I often would struggle to fall asleep or wake up in a panic.

Nurse practitioner Martha B describes her worries:

When I get home after seeing a day full of patients in an office, I worry about big and small things. I worry that I might have missed something important. I worry that the patient might not have completely understood instructions. I am making a mental list of what to follow up on the next day. I may worry about small tasks left undone in the electronic medical record and know they are piling up and will impede my progress the next day.

Unmanaged stress, whether external or internal, can affect "personal wellness and the capacity to provide professional and compassionate patient care."[37] Unmanaged stress can result in depression directly or can cause burnout, leading to depression indirectly; stress is also associated with increased anxiety.[38] Other personal consequences of stress include substance abuse, strained relationships, and suicide.[39] The consequences of unmanaged stress in HCPs extend to their patients. Krasner et al. cites the following common sequelae of burnout in HCPs: decreased quality of care, patient dissatisfaction, increased medical errors, increased lawsuits, and decreased ability to express empathy.[40]

A valuable metaphor to HCPs is this common instruction to airplane passengers—put the oxygen mask on yourself first before trying to help others. Caring for others, especially for patients who are anxious and in pain, requires first caring for yourself and cultivating a sense of balance and calm that can withstand the many stressors of work and personal life. Mindfulness training has been shown to cultivate equanimity and promote mental health. "The results of several systematic reviews and meta-analysis of mindfulness-based interventions suggest that [Mindfulness-based Stress Reduction and Mindfulness-based Cognitive Therapy]

significantly improve stress, anxiety, depression, quality of life and emotional regulations across a range of psychiatric and medical populations."[41]

Several studies have investigated the benefits of mindfulness for HCPs. A 5-year study of second-year medical students at Jefferson Medical College compared students who took an MBSR course with a control group. It found significant differences in total mood disturbance (TMD) as well as tension-anxiety and several other mood states; interestingly, these differences were noted despite a higher baseline TMD in the test group (mindfulness).[37] A randomized controlled trial of medical students found significant differences between control and test subjects in the areas of depression and anxiety even though the post-tests were during exam time, a particularly stressful period.[39] A 2011 randomized controlled trial of medical students found significant reductions in the mindfulness group on perceived stress scales (PSSs) and anxiety, and the benefits were constant at 8 weeks post trial.[42] Similarly, a study of primary care health professionals found increased mindfulness correlated with decreased perceived stress.[43]

How does mindfulness reduce stress and increase equanimity? Mindfulness has been found to induce changes in the amygdala, a part of the limbic system and the area where the stress reaction originates.[3,4] "Mindfulness training reduces the reactivity of the amygdala, which is overactive in people with stress, anxiety, and depression."[10] Mindfulness meditation has also been shown to activate areas of the prefrontal cortex involved in emotional regulation.[44]

In addition to the research findings, my own personal experience with mindfulness has convinced me of its value for cultivating equanimity, especially in the face of stress. Over time, the practice has allowed me to notice difficult thoughts and emotions, such as anxiety or self-judgment, and to experience them like clouds in the sky. Like any weather pattern, this too shall pass.

Parasympathetic Primer Experience: Progressive Muscle Relaxation

The value of simply relaxing the body cannot be understated. Put simply, one cannot be physically relaxed and anxious at the same time—the two are mutually exclusive.[45] Unfortunately, it is hard to relax the body on command, and sometimes, trying to relax can make one even more tense! Often, we are not even aware of tension.

The practice of progressive muscle relaxation (PMR) trains us to recognize the feel of tension and relaxation and, by doing so, promotes the ability to relax effectively and efficiently. PMR is a well-established, simple technique proven to treat anxiety, insomnia, and a host of other conditions.[46] It consists of two basic steps: (1) creating tension in specific muscles and (2) releasing the tension. The breath accompanies the two steps for each body part: inhaling on the tension, holding for about 5 seconds, and then exhaling on the release for about 5 seconds. The emphasis is on feeling the sensations of tension and relaxation.

The order of the body parts does not matter. You can practice part by body part or bundle several parts together. With just a few days of practice, you will be able to recognize tension and let it go. *Relaxed body, relaxed mind*. Video 2.1 provides a brief introduction followed by Video 2.2 which is a guided practice.

Formal Practice for Equanimity: BODY SCAN

"Out of the head, into the body": this is a recurrent theme in mindfulness practices and the path to mindfulness. Although we can think thoughts in the past and the future, we can only feel sensations in the present. So, by tuning into the body as we do in the *Body Scan* practice, we can tune into the present moment and find equanimity. There is no goal in this practice, such as relaxation or peace, although those may arise at times. Real equanimity does not come from chasing after it. Rather, it comes from being with what is. We start by being with the body as it is and simply notice any sensations in the body in the moment. We get out of the head by getting into the body.

A student once complained to his meditation teacher, reporting frustration that he could not feel any body sensations. As he was speaking, he was scratching his head. His teacher noticed this and asked why he was scratching his head. "Because I have an itch," the student replied. "Aha," the teacher pointed out, "see, you DO have sensations!" The body is constantly generating sensations, but many sensations fall under the radar, especially when we are lost in thought. With practice, these sensations can be more easily felt and tolerated. With practice, "we increase the distance between the itch and the scratch," as one of my meditation teachers David Nichtern used to say.

Emotions and our reaction to them are the psychological version of the itch and the scratch. Meditation teacher Ezra Bayda explains that stressful emotions consist of mainly two elements: *believed thoughts* and uncomfortable *physical sensations*.[47] In other words, challenging emotions are accompanied by an "itch" in the body—an uncomfortable physical sensation. When we are not mindful, these transient physical sensations provoke us to react unconsciously to avoid feeling them. However, if we can be mindful—simply notice these body sensations and allow them space—we develop equanimity and something more.

When we notice and allow space for the uncomfortable physical sensations associated with emotions, we experience a *gap* between the stimulus and our response, and by doing so, we actualize the power to choose. In this gap, we can choose whether or not to eat the whole box of donuts or reach for the bottle when we feel anxious. In the gap, we can choose whether or not to hit the send button for that nasty email written in anger. In the gap, even when we are rushed and frustrated during a medical procedure, we can choose whether or not to stop when the patient complains of pain. Simply by noticing and allowing the felt sense of the emotion in the moment—the tightness in the chest, the clenched jaw, the shallowness of the breaths—we can experience this gap. Author Steven Covey (inspired by holocaust survivor Viktor Frankl) writes:

> Our unique human endowments lift us above the animal world. The extent to which we exercise and develop these endowments empower us to fulfill our uniquely human potential. Between stimulus and response is our greatest power—the freedom to choose.[48]

So, although the body scan may seem ridiculously simple and stupid, know that this is a gateway to freedom from slavery to our emotions and the impulses they generate. This is a path to equanimity.

The next video provides a brief introduction to the body scan (Video 2.3) followed by two short body scan practices, first seated (Video 2.4), then lying down (Video 2.5).

Informal Practice: Gratitude

Informal practices are short practices that can be woven into your daily activities without requiring extra time or a special place. These practices will help you notice how you are feeling in the moment and restore mindfulness. For many of us, it can be hard to remember to stop and check in with ourselves during the whirlwind of daily life.

There have been many times when I felt like I went under water at the beginning of the workday and did not come up for air until the day was over! Setting aside a few minutes each day to formally practice mindfulness makes it possible to remember to "come up to the surface" and notice how you are feeling during activity.

Gratitude Practice

Throughout the course of human evolution, the humans who focused on the negative—the places where the saber-toothed tiger was last seen, the kinds of berries that are poisonous (i.e., not the humans who stopped to smell the flowers)—were more likely to survive long enough to pass on their genes. This resulted in the evolution of a human brain hard-wired to focus on the negative. Psychologist and author Dr. Rick Hanson describes our brains as "Velcro for negative experiences, but Teflon for positive ones."[49] A powerful antidote to this negativity bias, one that also reduces stress and cultivates equanimity, is *gratitude practice.*

How does gratitude practice decrease stress and increase equanimity? Similar to the way the biceps muscle sends inhibitory impulses to the triceps muscle so it can contract fully (called reciprocal inhibition),[50] practicing gratitude inhibits the stress response. In short, we cannot be grateful and stressed at the same time! Furthermore, by practicing gratitude, we are actually rewiring the brain to be more positively focused—because of our innate capacity for neuroplasticity, "neurons that fire together, wire together."[51]

The most common gratitude practice studied by researchers is the *gratitude list* practice described by Emmons and McCullough—writing three to five things you were grateful for during the day.[52] Many benefits of this practice have been demonstrated, including increased positive mood and happiness and decreased negative mood and stress.[53]

Several other documented strategies that are helpful to cultivating gratitude include writing a list several times per week, being specific instead of general (e.g., "my partner" instead of "people in my life"), and focusing on people more than things.[54] I like to make alphabet gratitude lists with a theme, such as parts of my body that start with a, b, c, etc., or a list of people whose names start with a, b, c, and so on (including the challenging ones, who help me expand my horizons!). You can also do a gratitude body scan, thanking each body part for what it does for you every day. One final

important note: do not try to force any feelings; simply orient the mind toward gratitude, staying there a few moments, letting it sink in. By doing so, you are watering the seeds of gratitude and equanimity.

Experiment:
The next time you feel genuine gratitude about something, notice what that experience is like, especially in the body. Is there any change in body sensations such as relaxing or releasing? Is there any change in your perception (e.g., noticing other senses, emotions)?

THE "A" IN EASE: ATTENTIVENESS

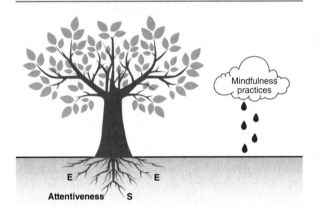

The faculty of voluntarily bringing back a wandering attention, over and over again, is the very root of judgement, character, and will.[55]
William James, father of modern psychology

One day, my lack of attentiveness at work resulted in an adverse outcome. As I sat down to prepare Mrs. Diaz's tooth #5 for a composite restoration (white filling), I noticed Joan, the hygienist, hovering behind me to request a hygiene check. We walked together toward her room as she described her patient, a college student named Susan, who had not been seen in more than 2 years and had a long list of new carious lesions (cavities). I examined Susan, confirmed the list Joan had made, and noted a couple more lesions. As I headed back to Mrs. Diaz, I was intercepted by one of my assistants, Stephanie, who informed me that another patient, Scott, had arrived for a restoration. She suggested anesthetizing Scott before continuing with Mrs. Diaz. "Hi Scott, what's new? Ready for a white filling in that front tooth?" "Well doc, I actually have a toothache on the other side and was hoping you could do something about it." I checked whether there was a recent radiograph and felt an internal tightening as I realized there was none. I asked Stephanie to obtain a radiograph of his painful tooth. My phone pinged; it was a text from my significant other alerting me of a change of plans requiring me to make dinner that evening. "Oh boy, what should I make?" Finally, I circled back to Mrs. Diaz, noticing I was way behind schedule. After a few seconds of preparing (drilling) her tooth, I realized, to my horror, that instead preparing of tooth #5, I had just started preparing tooth #4.

I was very shaken by this experience and took measures afterward to ensure it did not happen again—luckily, it has not. In health care, attentiveness not only ensures safe and accurate technical care, but it is also essential to patient-centered care. For example, attentiveness is fundamental to active listening.[1] Attentiveness allows the HCP to detect cues, both verbal and nonverbal, about patient needs,[56] such as a patient signaling their anxiety or pain by clutching the armrests or holding their breath. Unfortunately, attentiveness is becoming increasingly difficult to establish and maintain. Two main factors account for this difficulty: *hard-wired qualities of the human brain* and *modern culture*.

First, let's look at how the human brain functions. Have you ever driven somewhere and not remembered how you got there? Or perhaps you ate your favorite ice cream but did not taste anything until scraping the bottom of the bowl. Where were you? Most likely, you were on autopilot, mindlessly lost in thought. Scientists have mapped out the neural pathways of this mode of brain function and call it the DMN. This automatic default mode keeps us safe by constantly scanning for possible threats. This tendency to constantly look for problems enabled our ancestors to avoid predators and thus to survive. We scan memories of past threats, and we imagine future possibilities of threats. Unfortunately, the DMN, or inattention to the present, has the potential to compromise safety and quality of care, as the previous story illustrated.

If our hard-wired inclination for autopilot or mindlessness were not enough, modern culture magnifies this tendency. In his essay, "On Distraction," British philosopher Alain de Botton writes, "the past decade has seen an unparalleled assault on our capacity to fix our minds steadily on anything."[57] The most significant threat to our ability to choose our object of attention, and to stay there, is the internet—especially *social media*. The portability and thus ever-presence of our digital devices mean we are constantly being interrupted and distracted with texts, emails, and notifications. Neurologist Dr. Tarawneh reports, "Recent research suggests that excess use of the internet over prolonged periods of time may negatively affect some cognitive functions, particularly **attention** and short-term memory" (emphasis added).[58] Even worse, overuse of the internet bears addiction potential. A Harvard publication reports, "Every notification, whether it's a text message, a 'like' on Instagram, or a Facebook notification, has the potential to be a positive social stimulus . . . [Such stimuli] result in a release of dopamine, reinforcing whatever behavior preceded it."[59] This is the mechanism for addiction. What results is a human being who is anxious, restless, and distracted. What results in health care is an HCP who cannot listen, cannot make eye contact, cannot detect cues about patient pain or anxiety, and cannot empathize.

Despite the costs of internet overuse, tech companies want us to use their products more and more because our attention itself has become a priceless commodity. Recently, former high-level employees of tech companies and social media platforms, including Google, Facebook, and Twitter, have exposed the intentionality of their former companies to hijack and manipulate the attention of their users for economic gain.[60] By "leveraging the very same neural circuitry used by slot machines and cocaine to keep us using their products as much as possible,"[59] "users" (interesting how consumers of drugs and devices have the same name!) get hooked.

Evidence of the magnitude of this social phenomenon of digital distraction is everywhere. For example, recently as I rode a subway packed with passengers: every single person, as far as my eyes could see, was head-down, buried in their cell phone. Even people working in operating rooms cannot resist the pull of their cellphones, resulting in adverse outcomes such as a wrongful death of a patient during a low-risk cardiac procedure (the anesthesiologist admitted to texting, accessing websites, and reading e-books during procedures) and paralysis of a neurosurgery patient (the neurosurgeon had made 10 phone calls while operating[61]). A study of perfusionists (HCPs responsible for keeping patients alive during cardiopulmonary bypass surgeries) found that, although "the majority of perfusionists believe cell phones raise significant safety issues while operating the heart-lung machine," 55.6% reported using cell phones during cardiopulmonary bypass.[62]

A study of medical students found smartphone addiction in 60.3% of students based on the Smartphone Addiction Scale-Short Version.[63] We have been taken hostage. How do we shield ourselves from this onslaught? (If you would like to rate yourself for smartphone addiction, you can find a scale at https://www.researchgate.net/publication/259589326_The_Smartphone_Addiction_Scale_Development_and_Validation_of_a_Short_Version_for_Adolescents.)

Without making conscious choices about technology use and training our minds to be attentive to the present, we are unlikely to escape the consequences of internet overuse and addiction (Fig. 2.2). HCPs, especially, must find ways to set limits on internet use to protect their own well-being and that of their patients. Here are some suggestions:

- Turn off notifications, auditory signals, etc.
- Limit unnecessary screen time (set a timer)
- Schedule time to triage emails and to reply
- Establish tech-free zones and times (e.g., leaving devices out of the bedroom or patient treatment areas)
- Keep the device display on black and white (grayscale mode)[64]

As you try to distance yourself, you will notice the increased pull toward your devices. Be patient, and be creative in finding what works for you, given your work and family needs.

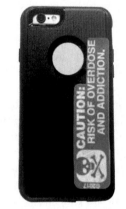

Fig. 2.2 Cell Phone With Warning.

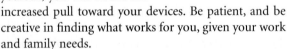

Questions for Reflection
1. My personal test of addiction to cell phone use (or any other behavior) is asking questions like: "Do I have a choice whether to pick up my phone or not right now?" or "Am I choosing not to put my phone down right now, or am I stuck doomscrolling again?" or "What's in control right now, me or my phone?" Our level of ability to choose or not helps gauge the need to take measures to treat our addiction. Try asking yourself questions in the moment as you interact with your devices.
2. Consider possible ways you can limit internet use in your daily life. Write down your ideas. Commit to them, and reassess over time.

Mindfulness helps cultivate attentiveness. Recent research has found evidence that mindfulness practice induces changes in brain anatomy and function pertaining to attention. Lazar, Kerr, and Wasserman showed that brain regions associated with attention, interoception, and sensory processing were thicker in meditation participants than in matched controls.[65] One randomized controlled trial demonstrated benefits to the anterior cingulate cortex, a region associated with attention, after only *1 month* of practicing 30 minutes per day.[66] Another randomized controlled trial investigated the effects of as few as *10 minutes* of daily mindfulness practice and showed better performance on all measures of electroencephalograph.[67]

Parasympathetic Primer Experience: Mindful Movement

In the practice of mindful movement, we align with the original intention of yoga, which is to unify the body and mind and to prepare the body for long periods of sitting meditation. (Modern yoga practice has evolved into another form of exercise, with the goal of improving physical strength and flexibility.) To begin mindful movement, first, set an intention of care for yourself and acceptance of whatever arises. Then, follow along as instructed in Video 2.6, and simply feel the sensations of the body as you move. Notice whatever thoughts arise—thoughts of the past (what I should have done), present (judgments of how bad I am doing this pose), and future (what I will have for dinner). Gently redirect the attention to the direct, moment-to-moment sensations in the body. Audio tracks 2.1 and 2.2 provide longer guided mindful movement.

Formal Practice: Awareness of Breath

Awareness of breath is a core practice of mindfulness. Meditation teacher Pema Chödrön summarizes the practice in three simple steps:
- Taking your seat
- Placing your attention on your breathing
- Labeling thoughts as thinking[68]

Try the practice as guided in Video 2.7 for a few minutes each day. You will notice that your mind tends to wander from the breath. This is totally normal because the mind is hard-wired to wander. Trying to stop the mind from thinking is like trying to stop the nose from smelling! The practice is simply to notice this has happened and to return your attention to the sensations of the breath in the moment. Simple, but not easy.

At times, especially in the beginning, it may be hard to stay with the focus of attention for even 2 seconds. You may catch only short glimpses of the breath because your mind is so busy. Meditation teacher Sharon Salzberg suggests following the breath like watching a friend through a crowded room—you do not need to beat down or push away what gets in the way. So, when you practice awareness of the breath, *you do not need to push thoughts away or try to stop thinking.* Once more . . . **you do not need to push thoughts away or try to stop thinking**. (This is the most common misunderstanding, so this point needs emphasis!) Thinking is what the mind does; trying to stop it only magnifies the mental activity. Allow whatever arises to be in the background—allow the judging thoughts such as "I'm not doing this right" or "I'm not good at this" or "This is a waste of time." Allow the thoughts of the past, such as what you wish you had said to your partner. Allow thoughts of the future, such as what you will have for dinner. Every time you notice your mind has wandered from the breath, simply guide it back with the same attitude as you would guide a puppy back onto the trail. Be kind, be patient, and be forgiving of yourself.

Just being able to notice that your mind has wandered is itself a profound insight because as soon as you notice you have wandered, you are already present again. Even more, each time you come back to the breath, you are exercising the "letting go" muscle.[69] Just like exercising any muscle, we start with a light weight and gradually build. Set a timer for just a few minutes if that is all you can do, and then build from there as you are ready. We must start where we are.

You might at times experience restlessness or irritation sitting still, and if you do, be gentle with yourself. (If you have a history of trauma, see the Cautionary Note at the end of the chapter for guidance.) Many of us spend a lot of time on digital devices, and as we sit, we might experience the effects of internet addiction and withdrawal. If you do, you will have much to gain from this practice because mindfulness-based interventions are being used increasingly to treat many addictions.[70] See if you can stay with the practice as you notice the pull of your devices and the momentum of your mind. Notice what the pull of the device feels like in the body. Be patient. Take baby steps. Again, we must start where we are.

Formal Practice: Walking Meditation

Like awareness of the breath, walking meditation, shown in Video 2.8, features a very specific object of attention to focus the mind. Instead of focusing on the breath, now we focus on the sensations of walking. Identify a space in which you can walk 10 to 15 paces. Walk slowly enough that you can notice each time you lift, move, touch, and step; as Jon Kabat-Zinn taught me, try saying silently to yourself, "lift, move, touch, step." Walk fast enough that you do not teeter off balance. Each time you reach the end of your path, pause for a few moments then turn around and walk back to the other end of your path. I like this practice when I am feeling too restless to sit still or when I cannot sleep. The movement helps to dissipate excess energy and settle the mind.

One of the fathers of the mindfulness movement in the West, a Vietnamese Buddhist monk named Thich Nhat Hanh, teaches walking meditation as a fundamental practice. He suggests pairing awareness of walking with awareness of the breath by counting the number of steps as you breathe in and as you breathe out. In his words,

> *"When we walk mindfully on the face of the earth, we are grounded in her generosity and we cannot help but be grateful. All of the earth's qualities of patience, stability, creativity, love, and non-discrimination are available when we walk reverently, aware of our connection."*[71]

Informal Practices: Mindfulness of Daily Activities

You can practice mindfulness as you go about your daily activities, without taking any extra time, simply by feeling the sensations in the body in the present moment. As you wash your hands at work, feel the sensations of the water and the soap on your hands as shown in Video 2.9. As you brush your teeth, feel the brush on the gums and taste the toothpaste. As you listen to a patient speak, feel the flow of your breath. Jessie, our dental hygienist friend, describes her experience of this informal mindfulness practice:

> *I have learned to do this especially when I get ready in the morning and get ready for bed. When I brush*

my hair, I always do it with such urgency and strength. I have to remind myself that I don't need to brush my hair so fast and hard. And when I reminded myself of this, I began brushing my hair slowly and gently. And I actually enjoyed the feeling of brushing my hair for what felt like the first time. I couldn't believe I had been brushing my hair this way for as long as I could remember.

Consider placing a sticker or other visual cue at key places in your surroundings to remind you to tune into the present moment in the body and the senses. For example, you could place a sticker on the dashboard of your car, next to your toothbrush, or at your computer. Make your smartphone an ally by setting it to provide regularly or randomly timed auditory signals, cueing you to rest in mindfulness.

THE "S" IN EASE: SELF-AWARENESS

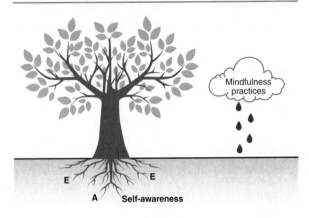

One of my patients, Maria, a recent immigrant from Italy (and owner of a fine pizzeria) needed a root canal that was too difficult for me, so I gave her a referral to a trusted endodontist. When she returned to my office next for treatment, she told me she had gone to a different endodontist (one I did not know) and presented me with the radiograph of her root canal. On the radiograph the root canal looked perfect—impressive considering the difficulty of her case, but when I asked Maria how the root canal went, her response surprised me. With her limited English she described her experience: "I will never have another root canal in all my life! The dottore ignore me for whole hour. Never ask me how I was doing. I could no breathe. I could no swallow with that rubber sheet they

put on my mouth. Plus, my mouth so tired open so big for so long time. It was nightmare. Never again!"

Maria's endodontist had performed a beautiful root canal and was clearly a technically skilled dentist. Unfortunately, he was so intent on the procedural aspects of the root canal that he neglected the patient. This reflects a challenge for many HCPs: to maintain awareness of the patient while performing a difficult or new procedure. Here again, my dental hygienist friend Jessie shares her experience:

I sometimes have to remind myself of this . . . especially during long . . . appointments... I either get so caught up in making sure I'm removing the calculus, or I start to daydream and then have to remind myself to check in on my patient and make sure they are still okay. Wearing loupes does not help with this either! I love my loupes and could not imagine working without them, but they have a way of making me only see the mouth and forgetting that there is a person attached to the tooth!

Neuroscience provides an interesting explanation for the challenge of maintaining awareness of both the procedure and the patient during the procedure. Neural networks governing empathy and cognitive problem solving are anticorrelated so that "increases in one network necessitate decreases in the other."[72] So, HCPs must somehow find a way "to be able to move back and forth from objective observation to empathetic identification."[73] This ability to toggle between thinking and feeling is made possible by self-awareness.

Self-awareness: Good for the Patient

Self-awareness benefits patients by enhancing both the technical quality of care and the quality of our relationships. First, self-awareness limits "cognitive bias" that is caused by "the unconscious assumptions taken into clinical interactions."[10] Self-awareness promotes the opposite, "cognitive flexibility": "Self-observation allows disengaging the automatic pathways and enables present-moment input to be integrated in a new way."[74] For example, what may look like a common lesion actually could be a rare pathologic condition; self-awareness allows one to devise an accurate differential diagnosis instead of allowing previous experiences to bias one's judgment.

Self-awareness also enriches our relationships. Perhaps you recall a time when you reacted to a patient unskillfully, maybe by interrupting them as they described their symptoms or forcing them through a difficult procedure despite their complaints of pain. You may have been reacting to something under the radar, like irritation or impatience. When we are unaware of our own thoughts, emotions, and impulses, we react unconsciously, without freedom to choose. Mindfulness practice increases self-awareness, making it possible to notice "irritation is here," or "impatience is here" and to notice what it feels like in the body in the moment without reacting—without itching the scratch. In this way, we avoid unconscious *reactions* and instead get to choose a skillful *response.*

Finally, self-awareness also enhances relationships with patients by exposing our prejudices. I work in a public health clinic with patients who are predominantly poor, uneducated, and Black. One day, I had a new patient who was a White woman my age, and—to my dismay—I caught myself explaining treatment options in more detail than I normally would have with a Black patient. This exposed my assumption that a dark-skinned patient will choose a cheaper option, such as tooth extraction, and therefore not be interested in hearing about other treatment options. Self-awareness of prejudices like these enables us to not be confined by them and to remember to offer all reasonable options to all patients, regardless of their skin color. (If you think you do not have racial biases, I encourage you to take an implicit bias test at https://implicit.harvard.edu/implicit/selectatest.html. You may be surprised at what you uncover!)

Self-awareness: Good for the Professional

Finally, self-awareness also enhances the HCP's well-being. Psychologist and mindfulness teacher Patricia Dobkin asserts, "the doctor that is self-aware is more likely to engage in self-care activities and manage stress better."[13] For example, awareness helps me notice fatigue, providing the option to take a break, when I can. Self-awareness makes it possible to notice tension in the body and to release it. Self-awareness highlights poor working posture, allowing one to reposition.

Mindfulness Practice Builds Self-Awareness

Self-awareness is at the heart of mindfulness practice, and research is uncovering a link between mindfulness practices and objective measures of awareness. A review of 21 neuroimaging studies examining approximately 300 meditation practitioners identified eight brain regions consistently altered in meditators, and three of these regions govern awareness.[75] In summary, "formal training in self-awareness has been recommended to potentially enhance evidence-based decision making, patient-centered care, communication, cultural competency, team-building, professionalism, personal development, and self-care."[1]

Parasympathetic Primer Experience: Diaphragmatic Breathing

In Chapter 5, we will discuss the benefits and mechanism of deep belly breathing or diaphragmatic breathing in more depth. For now, you are invited to follow along with the guided practice in Video 2.10 as a way to calm the body and mind in preparation for formal practice.

Formal Practice: Choice of Anchors

Many years ago, when I was teaching mindfulness meditation to a group of oral surgery residents, a hulking male resident blurted, "I don't like feeling my breath." At first, I was taken aback by his bluntness, but I quickly realized he was sharing his reaction in earnest. At the time, I did not have an answer for him, but since then, research findings have elucidated a few reasons why some individuals find awareness of the breath meditation aversive. For example, people who struggle with breathing due to asthma or allergies may find focusing on the breath difficult. Others, particularly those with a history of trauma, may find increasing anxiety or agitation when focusing on the breath. If the breath does not work for you for whatever reason, there are two other anchors recommended for practice:

1. Sounds: this can feel more spacious when the breath feels confining or uncomfortable
2. Body sensations, especially the contact points of the feet on the floor or the hands resting on the legs

In this next practice shown in Video 2.11, you will have a chance to try all three options one at a time. The practice in Video 2.12 shows a way to work with multiple anchors at once. See which anchor is most stabilizing for you—which one brings a sense of ease. Each time you notice your mind wandering from your anchor, gently but firmly return, with patience. If you notice impatience, bring patience to that! Afterward, you can journal your experience.

See Table 2.1.

Informal Practices: Three Breaths and STOP

Throughout the day, simply stopping to take *three conscious breaths* can help to short-circuit the DMN (autopilot) and create space in the mind and the body. This practice, shown in Video 2.13, can be done any time, including at work.

Two dental hygienist friends describe the value of this practice at work:

Simple, yet so effective . . . Our job has many stressors. Whenever I find myself getting worked up, I focus on my breathing. It helps to center me and helps me to relax, thus making the appointment go a bit smoother.

Kevin T, RDH

I have really started to implement this into my day-to-day life in the past year or so. It was surprising how hard it was to do, yet so relieving at the same time. It gets easier with practice. However, sometimes stress catches up to me and I forget to decompress. It's amazing how fast negative emotions can take over your body. Trying to make myself be mindful again can feel like starting over. And something as simple as breathing, moving slowly, unclenching my jaw, and stretching can feel like huge tasks again. Until I repeat it for a couple days and it comes naturally again.

Jessie M, RDH

Meditation teacher Pema Chödrön recommends, "Let your mind relax and drop for just a few breaths the story line you are working so hard to maintain."[76] Remembering to take three breaths during the workday becomes easier by practicing mindfulness formally on a regular basis.

Another informal practice is STOP as described by Stahl and Goldstein[77]:

- S: **Stop**. Be physically still.
- T: **Take** a breath. Feel the sensations of the breath. (The direct experience of the breath can immediately bring us into the present because it is not possible to feel the breath in the past or the future—only in the present!)
- O: **Observe** sensations in the body and any senses including sounds, sights, smells, and touch.
- P: **Proceed** with activity.

This practice can be woven into the workday very easily. Some possible opportunities to practice STOP include:

- During hand hygiene (feeling sensations of water or hand sanitizer)
- While waiting (for local anesthesia to take effect or dental impression to set)
- Before greeting a patient

Consider placing stickers or sticky notes in places where you go every day as a cue to practice STOP.

Video 2.14 illustrates STOP before entering a treatment room. Also, you can find a brief video illustrating more opportunities for practicing STOP, courtesy of the University of Wisconsin Department of Family Medicine and Community Health at https://youtu.be/vhlv3cntCr4.

THE LAST "E" IN EASE: EMPATHY (AND COMPASSION)

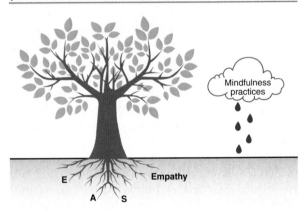

Open wide.

A tense silence, no response. Little Josh sits frozen in the dental chair, his worn sneakers barely reaching halfway down the dental chair. "Joshua, I need you to open your mouth, or we can't do your filling." I feel an internal tightening in my chest as I wonder if or when Josh will cooperate. Time is running out, and my schedule is packed. My mind flashes forward—I imagine Josh's mom being angry at me for not getting anything done and having to refer her to a pediatric dentist. Then I notice Joshua's hands wringing each other, and this touches something inside me. "Are you scared, Josh?" He nods in affirmation, tears welling up in his dark eyes. "Are you afraid it's going to hurt?" He nods again, now the tears overflow and stream down his pale cheeks. "I see that you're scared, and I understand why this is scary for you!" I sit quietly with him for a few moments more, breathing with his fear. His tears flow, and after a few moments, his face relaxes, seeming more reassured, more receptive. "I promise to do my very best to make it very easy, and you can stop me anytime you need a break." Within just a few minutes, the procedure is complete, and we end the visit with a high five.

This true scenario illustrates how empathy creates connection and heals. Empathy opened the door to allow Joshua to receive the treatment he needed. In the medical and dental literature, empathy has been established as "a crucial element of the doctor-patient relationship."[39] Further, empathy is a "key factor in a patient's definition of quality of care."[78] Dental researchers report, "Patients value empathy above all else."[79]

Studies on malpractice trends confirm the importance of empathy to patients. Frankel's study of more than 400 letters to an Health Maintenance Organization over a 4-year period revealed that 70% of complaints were related to relationship issues and that "perceived absence of empathy in care is a strong motivation for patients to express their dissatisfaction through letters of complaint."[80] From patients' perspective, quality technical care does not compensate for lack of empathy; a study by Lester and Smith showed that even when there was no medical error, low empathy was associated with increased litigiousness.[81]

Empathy is defined in medicine as having two components: "appreciation of the patient's emotions and expression of that awareness to the patient."[82] The first component, "appreciation of the patient's emotions," is covered here; the second component, "expression of that awareness," will be discussed in Chapter 3. In health care literature, many benefits of empathy for both patients and providers have been noted. Psychiatrist and empathy researcher Dr. Helen Riess summarizes the benefits of "empathetic communication skills" in medicine as far-reaching: "Increased patient satisfaction, improved adherence to therapy, decreased medical errors, better outcomes, decreased burnout and increased physical well-being."[83] In dentistry, "The demonstration of empathy by dentists has been correlated with decreased dental fear, increased compliance with treatment, improved treatment success, and cooperation by patients."[84]

It is not surprising that provider empathy results in better health care, given recent findings about our evolution. Contrary to the previously held thought that ethical behavior is rooted in reason, evolutionary biology has found that altruistic behavior is actually rooted in empathy.[85] Furthermore, although empathy has historically been regarded as an inborn trait, research has found that, actually, empathy can be learned with practice[41] and "enhanced by educational interventions."[86] Before discussing a mindfulness approach to cultivating empathy, let's touch on two other paths, *narrative medicine* and *mirroring*.

First, empathy can be cultivated by maintaining a "natural curiosity about . . . patient's lives."[87] Research in narrative medicine has found that listening and telling patients' stories is an effective way for HCPs to cultivate empathy.[88] Imagine a patient who is angry about having to wait for their appointment. How much easier would it be to feel empathy if you knew they were a single mother of a special needs child who was recovering from their fifth surgery? An HCP can learn patients' stories by asking questions and by mindful listening—both communication skills that will be covered in Chapter 3.

Another way to cultivate empathy is through the simple practice of mirroring.

> **Experiment:**
> Smile for a few minutes, and try to feel angry. Then try the opposite—frown and try to feel happy.

If you found this challenging, you are not alone. Researchers have confirmed that simply adopting certain facial expressions affects mood.[89] (As you might have guessed, smiling induces happiness, while frowning induces sadness.) What if an HCP mirrors the facial expressions of their patient—can that help them attune to the patient's mood? Indeed, experts in doctor-patient relations assert that the simple act of mirroring a patient's expressions and words helps the doctor to "get in touch with the patient's basic emotions."[73] The attunement that comes from mirroring naturally gives rise to empathy.

Mindfulness Practice for Empathy

Several studies have documented increases in HCP empathy after mindfulness training.[90–92] The seminal study by Krasner et al. of primary care physicians who completed an 8-week intensive course with 10 months of maintenance training showed *improvement in empathy correlated with increases in mindfulness.*[40] Conducted by

Shapiro et al, a randomized controlled study of premed and medical students measured a statistically significant *increase in empathy* in the study group receiving mindfulness training.[39] Interestingly, empathy in the control group (no mindfulness training) actually declined during the same time period, highlighting a concerning trend.

The erosion of empathy during education and training has been documented in several studies including both medical and dental students.[84,93] Several theories have attempted to explain this downward trend. One explanation is the cultural belief that empathy is not an essential part of health care as compared with technological, surgical, or pharmaceutical interventions.[10] Helen Riess, an expert in empathy in health care, suggests that decreasing empathy may be a way to "buffer . . . from the psychological distress of performing painful procedures on patients."[83] Patricia Dobkin proposes a more physiologic explanation: the "vicarious stress" of dealing with patients who are stressed activates the amygdala, which results in impaired empathy.[10]

Is Too Much Empathy Harmful?

Health care provider burnout is a growing concern indicated by the increased use of terms like "empathetic distress" and "compassion fatigue." Is too much empathy harmful, and if so, how does the HCP balance their patients' need for empathy with their own need for self-preservation?

My own wide range of experiences helping patients cope with pain and anxiety has led me to explore this issue. At times, when I am caring for a patient who is anxious or in pain, the experience is heavy and depleting, leaving me feeling impatient and irritable. In contrast, other times it actually feels soothing and energizing, such as when I touch a patient during a procedure as I wish them well (more on *mindful procedural touch* in Chapter 4) or when I rest my hand on a patient's shoulder to soothe them (more on *expressive touch* in Chapter 5). These encounters usually result in a warm, soft feeling in my chest, a release of physical tension, and an uplifted mood. You may have experienced a similar reaction while petting an animal or holding a baby. Recent findings in the field of neuroscience, with important implications for all HCPs, are beginning to explain why the experience of caring for people in distress is at times a negative experience and at other times a positive one.

A look at the definitions of empathy and compassion starts to uncover an explanation for this apparent range of experiences. Empathy involves "vicariously experiencing another's emotions by recognizing, understanding, and resonating with their emotional state."[41] The focus of empathy is on the other's pain and suffering. Compassion, on the other hand, includes empathy as it "originates as an empathetic response to suffering,"[94] but compassion adds something more. The focus of compassion is highlighted in the following definitions of compassion (emphasis added):

- "The emotion one experiences when feeling concern for another's suffering and *desiring to enhance* that individual's welfare."[95]
- "A deep awareness of the suffering of another coupled with the *wish to relieve it.*"[96]
- "Compassion is not only about feeling touched by a person's suffering but also about *wanting to act to help them.*"[97]

Fig. 2.3 below highlights the relationship between empathy and compassion.

So, while the emphasis of empathy is on the suffering itself, compassion focuses on the desire/wish/want to help. Interestingly, a study of Canadian cancer patients found that patients prefer compassion to empathy or sympathy.[98] The more positive focus of compassion seems to have protective effects for the caregiver, as research in neuroscience is proving.

Compassion: An Antidote to Burnout

Compassion does not fatigue—it is neurologically rejuvenating![99]

Dr. Trisha Dowling

Interestingly, neuroscience has identified the brain networks activated after both empathy and compassion training and has found them to be "distinct and non-overlapping."[100] This research helps to explain why empathizing with others' pain can be so depleting, whereas compassion is "rejuvenating." When we empathize with a person in pain, the same neural networks are activated as when we experience pain firsthand.[101–103] In study subjects undergoing empathy training followed by viewing videos of people in distress,

Empathy + Well-wishes = *Compassion*

Fig. 2.3 Relationship of Empathy and Compassion.

increased activation was also noted in networks for negative emotions.[100]

In contrast to empathy, compassion training appears to engage a *positive* neural network. Researchers found compassion training increased activity in "a network previously associated with positive affect, affiliation, and reward."[100] (Affiliation networks involve oxytocin,[99] which is what gives "a feeling of connection and love" as when stroking a pet.[104] Reward networks involve dopamine,[99] which is the neurotransmitter producing pleasure as when eating chocolate.[104]) Several studies have found increased self-reported positive mood after compassion training.[100,105,106] Studies using functional magnetic resonance imaging (MRI) have shown that compassion training results in increased activity in the parts of the brain associated with positive mood and affiliation,[106] even while participants were observing videos of others in distress. Compassion training was associated not only with increased positive mood—it reversed the increased negative mood experienced after empathy training followed by viewing of videos of people in distress[100]; this is a great benefit to HCPs who regularly witness suffering. Studies have also found that compassion training is associated with increased altruistic or helping behaviors,[107,108] another relevant benefit to health care workers.

The Dalai Lama asserts that our true nature is gentleness and compassion, and the evidence lies in our physiology. "We can see how a calm, affectionate, wholesome state of mind has beneficial effects on our health and well-being. Conversely, feelings of frustration, fear, agitation, and anger can be destructive to our health."[109]

In summary, empathy, which is cultivated by the core mindfulness practices (body scan, awareness of breath, walking meditation), is fundamental to patients' definition of quality care. However, a focus on empathy can cause stress for the HCP and eventually result in burnout. Alternatively, compassion originates with empathy but has the more positive focus of wishing to enhance others' well-being. Perhaps because of this focus, compassion can decrease HCP suffering and enhance their well-being while also increasing their motivation to help others. Compassion is therefore a way of caring for oneself while also caring for others. So, what is the "compassion training" that allows HCPs to be empathetic to patients while also rejuvenating themselves?

Formal Practice: Lovingkindness/Metta

By far, the most investigated compassion practice is *lovingkindness*, an ancient meditation practice called "metta" in the Buddhist tradition. A systematic review of research on lovingkindness meditation found decreased depression and increased mindfulness, compassion, self-compassion, and positive affect.[110] Another review reported decreased negative affect and stress as well as increased positive affect, connectedness, and mindfulness.[41] Benefits of lovingkindness meditation appear to be dose-dependent, with increased time resulting in increased "physiologic, behavioral, or neural outcomes."[16] As beneficial as this practice is, it should come with a warning label for HCPs: "Potentially Aversive." (There have been times when this practice felt as appealing to me as drinking a gallon of maple syrup.) Perhaps the level of self-criticism, self-judgment, and perfectionism among many HCPs makes this practice difficult…but also particularly beneficial.

Lovingkindness practice consists of thinking of specific people and offering them well-wishes, usually in the form of phrases. These phrases are directed toward individuals with different roles in your life, starting with someone who has helped or loved you (my therapist always wins this position) followed by yourself, then a friend, a neutral person (e.g., store cashier), and finally, a difficult person (I can always think of a patient for this role!). The traditional phrases include, "May you be happy, may you be safe, may you be well, may you live with ease." You are encouraged to create other phrases that are meaningful to you.

Although this practice resembles intercessory prayer, the well-wishes in lovingkindness practice are not offered to seek the help of a higher power to obtain a particular outcome. Rather, the main intention is the well-being of the practitioner. Meditation teacher and lovingkindness expert Sharon Salzberg advises not worrying if you do not feel a swell of sentimental feelings or hear a choir of angels singing. Benefits come from just setting a kind intention and going through the steps as best you can. You will begin to notice subtle but profound shifts in your perception of yourself and others—more understanding, more kindness.

If you find this practice too aversive, try imagining each person as an innocent child (in reality, each of us has a little child inside wanting to be seen and loved). You could also explore an alternative practice to cultivate compassion, *forgiveness practice*. Sharon Salzberg writes, "In order to be released from deeply held aversion for ourselves and for others, we must be able to practice forgiveness."[111] Indeed, I have found forgiveness practice more accessible than lovingkindness, probably because it aligns with my persistent perception of being flawed. You can find the forgiveness meditation as taught by Salzberg in Chapter 4. In Video 2.15, you will find a guided lovingkindness meditation.

Formal Practice: Awareness of the Breath With Focus on Self-Compassion

Compassion for oneself is a powerful way to cultivate compassion for others, and Chapter 4 will feature self-compassion research and practices. The next mindfulness practice is awareness of the breath, described earlier, with the added focus of meeting whatever is in the present experience with self-compassion. As you practice now, whenever a difficult thought, emotion, or body sensation arises, notice it, name it, and bring an intention of kindness and acceptance to whatever arises. Try saying a variation of these words silently to yourself:

May there be care for this _____ (tightness in my forehead, impatience, worried thought, etc.).

I have found this practice very helpful in difficult times. The heart seems to soften, and so does the body and mind. With practice, your capacity to meet uncomfortable thoughts, emotions, and sensations—yours and others'—expands.

Question for Reflection about Empathy:
(1) Psychologist and mindfulness teacher Shauna Shapiro sums up the stress of training: "The reigning paradigm in medical education emphasizes performance under stress, competition, and self-denial."[112] The HCP's ability for self-denial is important at times and might manifest as sacrificing sleep to prepare for an exam, delaying a bathroom break to finish a procedure, or ignoring a worry about a family situation to stay focused during a medical procedure. In contrast, caring for patients, especially when they are afraid or in pain, requires acknowledging, validating, and attending to the physical and emotional needs of others. How do you reconcile the seemingly conflicting abilities of denial of needs versus attentiveness to needs?
(2) Education and training to become an HCP and successful clinician require being tenacious, defined as "persistent in maintaining, adhering to, or seeking something valued or desired."[113] In

---

contrast, caring empathetically for others requires nondoing, being present, and letting go of an agenda. Compare and contrast these two seemingly opposing skills of doing versus being, of persisting versus surrendering.

Parasympathetic Primer Experience: Emotional Freedom Technique Tapping

The emotional freedom technique (EFT), or EFT tapping, is a way to dial down the voltage and settle before a formal meditation practice or anytime you feel off balance. It is excellent for the times when you are experiencing acute stress but need to focus and rebalance quickly at work. For example, you might have heard bad news about your dad, who is in the hospital, but you are about to start a surgical procedure and need to calm and focus yourself immediately. Once you learn EFT, you just need a few seconds and a private place (a bathroom stall at work will do).

This practice carried me through a very turbulent time. Almost 20 years ago, I had major challenges in every area of my life. I had a short marriage fail, I changed home as a result, I was diagnosed with a serious medical condition, and I was overseeing the construction of a new dental clinic. Through all of this, I never missed a day of work and maintained sanity (although at times holding on by my fingernails!) with the help of this peculiar technique.

In EFT tapping, three main elements—acupressure, mindfulness, and self-compassion—combine to create a potent antidote for stress. The "basic recipe," as described by Gary Craig,[114] can be found online at https://www.emofree.com/eft-tutorial/tapping-basics/how-to-do-eft.html. There are five main steps and nine pressure points, as summarized in Fig. 2.4.
1. Identify the issue: Choose one issue to focus on for each round. It might be an emotional (e.g., anxiety), a physical (e.g., headache), or a performance issue (e.g., a deadline, dental/medical procedure at work).
2. Test the initial intensity: Rate the intensity on a scale of 1 to 10, with 10 being highest. This will serve as the baseline to compare with after each round of the technique.
3. The set-up: A simple reminder phrase is repeated during the sequence while tapping on the first point, "karate chop point" (the fleshy part of the outside of either hand) shown in Fig. 2.5. The reminder phrase consists of two parts:

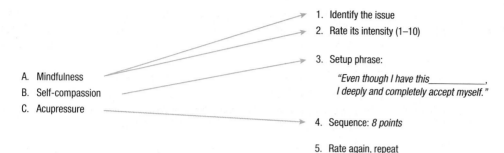

1. Identify the issue
2. Rate its intensity (1–10)

3. Setup phrase:
   "Even though I have this_____,
   I deeply and completely accept myself."

A. Mindfulness
B. Self-compassion
C. Acupressure

4. Sequence: *8 points*

5. Rate again, repeat

Fig. 2.4 Emotional Freedom Technique (EFT): A Combination of Three Elements.

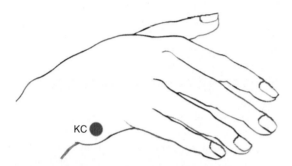

Fig. 2.5 Karate Chop *(KC)* Point for Setting Up Emotional Freedom Technique (EFT). (Graphic is from https://www. emofree.com/eft-tutorial/tapping-basics/how-to-do-eft.html.)

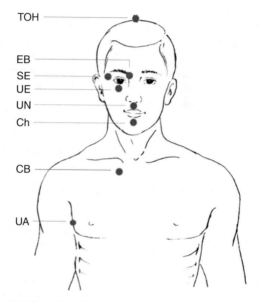

Fig. 2.6 The Eight Points of Emotional Freedom Technique (EFT). *CB,* Soft space between collar bone, breast bone, and the first rib; *Ch,* between chin and lower lip; *EB,* inner eyebrow; *SE,* side of the eye; *TOH,* top of the head; *UA,* under the arm; *UE,* under the eye; *UN,* under the nose. (Graphics is from https://www.emofree.com/eft-tutorial/tapping-basics/how-to-do-eft.html.)

a. "Even though I have this_____ (current issue),
b. "I deeply and completely accept myself." (self-compassion)

4. The sequence: This is the heart of the technique and consists of repeating the reminder phrase as you tap eight points on the body. You can tap the points on either side of the body with two fingers from the opposite side hand. The points are illustrated in Fig. 2.6 and include the top of the head (TOH); inner eyebrow (EB); side of the eye (SE); under the eye (UE); under the nose (UN); between chin and lower lip (Ch); soft space between collar bone, breast bone, and the first rib (CB); and under the arm (UA) on side of the body at the level of the breast.

5. Test the intensity again. Compare with baseline; note improvement. Repeat the sequence until you reach zero or a plateau.

The next video (Video 2.16) demonstrates the complete EFT sequence.

Research on EFT has found empirical evidence of its effectiveness for a variety of emotional and physical conditions. A systematic review and meta-analysis of 14 different randomized, controlled studies on EFT for anxiety showed "significant decrease in anxiety scores even when accounting for the effect size of control treatment."[115] Another systematic review and meta-analysis of 12 randomized, controlled studies and 8 outcome studies focused on the effects of EFT on depression. "The results showed that Clinical EFT were highly effective in reducing depressive symptoms in a variety of populations and settings," and "mean symptom reductions across all studies was -41 percent."[116] Finally, a study of 200 subjects measured both psychological and physiologic benefits of EFT, including significant improvement in resting heart rate, cortisol levels, and systemic and diastolic blood pressures—all objective measures of stress.[117] The importance of the tapping component of EFT was investigated in a review, which reported: "Meta-analysis indicated that the acupressure component was an active ingredient and outcomes were not due solely to placebo, nonspecific effects of any therapy, or nonacupressure components."[118]

A final note: The more precisely you can identify the issue, the more targeted and effective the technique. With each round of EFT, try to notice different aspects of the issue (check in with the triad of your experience—emotions, thoughts, or body sensations). For example, I might start a round of EFT for a bad headache and then notice tight breathing (then do another round for that), and then sadness (another round), and then frustration about falling behind schedule again (another round). In this way, you can penetrate what starts as a solid mass of experience and end up with workable parts of experience that quickly dissipate, allowing you to regain your balance.

Informal Practices for Compassion
Lovingkindness Meditation While Driving

This practice cultivates compassion while also improving driving safety. As shown in Video 2.17, simply notice the cars around you as you drive and send well-wishes to each of the drivers you see. Admittedly, there are times, such as when someone cuts you off on the road, when well-wishes might be the furthest thing from your mind, and you really want to offer your fellow motorist the one-finger salute! For these situations, try sending forgiveness (more on forgiveness practice in Chapter 4).

Compassion Practice at Work

As you walk toward your workplace, think of the patients you will see today—some you may already know and others will be new to you. Send them all well-wishes. Wish that you and your team will decrease their suffering in some way and increase their well-being.

You can also practice compassion by reviewing your schedule for the day and send well-wishes to each person listed. Remember that, just like you, each of them experiences anxiety and fear. Each of them wants to be safe and healthy. Each one wants to be happy. Set an intention to

not cause physical or emotional harm and to be of benefit to all. One of my favorite meditation teachers, Bob Stahl, once said on a retreat that when you set an intention, although you might forget about it, it comes back to find you. If you find it helpful to solidify your intention, you can place your hand on the schedule while setting your intention for compassion for the day, as illustrated in Video 2.18.

> **Note:** For confidentiality purposes, be sure to keep schedules (printed or electronic) posted/positioned in a place that is not visible to patients. Although my schedule is computerized, I like to have a printed copy of the schedule to which I add notes about each patient's key medical conditions, needed comfort measures, and personal/social issues. I keep this "cheat sheet" in my pocket for easy access all day.

INTEGRATING EASE: THE PRACTICE OF RAIN

Until I started a regular meditation practice, most of my challenging feelings stemmed from low self-esteem. I was constantly judging myself harshly. My favorite question was a version of the age-old nature versus nurture dilemma, with a self-critical twist: "Was I born stupid, or am I just being lazy?" The self-criticism was relentless, even as awards and accolades piled higher from school and piano performances. The practice of Recognize, Allow, Investigate, Nurture (RAIN) has been very helpful to me and many others in cooling the heat of difficult emotions, especially the guilt and shame created by harsh self-criticism. It incorporates all of the formal mindfulness practices we have learned so far, including awareness of the breath, body, thoughts, and emotions as well as compassion practice. The following is a true story illustrating how the mindfulness practice of RAIN benefitted me and my ability to care for patients:

It was a hectic day in the dental clinic, and I found myself running behind early in the day, trying to juggle everything—my scheduled patients, the hygiene patients, walk-in emergency patients, and a new resident from the nearby hospital needing orientation. On top of everything, we were in the middle of a major clinic expansion project, and dental supply representatives and contractors frequently were soliciting my input by phone and email. The treadmill was going faster than I could run. Soon, I began to notice difficulty breathing and frustration. Then came the headache, like a vice grip on my temples. I wondered if I would make it through the day and fantasized about fleeing the clinic. I told the receptionist I wasn't feeling well and to prepare for the possibility of canceling patient appointments.

Fortunately, I had a break at lunch, so I closed my office door and turned out the lights. Sitting relaxed and upright, I focused on my breath. At first, my breath was short and shallow, but then I noticed it deepening and elongating. I spent a couple minutes just feeling the movement of air through my nose and the rising and falling of my belly. As my attention settled on the breath, I expanded my attention to include what was bothering me. I opened to the headache and allowed it space. After a few moments, I began to investigate the **sensations** of the headache. What is it? Pressure. Where is it? Temples. Forehead, too, on the surface. How is it? Metal hard. As I breathed with the intense sensations, I found them slowly easing. Then, I widened the attention more to include any **thoughts** underlying the headache. I breathed for a while, and suddenly a thought bubbled up—the main thought that had been jabbing me all morning: "The reason you are falling behind is because you are such a bad dentist." The awareness of this belief made its **emotional** imprint clear . . . the sense of shame, the sadness, the weight of it all. Tears rolled down. As I placed my hand on my heart, I felt the grip of this thought loosen. Soon, I felt a sense of ease and calm arising. I emerged from my office with renewed energy and met the rest of the day feeling fine.

Psychotherapist, meditation teacher, and author Tara Brach has become an authority on RAIN and has created web resources and written books on this practice. She recommends RAIN as a meditation, or simply moving "through the steps whenever challenging feelings arise."[119] If you are practicing RAIN as a meditation, start by asking yourself, "What is bothering me right now?"

R is for **recognize.** Notice that a difficulty is here. Maybe the difficulty is something you do not want (headache) or an unmet expectation (being on time with the schedule). If possible, label the hardest thing silently to yourself—the believed thought ("I'm so far behind, my day is ruined"), the emotion ("anger is here"), or the body sensation ("tightness in the forehead"). When that is not possible, simply acknowledge difficulty: "This is hard for me right now."

A is for **allow.** Give some space for the experience to be there, as it is, "without trying to fix or avoid anything."[119] Allowing does not mean approving of your circumstances. (For example, in the previous example, I might need to find ways to reduce the patient load or the number of interruptions to my work.) Allowing means letting the *experience* of the present moment conditions be as it is—the emotions, the thoughts, the body sensations. Breathe with them. Offer a word of welcome: "Hello, headache, I see you."

I is for **investigate with interest and care.** Tune in to the specific body sensations that capture the difficulty rather than ideas or commentary about the experience. Perhaps there is a sense of bracing, tightness, or clenching. Maybe your breath is constricted. Feel the sensations directly. Notice any shifts in the sensations as you observe. In addition, notice any thoughts or emotions that are present. In the previous story, I noticed the various sensations in my head, the thought behind the headache ("I'm a bad dentist"), and the emotions of shame and sadness.

N is for **nurture with self-compassion.** Give yourself a word or a gesture of kindness. You might say silently to yourself, "This is hard for you right now," or gently place your hand on your heart. Summon up a caring attitude toward yourself or, if it feels more natural, an intention of self-forgiveness.

Formal mindfulness practice will make the practice of RAIN more possible amid a stressful moment. See the work of Tara Brach for more guidance on RAIN and other practices for managing stress and increasing EASE in your life.

CAUTIONARY NOTE: TRAUMA SENSITIVITY AND MINDFULNESS PRACTICE

While the benefits of mindfulness have been well established, mindfulness practice can be problematic for some individuals with a history of trauma. Mindfulness helps us deal with difficulties by turning our attention toward the present moment with a sense of kindness and acceptance. For those who experience traumatic stress or post-traumatic stress disorder (PTSD), turning toward experience can result in "contact with traumatic stimuli—thoughts, images, memories, and physical sensations that may relate to a traumatic event," and this brings the potential to "aggravate and intensify symptoms of traumatic stress."[44]

Several possible sources of trauma threaten HCPs, including personal life, professional education/training, and work. According to Dr. Albert Wu, professor of health policy and management at Johns Hopkins, "It's not a matter of if clinicians are going to experience trauma while providing care, but when and how often."[120] Potentially traumatic aspects of work include witnessing and, especially, inducing pain and anxiety. Such situations bear the potential for causing secondary and vicarious traumatic stress.

Learning to recognize the symptoms of traumatic reactions is pivotal to staying in your window of tolerance as you practice mindfulness meditation. Reactions can manifest as *hyperarousal* (fight or flight reactivity) or *hypoarousal* (freeze reaction).[44] Psychologist, author, and expert on trauma-sensitive mindfulness Dr. David Treleaven describes hyperarousal as feeling "hypervigilant and anxious" and hypoarousal as "feeling foggy, listless, and numb."[44] Between these two extremes lies the "window of tolerance" described by Siegel.[121] As we practice mindfulness, we aim to stay within the window tolerance: the place where we feel safe and balanced.

If you find any such symptoms arising during your meditation practice, know that you always have the option to modify the practice in the way that feels right to you, as discussed at the beginning of this chapter. Choose the anchor that feels right to you. The three recommended options for anchors include the breath, the body sensations, and sounds. Choose a position that supports calming and focusing, whether it be standing, sitting, or lying down. You may also choose to keep your eyes open or closed. In addition, there are specific ways to "apply the brakes" during meditation practice, as described by Treleaven:

- Open one's eyes during meditation practice
- Take a few slow, deep breaths
- Focus on a resourceful, external object in one's environment
- Engage in shorter practice periods[44]

If the formal mindfulness practices are simply not accessible for you, honor your limits and allow the PPEs to be your main diet for now. These practices will bring you closer to the sensations of your body and cultivate presence. Finally, many of us with a trauma history need a teacher or therapist in the beginning to provide one-on-one support to find a sense of balance, as was the case for me. Again, the bottom line is to honor your limits and follow your own innate wisdom.

CONCLUSION

Mindfulness can be thought of as "preventive medicine" for future doctors, helping them cultivate a "way of being" that may foster healing and growth in their own lives as well as skills to effectively help others heal and grow in the future.[39]

Returning to the previous metaphor (see Fig. 2.1), remember that the mindful HCP is a like a strong tree. The roots represent the qualities of mindfulness: EASE. Water nourishes the roots of the tree and represents mindfulness practices cultivating the qualities of the patient-centered professional. The branches and fruits of the tree represent the actions and words that express care and respect. Rooted in mindfulness, we can notice and understand what is needed. Rooted in mindfulness we can meet the needs of the patient in the moment with our words and actions in a way that brings connection and healing. You now have the tools to cultivate EASE; however, they are only effective when they are practiced regularly over time. Many of these same practices can also help patients when they are anxious or in pain, as we will explore in Chapter 5.

While mindfulness guides the HCP's words and actions moment-to-moment, research on patient preferences and perceptions may also serve as a guide. Are there specific words or behaviors that patients are most likely to interpret as caring and respect? Indeed, a review of the literature has identified 6 core categories of communication skills. These are unveiled in the next chapter.

REFERENCES

1. Lovas JG, Lovas DA, Lovas PM. Mindfulness and professionalism in dentistry. *J Dent Educ.* 2008;72:998–1009.
2. Nanticoke Indian Association. *The Tale of Two Wolves.* Available at: https://www.nanticokeindians.org/page/taleof-two-wolves. Accessed May 6, 2020.
3. Hölzel BK, Carmody J, Evans KC, et al. Stress reduction correlates with structural changes in the amygdala. *Soc Cogn Affect Neurosci.* 2010;5:11–17.
4. Chiesa A, Brambilla P, Serretti A. Neuro-imaging of mindfulness meditations: implications for clinical practice. *Epidemiol Psychiatr Sci.* 2011;20:205–210.
5. Goldstein J. *Mindfulness: A Practical Guide to Awakening.* Boulder: Sounds True; 2013.
6. Kabat-Zinn J. Mindfulness-based interventions in context: past, present, and future. *Clin Psychol Sci Pract.* 2003;10:144–156.

7. Bishop SR, Lau M, Shapiro S, et al. Mindfulness: a proposed operational definition. *Clin Psychol Sci Pract.* 2004;11:230–241.

8. Sharma M, Rush SE. Mindfulness-based stress reduction as a stress management intervention for healthy individuals: a systematic review. *J Evid Based Complementary Altern Med.* 2014;19:271–286.

9. Praissman S. Mindfulness-based stress reduction: a literature review and clinician's guide. *J Am Acad Nurse Pract.* 2008;20:212–216.

10. Dobkin PL, Hassed C. *Mindful Medical Practitioners: A Guide for Clinicians and Educators.* Switzerland: Springer International; 2016.

11. Zoppi K, Epstein RM. Is communication a skill? Communication behaviors and being in relation. *Fam Med.* 2002;34:319–324.

12. *Mindfulness: Good for Patients, Good for Nurses.* 2019. Available at: https://degree.louisiana.edu/online-programs/nursing/rn-to-bsn/mindfulness-for-patients-and-nurses/. Accessed September 21, 2021.

13. Dobkin PL, Hutchinson TA. Teaching mindfulness in medical school: where are we now and where are we going? *Med Educ.* 2013;47:768–779.

14. Hick SF, Bien T. *Mindfulness and the Therapeutic Relationship.* New York: Guilford; 2010.

15. Pradhan EK, Baumgarten M, Langenberg P, et al. Effect of Mindfulness-Based Stress Reduction in rheumatoid arthritis patients. *Arthritis Rheum.* 2007;57:1134–1142.

16. Pace TW, Negi LT, Adame DD, et al. Effect of compassion meditation on neuroendocrine, innate immune and behavioral responses to psychosocial stress. *Psychoneuroendocrinology.* 2009;34:87–98.

17. *Dental Student's Father Bemoans Privacy Laws.* Available at: https://ssristories.org/dental-students-father-bemoans-privacy-laws-voices-of-ny/. Accessed January 18, 2019.

18. *Body Found in Hudson River is Identified as that of Missing Columbia University Student Jiwon Lee.* Available at: https://www.nydailynews.com/new-york/body-hudson-river-missing-columbia-student-article-1.1779450. Accessed January 18, 2019.

19. Insight Meditation Center. *Equanimit.* Available at: https://www.insightmeditationcenter.org/books-articles/equanimity/. Accessed March 11, 2020.

20. Rodin AE, Key JD. William Osler and Aequanimitas: an appraisal of his reactions to adversity. *J R Soc Med.* 1994;87:758–763.

21. Stagman-Tyrer D. Resiliency and the nurse leader: the importance of equanimity, optimism, and perseverance. *Nurs Manage.* 2014;45:46–50.

22. Corah NL, O'Shea RM, Bissell GD, et al. The dentist–patient relationship: perceived dentist behaviors that reduce patient anxiety and increase satisfaction. *J Am Dent Assoc.* 1988;116:73–76.

23. Irving JA, Dobkin PL, Park J. Cultivating mindfulness in health care professionals: a review of empirical studies of mindfulness-based stress reduction (MBSR). *Complement Ther Clin Pract.* 2009;15:61–66.

24. Azimi S, AsgharNejad Farid AA, Kharazi Fard MJ, et al. Emotional intelligence of dental students and patient satisfaction. *Eur J Dent Educ.* 2010;14:129–132.

25. Rada RE, Johnson-Leong C. Stress, burnout, anxiety and depression among dentists. *J Am Dent Assoc.* 2004;135:788–794.

26. Shanafelt TD. Enhancing meaning in work: a prescription for preventing physician burnout and promoting patient-centered care. *JAMA.* 2009;302:1338–1340.

27. Prasad K, McLoughlin C, Stillman M, et al. Prevalence and correlates of stress and burnout among U.S. healthcare workers during the COVID-19 pandemic: a national cross-sectional survey study. *EClinicalMedicine.* 2021;35:100879.

28. Roberts R, Grubb PL, Grosch JW. *Alleviating Job Stress in Nurses.* Medscape; 2012. Available at: https://www.medscape.com/viewarticle/765974_2. Accessed January 28, 2021.

29. New Zealand Dental Association and Dental Council of New Zealand. *Self Care for Dentists.* Available at: https://www.dcnz.org.nz/assets/Uploads/Publications/SelfCareForDentists.pdf.

30. Epstein EG, Haizlip J, Liaschenko J, et al. Moral distress, mattering, and secondary traumatic stress in provider burnout: a call for moral community. *AACN Adv Crit Care.* 2020;31:146–157.

31. Sancho FM, Ruiz CN. Risk of suicide amongst dentists: myth or reality? *Int Dent J.* 2010;60:411–418.

32. Baile WF, Buckman R, Lenzi R, et al. SPIKES—a six-step protocol for delivering bad news: application to the patient with cancer. *Oncologist.* 2000;5:302–311.

33. Beck J. *The Concept Creep of 'Emotional Labor'.* The Atlantic; 2018. Available at: https://www.theatlantic.com/family/archive/2018/11/arlie-hochschild-housework-isnt-emotional-labor/576637/. Accessed January 26, 2021.

34. Sanders MJ, Turcotte CM. Occupational stress in dental hygienists. *Work.* 2010;35:455–465.

35. Siwicki B. *Pandemic-Era Burnout: Nurses in the Trenches Say Technology Hurts and Helps.* Healthcare IT News; 2020. Available at: https://www.healthcareitnews.com/news/pandemic-era-burnout-nurses-trenches-say-technology-hurts-and-helps. Accessed September 02, 2021.

36. Shumake K. *The Benefits of Self-Forgiveness.* BeWell Stanford; 2019. Available at: https://scopeblog.stanford.edu/2019/08/02/the-benefits-of-self-forgiveness/. Accessed September 22, 2020.

37. Rosenzweig S, Reibel DK, Greeson JM, et al. Mindfulness-based stress reduction lowers psychological distress in medical students. *Teach Learn Med.* 2003;15:88–92.

38. LaPorta LD. Occupational stress in oral and maxillofacial surgeons: tendencies, traits, and triggers. *Oral Maxillofac Surg Clin North Am.* 2010;22:495–502.

39. Shapiro SL, Schwartz GE, Bonner G. Effects of mindfulness-based stress reduction on medical and premedical students. *J Behav Med.* 1998;21:581–599.

40. Krasner MS, Epstein RM, Beckman H, et al. Association of an educational program in mindful communication with burnout, empathy, and attitudes among primary care physicians. *JAMA.* 2009;302:1284–1293.

41. Luberto CM, Shinday N, Song R, et al. A systematic review and meta-analysis of the effects of meditation on empathy, compassion, and prosocial behaviors. *Mindfulness (N Y).* 2018;9:708–724.

42. Warnecke E, Quinn S, Ogden K, et al. A randomised controlled trial of the effects of mindfulness practice on medical student stress levels. *Med Educ.* 2011;45:381–388.

43. Atanes AC, Andreoni S, Hirayama MS, et al. Mindfulness, perceived stress, and subjective well-being: a correlational study in primary care health professionals. *BMC Complement Altern Med.* 2015;15:303.

44. Treleaven DA. *Trauma-Sensitive Mindfulness: Practices for Safe and Transformative Healing.* New York: WW Norton; 2018.

45. Healthwise Staff. *Stress Management: Doing Progressive Muscle Relaxation.* University of Michigan Health; 2020. Available at: https://www.uofmhealth.org/health-library/uz2225. Accessed July 07, 2020.

46. Mirgain S, Singles J. *Whole Health: Change The Conversation, Progressive Muscle Relaxation.* Available at: http://projects.hsl.wisc.edu/SERVICE/modules/12/M12_CT_Progressive_Muscle_Relaxation.pdf. Accessed July 07, 2020.

47. Bayda E. *Being Zen: Bringing Meditation to Life.* Boston: Shambhala; 2002.

48. Covey SR. *The Seven Habits of Highly Effective People: Restoring the Character Ethic.* New York: Simon and Schuster; 1989.

49. Hanson R. *Take in the Good.* Available at: https://www.rickhanson.net/take-in-the-good/. Accessed June 10, 2021.

50. Oxford Reference. *Reciprocal Inhibition.* Available at: https://www.oxfordreference.com/view/10.1093/oi/authority.20110803100408294. Accessed June 10, 2021.

51. Hebb DO. *The Organization of Behavior.* New York: Wiley & Sons; 1949.

52. Emmons RA, McCullough ME. Counting blessings versus burdens: an experimental investigation of gratitude and subjective well-being in daily life. *J Pers Soc Psychol.* 2003;84:377–389.

53. Cunha LF, Pellanda LC, Reppold CT. Positive psychology and gratitude interventions: a randomized clinical trial. *Front Psychol.* 2019;10:584.

54. Greater Good in Action. *Gratitude Journal.* Greater Good Science Center Magazine. Available at: https://ggia.berkeley.edu/practice/gratitude_journal. Accessed June 10, 2021.

55. James W. *The Principles of Psychology.* New York: H. Holt and Company; 1890.

56. Leebov W, Rotering C. *The Language of Caring Guide for Physicians: Communication Essentials for Patient-Centered Care.* 2nd ed. USA: Language of Caring LLC; 2014.

57. de Botton, A. *On Distraction: Our Minds Need to go on a Diet.* City Journal; 2010. Available at: https://www.city-journal.org/html/distraction-13292.html. Accessed February 24, 2022.

58. Tarawneh R. *"How Does the Internet Affect Brain Function?" Wexner Medical Center.* The Ohio State University; 2020. Available at: https://wexnermedical.osu.edu/blog/how-internet-affects-your-brain. Accessed January 15, 2021.

59. Haynes T. *Dopamine, Smartphones & You: A Battle for Your Time.* Science in the News, Harvard University; 2018. Available at: http://sitn.hms.harvard.edu/flash/2018/dopamine-smartphones-battle-time/. Accessed January 15, 2021.

60. Orlowski J. *A Social Dilemma.* [Video Documentary] USA; 2020.

61. Buckwalter-Poza R. *Treat, Don't Tweet: The Dangerous Rise of Social Media in the Operating Room—Pacific Standard.* Pacific Standard. Available at: https://psmag.com/social-justice/treat-dont-tweet-dangerous-rise-social-media-operating-room-79061. Accessed March 31, 2022.

62. Smith T, Darling E, Searles B. 2010 Survey on cell phone use while performing cardiopulmonary bypass. *Perfusion.* 2011;26:375–380.

63. Alsalameh AM, Harisi MJ, Alduayji MA, et al. Evaluating the relationship between smartphone addiction/overuse and musculoskeletal pain among medical students at Qassim University. *J Family Med Prim Care.* 2019;8:2953–2959.

64. Nield D. *Try Grayscale Mode to Curb Your Phone Addiction.* Wired; 2019. Available at: https://www.wired.com/story/grayscale-ios-android-smartphone-addiction/. Accessed February 19, 2021.

65. Lazar SW, Kerr CE, Wasserman RH, et al. Meditation experience is associated with increased cortical thickness. *Neuroreport.* 2005;16:1893–1897.

66. Tang YY, Lu Q, Geng X, et al. Short-term meditation induces white matter changes in the anterior cingulate. *Proc Natl Acad Sci U S A.* 2010;107:15649–15652.

67. Moore A, Gruber T, Derose J, et al. Regular, brief mindfulness meditation practice improves electrophysiological markers of attentional control. *Front Hum Neurosci.* 2012;6:18.

68. Chodron P. *Start Where You Are: A Guide to Compassionate Living.* Boston: Shambhala; 2003.

69. Salzberg S. *Week One of the 2019 Challenge.* Sharon Salzberg; 2019. Available at: https://www.sharonsalzberg.com/week-one-of-the-2019-challenge/. Accessed October 30, 2020.

70. Garland EL, Howard MO. Mindfulness-based treatment of addiction: current state of the field and envisioning the next wave of research. *Addict Sci Clin Pract.* 2018; 13:14.

71. Hahn TN. *Thich Nhat Hanh on Walking Meditation.* Lion's Roar. Available at: https://www.lionsroar.com/how-to-meditate-thich-nhat-hanh-on-walking-meditation/. Accessed February 24, 2022.

72. Haque OS, Waytz A. Dehumanization in medicine: causes, solutions, and functions. *Perspect Psychol Sci.* 2012;7:176–186.

73. Virshup BB, Oppenberg AA, Coleman MM. Strategic risk management: reducing malpractice claims through more effective patient-doctor communication. *Am J Med Qual.* 1999;14:153–159.

74. Davis DM, Hayes JA. What are the Benefits of Mindfulness? *Am Psychol Assoc Monitor Psychol.* 2012;43:64.

75. Fox KC, Nijeboer S, Dixon ML, et al. Is meditation associated with altered brain structure? A systematic review and meta-analysis of morphometric neuroimaging in meditation practitioners. *Neurosci Biobehav Rev.* 2014;43:48–73.

76. Chödrön P. *Take Three Conscious Breaths.* Lions Roar; 2017. Available at: https://www.lionsroar.com/take-three-conscious-breaths/. Accessed July 08, 2020.

77. Stahl B, Goldstein E. *A Mindfulness-Based Stress Reduction Workbook.* Oakland: Bob Stahl and Elisha Goldstein; 2010.

78. Mercer SW, Maxwell M, Heaney D, et al. The consultation and relational empathy (CARE) measure: development and preliminary validation and reliability of an empathy-based consultation process measure. *Fam Pract.* 2004;21: 699–705.

79. Vergnes JN, Apelian N, Bedos C. What about narrative dentistry? *J Am Dent Assoc.* 2015;146:398–401.

80. Frankel RM. Emotion and the physician-patient Relationship. *Motiv Emot.* 1995;19:163–173.

81. Lester GW, Smith SG. Listening and talking to patients: a remedy for malpractice suits. *Western Journal of Medicine.* 1993;158:268–272.

82. Haslam N. Humanizing medical practice: the role of empathy. *Med J Aust.* 2007;187:381–382.

83. Riess H, Kelley JM, Bailey RW, et al. Empathy training for resident physicians: a randomized controlled trial of a neuroscience-informed curriculum. *J Gen Intern Med.* 2012;27:1280–1286.

84. Yarascavitch C, Regehr G, Hodges B, et al. Changes in dental student empathy during training. *J Dent Educ.* 2009;73:509–517.

85. Nash DA. Ethics, empathy, and the education of dentists. *J Dent Educ.* 2010;74:567–578.

86. Rosenzweig J, Blaizot A, Cougot N, et al. Effect of a person-centered course on the empathic ability of dental students. *J Dent Educ.* 2016;80:1337–1348.

87. Halpern J. What is clinical empathy? *J Gen Intern Med.* 2003;18:670–674.

88. Chen PJ, Huang CD, Yeh SJ. Impact of a narrative medicine programme on healthcare providers' empathy scores over time. *BMC Med Educ.* 2017;17:108.

89. Mori H, Mori K. A test of the passive facial feedback hypothesis: we feel sorry because we cry. *Percept Mot Skills.* 2007;105:1242–1244.

90. Lamothe M, Rondeau É, Malboeuf-Hurtubise C, et al. Outcomes of MBSR or MBSR-based interventions in health care providers: a systematic review with a focus on empathy and emotional competencies. *Complement Ther Med.* 2016;24:19–28.

91. Conversano C, Ciacchini R, Orrù G, et al. Mindfulness, compassion, and self-compassion among health care professionals: what's new? A systematic review. *Front Psychol.* 2020;11:1683.

92. McConville J, McAleer R, Hahne A. Mindfulness training for health profession students-the effect of mindfulness training on psychological well-being, learning and clinical performance of health professional students: a systematic review of randomized and non-randomized controlled trials. *Explore (NY).* 2017;13:26–45.

93. Sherman JJ, Cramer A. Measurement of changes in empathy during dental school. *J Dent Educ.* 2005;69: 338–345.

94. Perez-Bret E, Altisent R, Rocafort J. Definition of compassion in healthcare: a systematic literature review. *Int J Palliat Nurs.* 2016;22:599–606.

95. Keltner D, Goetz J. Compassion. In: Baumeister R, Vohs KD, eds. *Encyclopedia of Social Psychology.* Thousand Oaks: Sage Publications; 2007:159–161.

96. Gilbert P. *The Compassionate Mind: A New Approach to Life's Challenges.* London: Constable and Robinson; 2009.

97. Strauss C, Lever Taylor B, Gu J, et al. What is compassion and how can we measure it? A review of definitions and measures. *Clin Psychol Rev.* 2016;47:15–27.

98. Sinclair S, Beamer K, Hack TF, et al. Sympathy, empathy, and compassion: a grounded theory study of palliative care patients' understandings, experiences, and preferences. *Palliat Med.* 2017;31:437–447.

99. Dowling T. Compassion does not fatigue! *Can Vet J.* 2018;59:749–750.

100. Klimecki OM, Leiberg S, Ricard M, et al. Differential pattern of functional brain plasticity after compassion and empathy training. *Soc Cogn Affect Neurosci.* 2014;9: 873–879.

101. Singer T, Seymour B, O'Doherty J, et al. Empathy for pain involves the affective but not sensory components of pain. *Science.* 2004;303:1157–1162.

102. Fan Y, Duncan NW, de Greck M, et al. Is there a core neural network in empathy? An fMRI based quantitative meta-analysis. *Neurosci Biobehav Rev.* 2011;35: 903–911.

103. Lamm C, Decety J, Singer T. Meta-analytic evidence for common and distinct neural networks associated with directly experienced pain and empathy for pain. *Neuroimage.* 2011;54:2492–2502.

104. Knox M. *6 Ways Dogs Teach Us Self-Compassion.* Center for Mindful Self-Compassion; 2019. Available at: https://centerformsc.org/how-dogs-teach-us-self-compassion/. Accessed November 19, 2020.

105. Fredrickson BL, Cohn MA, Coffey KA, et al. Open hearts build lives: positive emotions, induced through loving-kindness meditation, build consequential personal resources. *J Pers Soc Psychol.* 2008;95: 1045–1062.

106. Klimecki OM, Leiberg S, Lamm C, et al. Functional neural plasticity and associated changes in positive affect after compassion training. *Cereb Cortex.* 2013;23: 1552–1561.

107. Leiberg S, Klimecki O, Singer T. Short-term compassion training increases prosocial behavior in a newly developed prosocial game. *PLoS One.* 2011;6:e17798.

108. Weng HY, Fox AS, Shackman AJ, et al. Compassion training alters altruism and neural responses to suffering. *Psychol Sci.* 2013;24:1171–1180.

109. Dalai Lama, Cutler HC. *The Art of Happiness.* London: Hodder Paperback; 1999.

110. Galante J, Galante I, Bekkers MJ, et al. Effect of kindness-based meditation on health and well-being: a systematic review and meta-analysis. *J Consult Clin Psychol.* 2014;82:1101–1114.

111. Salzberg S. *Loving-Kindness: The Revolutionary Art of Happiness.* Boston: Shambhala Publications; 1997.

112. Shapiro SL, Shapiro DE, Schwartz GE. Stress management in medical education: a review of the literature. *Acad Med.* 2000;75:748–759.

113. Merriam-Webster. *Tenacious.* Available at: https://www.merriam-webster.com/dictionary/tenacious. Accessed October 15, 2020.

114. Craig G, Craig T. *How to do the EFT Tapping Basics—The Basic Recipe.* The Gary Craig Official EFT Training Centers; 1995. Available at: https://www.emofree.com/nl/eft-tutorial/tapping-basics/how-to-do-eft.html. Accessed October 12, 2020.

115. Clond M. Emotional freedom techniques for anxiety: a systematic review with meta-analysis. *J Nerv Ment Dis.* 2016;204:388–395.

116. Nelms JA, Castel L. A systematic review and meta-analysis of randomized and nonrandomized trials of clinical emotional freedom techniques (EFT) for the treatment of depression. *Explore (NY).* 2016;12:416–426.

117. Bach D, Groesbeck G, Stapleton P, et al. Clinical EFT (Emotional Freedom Techniques) improves multiple physiological markers of health. *J Evid Based Integr Med.* 2019;24:2515690X18823691.

118. Church D, Stapleton P, Yang A, et al. Is tapping on acupuncture points an active ingredient in emotional freedom techniques? A systematic review and meta-analysis of comparative studies. *J Nerv Ment Dis.* 2018; 206:783–793.

119. Brach T. *True Refuge.* New York: Bantam Books; 2013.

120. Paturel A. *When Physicians are Traumatized.* Association of American Medical Colleges; 2019. Available at: https://www.aamc.org/news-insights/when-physicians-are-traumatized. Accessed July 02, 2020.

121. Siegel D. *The Developing Mind.* New York: Guilford Press; 1999.

The Branches: What We Say

Continued

Patients reported that doctors needed both technical competence and a clear interest in the patient, demonstrated by good communication.[1]

The successful… practitioner needs to have not only technical skill and knowledge but also the ability to create rapport and a therapeutic relationship.[2]

It would be so convenient to have a script for "creating rapport and a therapeutic relationship" in every clinical situation—what to say when a patient confesses their fear of their upcoming procedure, what to do when the patient cries "ouch!" during a procedure. While there is no formula for what to say or do that will work with every patient every time, there are several essential behaviors and skills that research has found foster a trusting, respectful relationship. These core behaviors are captured by several models for communication, such as the 4E model, developed by the Bayer Institute for Health Care Communication[3]; the SPIKES Model for delivering bad news in medicine and dentistry[4]; and the 4 Habits Coding Scheme (4HCS).[5] Unfortunately, these models, while helpful for many health care professionals (HCPs), have limited value for the procedure-oriented HCP, and here's why: communication models in health care focus on the *consultation* mode and, therefore, omit the many aspects of care that arise before, during, and after hands-on *procedures*. Dental researchers have noted that "models of clinical dental communication are almost non-existent."[6] The communication model presented in this chapter (and applied to clinical challenges in Chapter 4) aims to fill this void.

The ISLEEP model includes the core skills needed for patient-centered care during the consultation AND procedures. ISLEEP stands for: *introduce/interconnect, solicit, listen, empathize, explain,* and affirm *power* of the patient. (Just remember, *I sleep better when I*

communicate well!) Each element of ISLEEP represents a category of observable behaviors. They may be applied chronologically, but this is neither necessary nor always desirable.

Returning to the tree metaphor shown in Fig. 3.1, now we focus on the branches and fruit, which represent each of the ISLEEP behaviors. The ability to discern the skillful response to each patient moment by moment is the fruit of mindfulness. Rooted in mindfulness, the HCP can express respect and care with their words, employing the ISLEEP skills.

BACKGROUND OF ISLEEP

The ISLEEP model is the product of many years of informal, incidental interviews of many patients as well as observation of HCPs with patients known to be either satisfied or dissatisfied with their care. Patients generally shared information with me spontaneously, but some was elicited through more pointed inquiry. My questions have been very simple: "What makes an HCP a good one to you?" Or conversely, "What makes an HCP a bad one to you?" Other questions include, "What makes a procedure difficult?" And conversely, "What makes a procedure comfortable for you?" In addition, many research studies on patient satisfaction, patient-centered care, and malpractice trends have informed the ISLEEP model and are referenced throughout this chapter.

Videos of live patient encounters accompany each skill. These videos are all real patient encounters, not simulations, unless indicated otherwise. All are shared with the generous consent of the patients, and most of the videos feature a particular HCP, a dentist—myself! How would videos in dentistry be helpful to other HCPs? Dentistry represents the quintessential health care specialty that evokes pain and anxiety for patients. For example, imagine

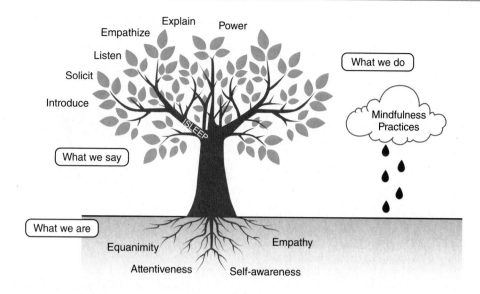

Fig. 3.1 The Communication Skills of the Patient-centered Provider.

meeting a fearful patient for the first time, having to give them an injection in one of the most sensitive and personal parts of their body, and then extracting their tooth—all in a matter of minutes! Such experiences require skillful communication to navigate. Further, most HCPs have experienced dentistry as a patient and therefore can relate to this setting at least from the patient perspective if not the professional.

Note: Most of the videos were filmed pre-Covid-19 pandemic, as reflected in the PPE used.

Note to Educators
Expressing care and respect during a patient interaction is a highly complex skill and art that defies methodology and objective standards. Attempts to teach and evaluate bedside/chairside manner without attention to cultivating therapeutic presence can easily devolve into a pedantic checklist approach. This is why education in patient-centered communication must start with cultivating mindfulness, which will guide wise, compassionate responses to each patient, moment by moment.

Although mindfulness is essential to skillful communication in health care, a systematic approach to education in communication is supported by the consistency of patient preferences documented by research. Furthermore, "adoption of a common set of evaluation tools between institutions would foster a more rigorous standard in behavioral science and communication skills."[7] A comprehensive, practical model such as the ISLEEP model will help advance a professional standard for education and practice. The ISLEEP model provides an objective, clear, finite framework for attuning trainees to evidence-based, core behaviors that foster patient-centered care. While some models include important elements such as respect and trust, this model captures the *observable behaviors* that give rise to respect, trust, and other hallmarks of therapeutic relationships.

Communication skills, like any other skill, are not learned by reading about them or hearing a lecture about them. Simply reading this book without experiencing the skills would be analogous to reading a musical score without ever picking up an instrument and then expecting to play the piece well. Skills are learned by doing them and by reflecting on how we did them. For this reason, many experiential exercises and reflection questions are included throughout this chapter. Some reflection questions that can accompany discussion of stories and videos depicting each ISLEEP skill include:

1. What thoughts and feelings arise for you?
2. How did the patient respond?
3. What obstacles (internal/external) do you face in trying to practice this ISLEEP skill?
4. What alternative ways or words can you find to implement this skill in this situation?

Consider establishing a shared, online platform where learners can share their reflections to the readings, videos, and experiential exercises as well as their answers to reflection questions. This allows an opportunity to build community and mutual support on the issues surrounding patient-centered care.

In alignment with the **K.O.S.E.** pedagogical model described by Lanning[8] (which has its underpinnings in the work of Miller[9]), first, trainees gain **knowledge** of ISLEEP behaviors by reading the text. Second, they **observe** each ISLEEP skill in the video recordings, allowing them to recognize the core ISLEEP behaviors. Third, **simulation** through many experiential exercises and role plays offers trainees the chance to practice each individual behavior. Finally, **experience** of ISLEEP skills in a live, clinical setting solidifies the skills learned.

Videorecording trainees to promote communication skills development is highly recommended and, thanks to widespread availability of smart phones, very workable. The experience of videorecording to improve communication skills has been rated highly by pre-professional students[10] as well as clinicians in practice.[11] Let the videos contained here be a springboard to creating your own collection. Learners can have fun producing videos that demonstrate both skillfulness and unskillfulness (on purpose!—for comic relief). Channel the creative and competitive spirit of HCPs by hosting an "Academy Awards," granting awards for the best skillful examples and best unskillful examples of the different ISLEEP skills.

This chapter serves as a primer for the six communication skills while Chapter 4 includes many examples of how to apply the ISLEEP skills in common clinical challenges, such as delivering bad news and adverse outcomes. A summary chart of the ISLEEP model is found in Table 3.1 as well as in Appendix B. Evaluation worksheets, found in Appendix C, are provided to guide instructor evaluation of trainees or for self-evaluation. Once practitioners can evaluate themselves, they can achieve a fundamental goal of education: self-efficacy.

Preparatory Question for ISLEEP Skill Introduce/Interconnect

How do you get to know a patient at the first visit and at subsequent visits to create personal connection?

ISLEEP: INTRODUCE AND INTERCONNECT

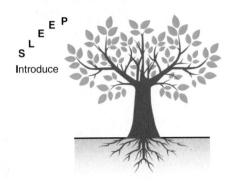

A crucial point in the encounter is the… first greeting of the patient.[3]

Huntington and Kuhn, Communication Gaffes: A Root Cause of Malpractice Claims

The very beginning of any health care encounter sets the tone of the visit—hopefully, a caring tone, and **introduce/interconnect** is the first core category of ISLEEP skills. Video 3.1 depicts Dr. Ronda, my colleague who was so highly revered that many of her patients wept at the news of her resignation. Notice how she conveys interest and care from her very first step into the treatment room.

Dr. Ronda sounds and looks so happy to see her patient, and the patient reflects her joy in his smile. There is no doubt that this doctor cares about the patient.

In addition to setting the general tone, the first ISLEEP element, introduce/interconnect, includes several facets. Video 3.2 shows a patient before dental extractions; the patient is preparing to receive dentures. Notice how the dentist connects with the patient (from 0 to 0:35, after that the dentist solicits the patient's concerns, the next ISLEEP skill).

In the previous video example, the dentist greets the patient with a general tone of warmth and interest. More specifically, she addresses the patient by name, asks how the patient is feeling (referring to his recent extractions), and reviews the plan for the visit.

These are the key components of **introduce/interconnect:**

1. Introduce yourself by name and title, address the patient by name
2. Interconnect: establish a personal connection
3. Introduce the agenda for the visit
   Let's explore each of these in more depth.

TABLE 3.1 ISLEEP Summary Chart

ISLEEP Behavior	Components
I. *Introduce/Interconnect*	a) Introduce self by name and title Address patient by name and title (Mr./Mrs.) or ask "how would you like to be called?" b) *Interconnect* with the patient as a person (e.g., not just a tooth problem) c) *Introduce* the planned procedure/purpose for visit
S. *Solicit*	*Before/after procedures*: solicit questions/concerns/fears using open-ended questions (why, what, where, when, how) *During procedures:* solicit comfort level using closed-ended questions (yes/ no)
L. *Listen*	• Focusing with Mindfulness: **S.T.O.P**. = Stop, Take a breath, Observe, Proceed • Demonstrating active listening sitting still, at eye level, making eye contact, leaning forward, nodding, mirroring words and body • Attire: without gloves and goggles, clean, professional Note: when possible, give the patient a chance to tell their story uninterrupted
E. *Empathize/ Validate*	• *NONVERBAL*—Body language mirrors the patient's emotions • *VERBAL:* "It must be hard to feel so _____." "It makes sense that you would feel _____."
E. *Explain/ reassure*	• *Before tx:* explain how you can address the need/want/fear, tx options, risks and benefits • *During exam:* what you are looking for • *During tx:* what sensations will be felt (**especially** discomfort) • After tx: what to expect Note: use language the patient can understand
P. *Power* of the patient	• *Before and after tx:* offer recommendations and suggestions (not commands) • *During tx:* a) make requests NOT commands—"could/would you, _____?" "when you're ready, please _____." b) ask permission—"I'm going to_____, is that alright/ok?" c) give options—"can you keep going or do you need a break?" esp. for pain during procedures: (i.e., "Would you like to try again, wait a moment, or more numbing medicine?")

Introduce Yourself by Name and Title, Address the Patient by Name

Martha B, Certified Nurse-Midwife, shared this story with me:

A busy labor and delivery hospital unit with a bustling nurse's station behind a counter. An orderly brings up a new patient in a wheelchair. She is uncomfortable and sitting in the wheelchair only able to see the walls of the counter and hear the loud voices of the nurses and doctors chatting on unaware of her. One nurse I observed always made a point of coming out from behind the counter immediately when aware of a patient arrival and would crouch beside the laboring woman in the wheelchair, look her in the face, call her by name, welcome her, and let her know she will be well taken care of. That contact set the tone of caring, provided a moment of connection between the patient and the nurse, and made such a difference when compared to the woman just waiting in the chair for someone to tell the orderly what room to bring her to.

As the story above illustrates, a warm welcome that includes names makes such a difference to patients. When providers address themselves by their first and last name, it reduces the sense of hierarchy and distance that a title confers and, by doing so, fosters a sense of connection. Also, stating your role (e.g., administrator, assistant, HCP) makes your relationship to the patient clear. Everyone on the team counts: experts on preoperative anxiety report, "Most patients like to be informed and introduced to all of the members of the surgical team. Patients like to know the role of each provider."[12]

Regarding the patient's name, make sure to use the name the patient prefers. In the words of Dale Carnegie, "A person's name is to him or her the sweetest and most important sound in any language."[13] To avoid mispronouncing a patient's name, you might simply ask, "How would you like us to call you?" If needed, *note the pronunciation and preferred name in the chart*. This will avoid the awkwardness (and possible disrespect) of repeatedly calling a patient Petunia when they hate that name and much prefer to be called Pat, for example. A study found that patients generally "preferred to use surnames at the first visit."[14] Addressing the patient by Mr., Ms., or Mrs., especially if they are older than you, conveys a sense of respect.

Whom do you address when the patient is accompanied by others? Experts say the "patient" is "anyone who has an interest in that sick person."[15] So, as you enter the reception room or the treatment room, introduce yourself to the patient *and to all those accompanying them*. Dental hygienist Jessie M described one of the possible challenges of this scenario:

> This is most challenging for me with pediatric patients. I always try my best to talk directly with the patient and include the parent in conversation whenever necessary. But sometimes, parents can be overbearing and try to take over the entire conversation, forcing me to ignore the patient, however little they may be.

Note that acknowledging everyone present does not preclude giving guidelines and setting limits about who is allowed to be present and what they can or can't do during treatment of the patient.

Interconnect: Establishing a Personal Connection

Here are some thoughts about **interconnecting** from dental hygienist Jessie M:

> There are some days at work I feel burnt out and don't have the energy to carry a conversation with patients past small talk. These days always feel less

> productive and lead to negative thoughts about myself as a hygienist. The days where I talk to patients about their lives and really connect with them makes me feel better about myself and my work. I always consider an appointment to be productive if I can write something in the notes that I have learned about the patient to help me better remember them.

Expressing interest in the patient as a person, not just a medical/dental problem, is one of the most effective ways to build trust and convey care. "Early in the interview the professional should be more interested in developing the relationship than obtaining factual information."[14] This recommendation is reinforced by the Consultation and Relational Empathy (CARE) measure, a 10-item patient questionnaire that has been found to be valid and reliable both for medicine[16] and dentistry.[17] One of the 10 questions on the CARE measure is, "How was the doctor at treating you as a whole person, asking/knowing relevant details about your life, not treating you as just a number."[16] (More on the CARE measure in the section on Evaluating Patient-centeredness in the Conclusion of this book.)

I try to make a habit of finding out something personal or unique about each person at each visit. Patient demographics are a gold mine of possible icebreakers. Here are some suggestions for employing basic demographics as a springboard for **interconnecting**:

1. ADDRESS: If the patient lives far away: "How was your drive today?"
2. DOB: If the patient's birthday just passed or is coming soon: "Happy birthday!" (I have a patient who was born 3 days after me and for the past 18 years we have delighted in that connection, referring to each other as "birthday sisters.")

My favorite way to connect is with open-ended questions: "How is your day going so far?" "What's new?" "How's your family?" I am especially glad I asked about a patient's life and family when it elicits an important event such as, "My father just died," "My husband was just diagnosed with cancer," or "I am going on a special vacation for my anniversary." Knowing important positive and negative events like these provides a window into the life of the person in the chair and allows for deepening connections. As with the patient's name, consider *noting personal details in the chart* so you can follow up at subsequent visits and continue building on your relationship. Some electronic health records provide a personal "sticky note" where a provider can store a personal detail to have available when the patient returns. Examples of personal notes include:

- drives a truck
- originally from New Jersey
- child in hospital
- going on vacation to Italy

As you inquire about patient's background and experience, be careful to avoid probing into potentially sensitive topics. For example, asking a person, "Where are you from?" could imply that you view the patient as foreign—as not belonging here. I once asked this question of an Asian man who spoke with a heavy accent and was embarrassed when the patient answered with an irritated "Thirty years!" Being culturally sensitive also avoids arousing discomfort in a patient who may have experienced discrimination due to race or ethnic background. All are welcome, and we want to convey this both explicitly and implicitly.

A final note about **interconnect**: while establishing a personal connection is included here in the first skill of ISLEEP, interconnection is not limited to the beginning of a health care visit; it can occur at any time. In Video 3.3, I inquired about Nicholas' family while waiting for topical anesthetic to take effect by asking, "Your family's doing okay?" The patient shares an update and expresses his appreciation for my interest.

Group Experiment Exploring Interconnect:

Each participant writes down their basic demographics (as much as they are comfortable divulging) on a blank card. Then, the participant and a partner take turns asking questions as if they were each other's patients. Looking for commonalities and interesting facts, participants should try to strike up a conversation that allows them to connect and get to know each other.

Introduce the Agenda for the Visit

An explanation of the agenda for the visit sets the patients expectations and aligns them with the physician's.[3]

Huntington and Kuhn, Communication Gaffes: A Root Cause of Malpractice Claims

The last component of the I in ISLEEP, introduce agenda, intends to verify that both the provider and the patient understand and agree on the agenda for the visit. Frequently, I find that patients don't know the plan for their visit. For example, they may be scheduled for a consultation but think they are going to have a procedure done. They may think they are having an amalgam *(silver)* restoration in their tooth, but I am set up to do a composite *(white)* one. The beginning of a visit is the time to clarify. Another reason to clarify the agenda for the visit is to ensure that the patient doesn't have a new complaint that calls for more urgent attention than the scheduled procedure. Whenever possible, address the chief complaint.

PATERNALISM VERSUS PATIENT-CENTEREDNESS

Before moving on to the next elements in the ISLEEP model, let's look at two vignettes depicting the same patient encounter but as they would unfold in two very different styles. The first vignette lacks mindfulness and ISLEEP skills. Following, the same scenario is described as it unfolded between a patient and myself, demonstrating mindfulness (how it manifests internally) and the remaining elements of ISLEEP, including *solicit, listen, empathize, explain,* and affirm *power* of the patient. The second scenario took only 5 minutes longer than the first, but it opened the door to dental care for Joyce after decades of dental avoidance due to fear. We will refer to this scenario several times again when we unveil the next few ISLEEP skills.

Dentures for Joyce: A Paternalistic Approach

The hygienist hovers behind Dr. M, who is busy adjusting dentures, signaling him to come check her patient. Walking together toward her operatory, she describes her patient. "Doc, I don't think you will have anything to do here, so it should be quick: seventy years old, no teeth, wants dentures, but too terrified. It took a major effort just to get her to sit in the chair." Dr. M looks at his watch, realizing he's behind schedule and walks faster. Standing over the patient with mask and gloves on he says, "What can I do for you?" She replies, "I have been missing my teeth for a long time and would like dentures but am too terrified." Dr. M proceeds to recline the chair and poke around in the patient's mouth to check for signs of oral pathology or any need for pre-prosthetic surgery before dentures can be made. He tells her she would need a minimum of five visits to fabricate the dentures and when she is ready, she can schedule her appointments at the front desk. He then rushes back to the denture adjustment. The patient never returns.

Dentures for Joyce: Mindfully and Patient-Centered (Demonstrating ISLEEP Skills)

Victoria, the hygienist, hovers behind me as I adjust a patient's denture, signaling me to come check her patient. Walking together towards her operatory, she describes who I will meet: "Doc, I don't think you will have anything to do here so it should be quick: seventy years old, no teeth, wants dentures, but too terrified. It took a major effort just to get her to sit in the chair." I become aware of a thought, "I don't want to deal with this," and a sense of irritation. At the moment of this awareness, an internal shift occurs. Noticing my own thoughts and emotions creates a space between the experience and my reactions to it, allowing me to choose my response (MINDFULNESS). I set an intention to show up fully and to help this person as best I can.

She sits on the edge of the seat as if poised for escape, trembling and tense, her blonde hair pulled back too tightly. Wide-rimmed glasses cover most of her face, and lips drape the toothless space underneath. "Hello Joyce, I'm Dr. D'Arro. Nice to meet you. Welcome to our office." I sit down next to her and smile (INTRODUCE/INTERCONNECT). "What brings you here today?" (SOLICIT and Listen). She tells me how much she wants to have teeth, that she has not had teeth for decades but that she is so terrified of the dentist, she almost cancelled her appointment today. "Can you share with me what frightens you?" (SOLICIT and LISTEN). I reassure myself how little time it takes to connect when I bring full attention, and I bring my attention to the area of my own heart (MINDFULNESS).

Sitting still and silent, I rest my focus on Joyce (LISTEN). "When I was a little girl, one day my grandmother said we needed to go visit a friend. We went for a bus ride and stopped at the dentist office. I was tied to a chair and my front teeth were ripped out. I haven't had teeth ever since." She trembles as she speaks. But above the dark clouds of terror, I sense a brightness and clarity, her clear and intense wish to move beyond. I look in her eyes, touching her cold hand, "Joyce, it makes total sense that you would be terrified after this experience. I really honor you for the courage it took to come here" (EMPATHIZE/VALIDATE). "I'm wondering what would make it possible to move forward. What if you knew you could stop at

any time?" (SOLICIT). She agrees that would be very reassuring. "If you are willing to try, I am willing to take a chance and try to get your smile back. We can take baby steps. I will explain everything you will feel (EXPLAIN) and most importantly, you can stop me whenever you want (POWER of the patient). This is my promise." She lets out a mini-exhale, as if a full exhale might collapse her loosely assembled pieces. I am saddened at the suffering that Joyce's traumatic dental experience caused her for so long and hopeful that, together, we can get her smile back. Over the next few months, Joyce is faithful to her appointments, always on time despite having her heart in her throat. She has a new smile now, but it's more than the denture teeth that make her smile so bright. Her eyes and entire face shine with confidence and joy.[18]

Preparatory Questions for ISLEEP Skill Solicit
1. Do you assess if a patient is anxious about their appointment or procedure? If so, how?
2. Do you feel soliciting fears and anxieties about procedures increases or decreases them?

ISLEEP: SOLICIT

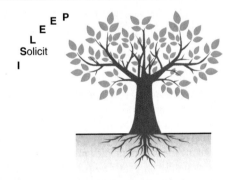

It is up to us, as doctors, to find commonalities and respect the differences between us and our patients. In that way, we can understand what they value, how best to communicate with them, and how to arrive at treatment plans that improve their health while respecting their wishes.[19]

Dr. Damon Tweedy, author of Black Man in a White Coat

Traditional medical and dental education and training prepares us well to **solicit** and listen for information about physical complaints. "What are your symptoms? How long have you had them? What medications have you taken for the pain?" These are the questions most HCPs know well. When it comes to patient emotions, on the other hand, we are not as well-versed in the skill of soliciting. A study of dental students found "identifying/labeling feelings" was one of three communication skills "not effective most often."[5] Many HCPs shy away from soliciting emotional issues surrounding illness and treatment for two main reasons: concerns about time and the fear of opening "Pandora's box" without the knowledge or ability to help.

Interestingly, research reveals that the process of **soliciting, listening,** and **empathizing** does not take significant time. One study of 335 patients and 14 doctors revealed a mean spontaneous talking time of *92 seconds,* and 78% of patients had finished their initial statement in *2 minutes.*[20] Yet, research shows it takes an average of only 22 seconds before a doctor in the United States will interrupt a patient.[21] Communication experts assert that soliciting and active listening actually *saves* time: "The time of an exam can be substantially reduced by a relaxed attitude, sitting down, asking about the patient's welfare, and listening to the answer. When you focus fully on your patients, you absorb what they're saying the first time they say it."[22] "It is primarily in situations where the physician appears rushed that the patient becomes uncomfortable and reaches out to hold him longer."[23]

Nurse practitioner Martha B reflects:

This is such an important point to remember. I am embarrassed to admit that I am afraid of "opening the floodgates" with questions that I ask patients during visits. I fear that their answers will be so long and emotional that I will fall hopelessly behind. I have found this especially true during the pandemic when patients (and everyone) have a lot to express.

In addition to possibly saving time, research also shows that **soliciting, listening**, and **empathizing** doesn't just open Pandora's box. It actually helps patients deal with the emotional issues surrounding illness and treatment, and empathy is the balm. "Empathy and related responses are...means by which physicians can reduce negative emotions such as anger, depression, and anxiety which are common reactions to illness."[24] Interestingly, there is some evidence that simply soliciting, without even responding, may benefit fearful patients. For example, one study showed "greater reduction in mean change of STAI-S scores" (state trait anxiety inventory) in patients who handed their dental anxiety scale to their dentist preoperatively compared to patients who handed the scale to the receptionist.[25] These findings suggest that patients find comfort in simply knowing that their provider is aware of their anxiety.

The Importance of Soliciting Patient Emotions: Focus on Fear and Anxiety

Fear and anxiety are common reactions to health care procedures, taking a toll on patients and providers alike. Fear is "a reaction to threatening stimuli," while anxiety is "an emotional state that precedes an actual encounter with the threatening stimuli, which sometimes is not even identifiable."[26] The quintessential fear-inducing specialty in health care is dentistry. Dental researchers estimate extreme fear in 11% to 22% of patients,[27] and others assert, "All patients may have some level of anxiety about their treatment."[28] "Fear not only prevents patients from seeking treatment but also interferes with the efficiency of treatment." In fact, one study showed that dental patients with high levels of fear required about 20% more time to treat.[14]

Fear and anxiety are especially common in people with a history of trauma or abuse. Because of the prevalence of trauma and abuse in our society and their impact on a person's experience of health care, patients should be solicited about their fear and anxiety early on. More on screening for procedural anxiety in Chapter 5.

Do Patients Want to Talk About Their Emotions?

A study by Hornung and Massagli found that "patients have two main goals in seeking health care services. The first goal is to obtain an accurate diagnosis and receive competent and appropriate treatment. The second goal is *relief of fear and anxiety* that accompanies illness" (emphasis added).[29] This applies not only to medicine but also to dentistry, as "Researchers in several studies have highlighted the importance that patients assign to dentists' willingness to discuss patient fears and perceived pain."[30]

Do Patients Volunteer Their Emotions?

Although patients value HCPs' support for managing emotions that accompany illness, they typically withhold their feelings from providers, as illustrated in the following vignette:

> *Mark is a kind, Black man who is preparing for his wedding. He and his fiancée would like to improve his smile for their big day. On the day of Mark's extractions, I enter the dental operatory and notice him clutching the armrests and smiling stiffly. I greet him with a smile and ask, "How are you doing," eager to aerate any fears he has about today's procedure. He replies with a perfunctory "Fine." We review the plan for the day. When I ask more pointedly, "Are you nervous?" he writhes tensely, and says "Maybe," laughing nervously. Finally, after I finish extracting several of his teeth, he confesses, "Actually, doc, I am terrified of needles and that's why I haven't been to the dentist for years."*

It saddened me that Mark withheld his fears from me, and it made me wonder how many others had withheld fears too. Was I doing something to make them feel judged, unsafe, uncomfortable? My self-doubt eased when I stumbled on many studies reporting that patient reticence is very common. "Patients often are unable or unwilling to express their expectations and needs."[30] "Patients often do not verbalize their anxieties directly, rather, they raise these issues indirectly by offering clues or hints about these psychological and social concerns."[31] Possible explanations for patients withholding their feelings include a passive or paternalistic view of their role in the relationship, anxiety and desire to finish as quickly as possible, and intimidation by professional terminology.[32]

Are Health Care Providers Good at Judging Patient Emotions?

Patients' reticence about their anxieties requires HCPs to assess patients' concerns and issues, but research indicates HCPs may not be the best judges of patient perceptions and feelings. "Studies indicate that there is disagreement between patient self-reported anxiety status and clinicians' rating of dental anxiety," and, because of this, "the practitioner should not rely exclusively on clinical judgment in assessing anxious patients."[26]

Not only is patient anxiety hard for HCPs to assess, so is patient satisfaction. A large-scale study of more than 5000 patients in about 200 dental practices found that "in cases in which patients were not satisfied, dentists seldom were aware."[30] In fact, of 726 cases of overall dissatisfaction with care in this study, dentists were unaware of dissatisfaction in 684 cases, amounting to 94%!

When we sum these factors—the prevalence of fear and anxiety surrounding many health care procedures, the value patients place on addressing it, the evidence of patient reticence, and the evidence that HCPs are not good judges of patient perceptions—we can see clearly the value of **soliciting** patient feelings and perceptions. Dental research has much to offer on the topic of managing fear and anxiety since "dental care has historically been characterized as generating more fear and anxiety than other forms of health care."[33] Experts in dental fear assert, "The health professional should raise the [fear] directly. The patient needs to know that you consider fear issues a part of 'normal' practice and that you have some knowledge about how to solve them."[34] In summary, "It is essential to the clinical management of the patient that the dental team assess the patient's level of anxiety and intervenes proportionately."[28]

How to Solicit Emotions and Who Should Do It

Soliciting patients' desires, expectations, perceptions, and fears is the responsibility of the entire health care team. Starting even before the first visit, the receptionist/scheduler can ask questions regarding previous health care experiences including "concerns or difficulties."[34] Before meeting with the HCP, support staff can solicit patient concerns and worries. This can be very helpful for patients who are reluctant to volunteer concerns with the HCP due to embarrassment or other reasons. So many times, patients disclose all manner of concerns to my dental assistant that I knew nothing about!

Once the patient arrives to the treatment area, the best way to solicit depends on the work mode. During "hands-on" care, such as procedures and clinical exams, the patient may not be able to talk. This underscores the importance of soliciting during consultations and immediately before and after procedures—or "hands-off" mode—when more conversation is possible. Since each of the two modes calls for a different way of soliciting, let's discuss each one on its own.

Soliciting While Hands Off

The basic empathetic approach is always to deal with the emotion first. Let the emotion out and let it be recognized.[35]

Pamela Schuster, Communication: The Key to the
Therapeutic Relationship

During a consultation and immediately before and after procedures—hands-off mode—the patient can talk, so this is the best time to solicit patient concerns and emotions. The types of questions asked will influence the answer. Critical care doctor and author Rana Awdish writes, "With the right question…each patient can be given a recommendation that fits their values."[36] Skillful soliciting is facilitated with *open-ended* questions, whereas "closed-ended questions can be answered with a simple 'yes' or 'no' response, and…don't tend to keep a conversation going."[32] Video 3.4 shows the conversation described earlier between me and Mark. When I ask Mark a closed-ended question, "Any questions, concerns?" he does not divulge his anxiety. Instead, he answers with a terse, "No…maybe." If I had asked an *open-ended* question such as, "*What* questions do you have," or "*How* is your anxiety level on a scale of 1 to 100," he probably would have shared more.

Let's return to the story of Joyce, the edentulous (toothless) patient who was terrified of dentistry because of her traumatic dental experience in childhood. My questions to her were more skillful and, as a result, more fruitful: "*What* brings you here today?" And, "Can you share with me *what* frightens you?" These invitational, open-ended questions opened the door to sharing the traumatic events that shaped not only her dental experience but also her life in general. Patients value this kind of interaction. In a study of patients' perception of dehumanization, "participants underscored the importance of providers asking open-ended questions and discussing confidentiality."[37]

Effective soliciting involves open-ended questions that start with "*what, how, when, where,* and *why.*" Compare the following pairs of questions, noticing how open-ended questions tend to keep the conversation going more than closed-ended ones.

Closed-ended: "*Are you feeling nervous about today's procedure?*"

Open-ended: "How *are you feeling about the procedure we are about to do?*" or "What *worries or concerns do you have about this procedure?*"

Here are more possible open-ended questions adapted from a dental hygiene text:
1. What dental hygiene procedures make you feel anxious?
2. What could I do as a hygienist to ease your anxiety?
3. What coping techniques have previously helped you feel more relaxed?[38]

Postoperatively, if the procedure was comfortable, soliciting feedback highlights to the patient the ease of the procedure, something good to reinforce for the fearful patient. If the procedure was uncomfortable, soliciting feedback provides the opportunity to be empathetic and to gather feedback to modify the technique in the future, for that patient and for others. In either case, soliciting after a procedure provides the fearful patient with what dental fear experts call "retrospective control"[34] and conveys care.

Compare and contrast the following postoperative questions:
- Closed-ended: "*Are you OK?*"
- Open-ended: "**How** *was that?*" "*What could I have done better?*" "*What would you like me to do differently next time?*"

Exercises

Scenario 1 (*pre*operative period): You are about to perform a procedure that could arouse anxiety or induce pain for the patient. Think of some open-ended questions you could ask to solicit the patient's emotions and needs.

Scenario 2 (*post*operative period): You have just completed a procedure that could arouse anxiety or induce pain for the patient. Think of some open-ended questions you could ask to solicit the patient's emotions and feedback.

Soliciting Beyond Patient Emotions

While patient anxiety and fear require understanding and care, patient-centered care requires understanding more than just emotions like anxiety and fear. The HCP must also understand the patient's "desires, expectations, perceptions."[30] The Four Habits Model of communication skills highlights the many patient issues that the HCP must understand and captures the paramount nature of the ISLEEP skill, **solicit**.[5,39] Here is a list of the Four Habits and issues from each habit that require soliciting:
- Habit 1: Invest in the beginning
  - Identify the problem, encourage expansion of the concern
- Habit 2: Elicit the patient's perspective
  - The patient's understanding of the problem, the patient's goals, impact on patient's life
- Habit 3: Demonstrate empathy
  - Identify/label feelings
- Habit 4: Invest in the end
  - Explore acceptability of treatment plan and barriers to implementation

Consider some questions you could ask in the consultation that would facilitate discussion about the above concerns, wants, needs, and issues. Here are some suggestions from Four Habits experts Drs. Stein, Krupat, and Frankel:

What would you like help with today?

I understand you're here for…could you tell me more about that?

How were you hoping I could help?

What do you think we could do to help overcome any problems you might have with the treatment plan?[40]

Remember to use "what, where, when, how" to frame open-ended questions and facilitate discussion.

A final note: not all open-ended questions facilitate patient-centered care. In fact, some questions, despite being open-ended, are designated by researchers as "empathic opportunity terminators" as opposed to "empathic opportunity continuers."[41] For example, for a patient presenting with a toothache, asking open-ended questions like, "How long have you had this pain?" and "What is the pain like?" may yield important diagnostic data, but it may not promote understanding the patient's emotions and needs. In contrast, the question, "How have the symptoms affected your daily life?" is an example of an "empathic opportunity continuer," creating an opening for empathy and connection.

Soliciting While Hands On

Let's return to the story of Maria and her root canal from Chapter 2. Despite receiving excellent technical care, her experience was so aversive that she vowed she would never have another root canal. Her main complaint was the dentist's lack of communication during the procedure. If the doctor had solicited her comfort level while working, for example, by asking "Are you doing okay? Are you still comfortable?" it would likely have made Maria's experience less traumatic and more comfortable.

Many medical and dental procedures don't allow patients to speak. For these procedures, the HCP must **solicit** the patient's comfort level frequently and in a way that doesn't require speech. **Soliciting** during procedures is usually best accomplished using

closed-ended questions. Here are examples of soliciting when hands on:

Are you doing okay?

Can you hang in there a little longer?

Do you need a break?

Closed-ended questions allow the patient to answer with a simple yes or no (or thumbs up or down), allowing them to communicate their physical or emotional discomfort during procedures. It is helpful to agree on a signal (for yes and no) *before* starting a procedure, especially one during which a patient cannot talk. HCPs who **solicit** frequently during procedures are highly rated by their patients. The following two short video clips demonstrate soliciting a patient's comfort level while "hands on"—first during an oral examination (Video 3.5) then during a dental extraction (Video 3.6).

Table 3.2 summarizes what to solicit during the different phases of care.

Appendices D, E, and F provide sample questions for soliciting in each of the phases of care, including the consultation (Appendix D), pre- and postoperative phases (Appendix E), and during procedures and clinical exams (Appendix F).

Final Note on Soliciting: Written Scales and Questionnaires

Written scales and questionnaires are a great way to quickly and easily solicit a patient's procedural anxiety. There are several advantages of written means of soliciting. First, questionnaires can be completed before procedures, thus saving procedure time and allowing the team a chance to prepare how to address the anxiety. Second, scales (such as the Visual Analogue Scale for Pain or Anxiety) and questionnaires (about specific fears or needs during procedures) can be administered by any member of the team. This can be especially helpful for patients who are uncomfortable divulging anxiety to their provider directly. We will discuss scales and questionnaires further in Chapter 5.

Whether done verbally or in writing, soliciting allows the HCP to respond to patient anxiety, concerns, and discomfort. This leads us to the next two elements of ISLEEP, which guide how to respond to the concerns you have solicited, **listening** and **empathizing**.

TABLE 3.2   Summary of Solicit During Different Phases of Care

ISLEEP Skill	HANDS OFF Consult/tx Plan	HANDS OFF Treatment Visit: Preop and Postop	HANDS ON Procedures and Clinical Exams

S. *Solicit*	• Chief complaint
	• Symptoms
	• Concerns/fears
	• Needs, wants, values
	• Beliefs about condition and tx options
	• How they experience(d) the condition or treatment
	• Questions about condition or treatment
	• Potential obstacles to care (social determinants)
		Preop:
		  • Questions
		  • Fears/concerns
		  • Requests for comfort measures
		Postop:
		  • Questions
		  • Feedback on experience
			• Comfort level (physical and emotional)
			• Details about discomfort

Preparatory Questions for ISLEEP Skill Listen

1. How do you focus your attention as you listen to a patient speaking?
2. How do you demonstrate to a patient that you are listening to them?
3. What helps/hinders your ability to listen to a patient?

ISLEEP: LISTEN

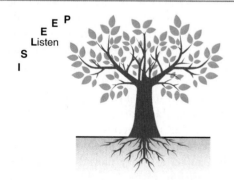

...the healing power of just being able to bear witness to someone's struggle.[36]

Dr. Rana Awdish, Author of In Shock:
My Journey from Death to Recovery and
the Redemptive Power of Hope

Listening is a key aspect of learning effective communication.[42] Listening is more than just waiting to talk—it is a mental and emotional stance. "An attitude of willingness to listen and be open to patient concerns...allowing the patient to tell his or her story" is key to developing therapeutic relations.[24] More specifically, "active listening establishes an empathic bond... a bond that leads to trust on the side of the patient and to compassionate understanding on the side of the physician"[23]

Unfortunately, "most people do not listen with the intent to understand, they listen with the intent to reply," says Stephen Covey, author of *The 7 Habits of Highly Effective People.*[43] From a study of patients' perceptions of their care: "When reflecting on negative aspects of care, many participants reported a sense of dehumanization that resulted from *not feeling listened to*, cared for, or seen as an entire human being" (emphasis added).[37]

Similar to the ISLEEP skill of soliciting, most HCPs are better trained at listening for clues about physical complaints than about emotions. For example, as a dentist, my ears are well-attuned for statements like, "The toothache wakes me up at night," or, "It hurts when I chew." But patient-centered care requires more than just listening for physical complaints—listening for cues about a patient's thoughts and emotions is also essential.

Remember that patients tend to share subtle clues about their concerns and fears rather than to volunteer them explicitly, so the HCP must listen carefully for these clues. For example, the statement, "My sister had a knee replacement and it failed," may indicate her worry that her knee replacement may fail, too. Similarly, a dental patient's comment, "I never smile anymore," may hint at shame about their appearance.

One of the challenges of listening for patient emotions, besides time pressure, is the challenge of tolerating negative emotions. Richard Frankel, an internationally recognized researcher on the doctor–patient relationship, describes the importance of "hearing, bearing, and tolerating expressions of painful feelings" to developing therapeutic relations.[24] I have noticed my own reactions to patients in response to statements like, "I am terrified of needles," or "I hate going to the dentist." Such expressions of negative emotions can arouse irritation or anxiety for me. In addition, many providers don't feel prepared or trained to handle the negative emotions that patients present in health care.[31] How does an HCP stay steady as they listen to a person expressing their anxiety or pain? How does an HCP convey they are listening, even when time is limited? The answers lie not in the *quantity* of time but in the *quality* of their presence as they listen—in other words, mindfulness.

Tuning In: Mindfulness and Listening

The quieter you become, the more you are able to hear.

Rumi[44]

In experimenting with different ways of quieting and focusing myself as I listen to a patient speak, I have discovered the value of quieting my whole self—not just my mouth but also my body. In the words of psychiatrist and best-selling author Scott Peck, "You cannot truly listen to anyone and do anything else at the same time."[45] Simply being quiet and physically still helps one listen more deeply, allowing for deep connection in a very short time. So, once you have solicited the patient's concerns with questions, try to simply STOP for a few seconds. Stop talking. Stop moving your body. Stop looking at a chart, clock, or computer. Stop everything.

When an HCP truly listens, they allow space—space for a patient to open. "An empty space in conversation may feel awkward at first, but it can send the essential message that it is ok—even preferred—that patients talk."[32] Clinician-educator, Dr. Paul Haidet describes,

I find that I am at my best when I can give patients space to say what they want to say…In this space, patients often either tell their story, allowing me to

understand the context around their symptoms, or ask the questions that allow me to tailor my explanations to their unique concerns.[46]

Exercise: STOP

The informal mindfulness practice STOP was described in Chapter 2 as way for the HCP to quiet and focus themselves. Here is it adapted slightly for listening to a patient:
- S- Stop
- T- Take a breath
- O- Open
- P- Proceed to listen

First, stop moving. Sit still and silent, resting your gaze on the patient. Next, take a breath. Since it is not possible to feel the breath in the past or the future, feeling the sensations of the breath immediately reconnects us to the present. Then, open. Open the heart to receive the patient's concerns, reconnecting to a caring intention. You might even tune into sensations in the area of your heart. Finally, proceed to listen—not just with ears but tuning in with all senses.

In the story of my encounter with Joyce, the denture patient with the traumatic dental past, the practice of STOP was so helpful. My initial irritation at the hygienist's interruption eased immediately when I remembered to **stop**, **take** a breath, and **open**. As I **proceeded** to listen to Joyce, I felt an immediate sense of calm and inner stillness. The entire first encounter with Joyce lasted only about 5 minutes, but it sparked something for us. Hearing her story allowed me to understand her better. Having her story heard created a connection that allowed her to trust enough to return, complete her treatment, and reach her goal of regaining her smile.

In addition to the informal mindfulness practice of STOP, mindfulness—awareness with an attitude of caring—is essential for deep listening. To review, as discussed in Chapter 2, simply allow the breath sensations to be your anchor to the present moment while connecting to an intention of care. Gather the attention and rest it on the patient as well as yourself, noticing your own thoughts and emotions. Meditation teacher and author Michael Carroll offers these instructions about mindful listening: "Observe how often you are thinking about what is being said…when you notice that you are distracted by your inner commentary, shift your attention back to the present moment. Listen fully to the words, body, language, and tone."[47] For example, as you listen, you may notice thoughts about the patient, such as, "I wish I didn't have to see her today," self-judgments, such as, "I am not doing a good job," or worries, such as, "I am going to be late."

Mindfulness makes it possible to notice what's present in ourselves and in the patient, to tolerate uncomfortable reactions (our own and our patient's), and to stay present. By doing so, the quality of listening is deep, and the presence is felt. In this space, much more can be exchanged in a very short time. I am often amazed at how deep a connection can be formed in just 1 or 2 minutes of deep, uninterrupted mindful listening! One last note: when you notice the patient starts to drag on or digress, mindfulness helps to discern when it is appropriate to interrupt and move on!

Listening Requires More Than Just Ears

Because patients often don't verbalize their concerns and fears, listening involves eyes as well as ears. Helen Riess, a leading researcher on empathy, reports, "Clinicians can better understand and attend to patients' emotions by decoding nonverbal behaviors and facial expressions," and further, "Neuroimaging studies reveal that empathy is related to the ability to decode these facial expressions."[48]

Dr. Riess describes a case in which her patient's emotions were conveyed only in nonverbal cues—which she unfortunately missed. This patient had been struggling with trying to lose weight. As part of a research study, the patient and Reiss were videotaped, and their stress levels were monitored using a common measure of sympathetic arousal called galvanic skin response (GSR). Reiss reports her shock on reviewing the results—although Reiss had not detected any anxiety in the patient during the session, the GSR tracings captured severe anxiety in her patient. Most importantly, she noticed that "The highest peaks of her tracings always coincided with these *subtle motor movements* such as just *flicking* her hair, or *looking down* in a way, or subtle *changes in her tone of voice*...as I paid attention to these signs and responded to them, our work went to a much deeper level. She unburdened herself emotionally and started to exercise for the first time in her life."[49]

Cues can sometimes be hard to decode, especially in the case of fear and anxiety. For example, dental fear experts report that anxiety may be expressed in the waiting room as fidgeting, pacing, and more movement; whereas in the chair, the anxious patient may be "quiet

and still...with hands clasped."[34] Dr. Rana Awdish, critical care physician and author, notes, "It's an easy task to recognize a crying person as sad. But a compulsively attentive patient...asking well-formulated questions is less easy to decode as anxious."[36]

While it may be difficult for the HCP to detect patients' emotions, research shows patients appreciate the effort it takes. A randomized controlled study of resident physicians investigating training in "decoding subtle facial expressions of emotion," found sustained *improvement in patient satisfaction ratings* for the doctors who received this training.[50] So, listen with ears and eyes, too. By doing so, you will find "empathic opportunities"— "statements that raised or alluded to concerns, emotions, or stressors,"[51] and these will provide an opportunity to express *empathy*, which is the next ISLEEP skill.

Demonstrating Mindful Listening

Even if the HCP listens mindfully, if they don't also *demonstrate* to the patient that they are listening, the patient might not feel heard, and the benefits of the mindful listening might be lost. So, listening requires not only the active process of learning and understanding the speaker but also conveying attention and care. Experts recommend the HCP should appear "interested and open to what the speaker has to say."[32] What are some ways to express interest while listening? Let's observe how two HCPs that are highly rated by patients demonstrate their deep listening to their patients in Video 3.7 and 3.8.

First is the previously mentioned Dr. Ronda, the primary care doctor who was so beloved that many patients cried when they heard the news that she was leaving our clinic.

Next, Dr. A, a general dentist, listens to a patient in an emergency consultation. (The sound has been omitted intentionally, to highlight nonverbal communication.)

Now, let's unpack the various ways both doctors demonstrate attention and care while listening.

Posture

Dr. Reiss reports, "Subtle differences in clinician posture have significant effects on ratings...so it is important that clinician posture convey mutual respect and openness."[48] A sitting posture doesn't take any more time than standing and conveys a much different message. From a study on malpractice trends and communication skills: "A sitting position demonstrates an interest and an unhurried attitude, while a standing position may give the impression of control, an authoritative attitude, and being rushed."[3] Avoid sitting directly face-to-face, which can be perceived as too direct, even confrontational. Rather, try sitting perpendicular and at eye level, as demonstrated by both Dr. Ronda and Dr. A.

Also, note the position of your hands and arms. Avoid fidgety hands as this might convey restlessness. Avoid crossed arms which could convey resistance. Whenever possible, try to have relaxed hands and uncrossed arms to convey calm and receptivity.

Eye Contact

Eye contact is important not only to convey attention and interest but also to detect the many subtle nonverbal cues to the patient's emotions. Unfortunately, the domination of computers in health care encounters increasingly detracts from HCPs' eye contact with their patients. For example, many primary care offices have a desk with a computer, so the clinician can take notes in real time. Such situations make it more challenging to convey attentiveness and care while listening. At times, electronic devices may even pose an actual physical barrier to seeing the patient. Also, the use of surgical loupes by many procedure-oriented HCPs—like myself—detracts from eye contact (and may appear intimidating to a patient). Whenever possible, set aside computers, loupes, faceshields, and goggles to allow for better eye contact.

Note that some cultures forbid direct eye contact between certain groups such as women and men or patients and doctors. So, sense if there is discomfort and adjust accordingly. More on the topic of eye contact as it relates to pain and anxiety management is presented in Chapter 5.

Nodding

As you listen, an occasional nod of the head can convey "Yes, I am with you. I hear you. I understand." This is also a way to validate the patient's experience and affirm them.

Clarifying and Facilitating Questions and Summaries

If what the patient is trying to express is not clear, assess a bit more. Facilitating questions, such as "Can you say more," can convey interest and encourage patients to speak.[32] If you miss something that the patient said, you might ask, "I'm sorry, could you repeat that please?" While this may seem like an embarrassing exposure of a lapse of attention, for many patients it actually conveys a desire not to miss anything and to understand.

Restatement and Paraphrasing

Many times when we think we are listening, we are actually preparing what we will say next. The practice of mirroring others' words really helps one to slow down and focus better on what one is hearing, as my experience has shown me countless times. Researchers affirm the value of restatement or paraphrasing, reporting that it "blocks the listener from rehearsing his or her next (magnificent) statement" while also blocking premature reassurances and premature problem-solving.[32] Finally, repeating the patient's words and thoughts such as "OK, let's summarize, I understand you want to…" can help confirm comprehension of what was shared[52] and gives the patient "the opportunity to correct any misinterpretations."[38]

Note: The practice of summarizing or mirroring emotion-laden words is a way to convey empathy and will be discussed more in the next ISLEEP skill, *empathize*.

Pairs Experiment: Unmindful Listening

I learned this exercise in an MBSR course at the Penn Program for Mindfulness, and it made a lasting impact, probably because unmindful listening felt so familiar to me! Find a partner and designate one person as the speaker and one as the listener. The speaker talks for 1 to 2 minutes about something bothering them in their life. Meanwhile, the listener counts backwards from 100 by 3. Switch roles and try again. Afterwards, reflect on your experiences as the speaker and as the listener. How did it feel? What did you notice? In contrast, try the following mindful listening exercise.

Pairs Experiment: Mindful Listening

Now we repeat speaking about something bothering us but this time with mindful listening. Recall the formal mindfulness practice of focusing on the breath. Previously, the instruction was to gather the attention and rest it on the sensations of breathing; each time the mind wanders, gently but firmly escort the attention back to the breath. In this pairs exercise, the listener focuses on the feel of their breath and also on the speaker. Pay attention to both verbal and nonverbal communications. Simply be present and receive what is shared without saying anything. You may convey attention and care nonverbally, but for now, resist the impulse to communicate verbally. This may feel unnatural, but it is an experiment in concentrated, mindful listening. Sometimes straightening a bent rod requires bending it first to the other side!

Reflect on your experiences as the speaker and as the listener. How did it feel to listen this way and to be heard in this way? Compare this experience to the previous unmindful listening exercise.

Try this practice at work. Remember the research finding that most patients stop speaking on their own in less than 2 minutes.[20] Mindful listening is a valuable skill not only for connecting with patients but with anyone you encounter in your life.

Preparatory Questions for ISLEEP Skill Empathize

1. Do you believe expressing empathy for a patient increases or decreases their distress?
2. Scenario: You are a patient who needs a dental restoration due to caries (decay), and you are anxious about the handpiece (drill) because of a past traumatic dental experience. You have two choices. The first choice is a robot dentist that would perform the procedure with mechanistic perfection but would not respond to you in the event you were anxious or in pain. The second choice is a human dentist who is imperfect but friendly and empathetic. Which would you choose and why?
3. How do you express empathy when a patient expresses anxiety or pain about a procedure?

ISLEEP: EMPATHIZE

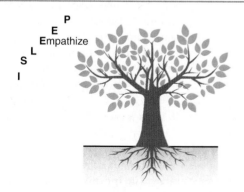

Note: Because of the paramount importance of empathy in patient-centered care, this section is a bit longer than others.

Imagine you have injured yourself working out at the gym and haven't been able to move or even sleep due to severe pain. You have waited a whole miserable week for an appointment with a doctor. As you hold back tears, the medical assistant calls you by name and leads you to a treatment room where they mechanically check your vital signs and leave. Next, the doctor enters, asks questions about your pain level and range of motion, examines the area, and prescribes you a pain medicine. Everyone did their job. But somehow you leave feeling disappointed, dissatisfied, alone. No one really saw you. No one acknowledged your suffering. No one showed empathy.

Unfortunately, this scenario is all too common, despite ample research demonstrating that expressing empathy to patients is essential for so many reasons. Empathy can actually *decrease pain* (which might have helped the patient above) and can also result in "increased compliance… reduced recovery time as well as increased patient satisfaction and decreased medical litigation."[53] "Despite differences in definitions, methods, and study populations, the finding that empathy leads to higher levels of patient satisfaction has been consistent."[24] In dentistry, "The demonstration of empathy…has been correlated with a decrease in dental fear."[53] Empathy benefits not only the patient but the provider as well; "studies suggest that providing empathy is one way to prevent burnout, reduce physicians' stress and make medical practice more rewarding."[51]

Obstacles to Expressing Empathy

Despite being considered "the backbone of the patient-centered approach,"[17] researchers report HCPs miss their cues for empathy: "The majority of the time physicians passed up opportunities presented by patients."[31] Morse's study of physicians and cancer patients noted that out of 384 empathic opportunities, physicians had responded empathically to only 39 (10%) of them."[51] Why would this be?

There are several possible explanations for lack of empathetic responses from HCPs. As we saw earlier, patients don't usually share their emotions clearly (which is why we need to solicit them). They may offer only clues, and these clues can be hard to detect. Burnout of the HCP is another contributor to the lack of empathy. We know that burnout rates are at an all-time high and that one of the hallmarks of burnout is dehumanization of the patient. Probably the main hindrance to expressing empathy is time pressures. Many HCPs are under pressure to be financially productive, which means completing procedures attached to billable codes, but unfortunately there are no billable codes for expressing empathy! Yet, research suggests that providers may overestimate the time cost. In fact, some evidence suggests empathy *saves time*, because when patients don't feel understood, "some patients attempted to raise the topic again, sometimes repeatedly and with escalating intensity."[41] Further, "Our data and those from other studies suggest that patients did not respond excessively when empathy was provided and suggests that visits with missed opportunities may be *longer* than visits with an empathetic response" (emphasis added).[51] Finally, HCPs may not express empathy due to lack of knowledge or training about how to express empathy in ways that are meaningful to patients. This is what we will focus on next.

Let's start with a scenario.

Imagine sitting with a patient just before a challenging procedure, such as a dental filling, having just demonstrated your mastery of the first three ISLEEP skills. So far, you have introduced yourself by name, asked how the patient would like to be called, asked the patient some questions to get to know them, and reviewed the plan for the visit (introduce/interconnect). You have asked them about their questions and concerns (solicit), and now you are listening mindfully. Oh, no! Now the patient is sobbing as they reveal their deepest fear: "I hate going to the dentist because I am terrified of needles!" It seems you have opened Pandora's box, and time is ticking. What should you do?

What Empathy Isn't

Because there is so much confusion about empathy, let's first talk about what NOT to do. Many common attempts at empathy are not reassuring and can actually increase rather than decrease a patient's distress.

The first example of how not to express empathy is offering *reassurances*. Illustrations of this include, "It's ok, it's nothing, everything is fine." Experts say, "Pat responses…should not be used because patients may interpret them as denying, minimizing, or ignoring their concerns."[38] This approach was demonstrated regularly by an oral surgeon I knew who practiced what he proudly termed "okay anesthesia"—whenever a patient expressed pain during procedures, he would respond with an "okay" and keep going! (Needless to say, his patients did not rate him highly.) A review study of

research with children and vaccination pain found that "repeated reassurances" like "you're okay" or "it's almost over" did not help with pain or distress.[54]

Another example of what empathy isn't is *explanations*. I have observed many HCPs responding to a fearful patient with information or advice—an impulse I continually struggle to curtail in myself. For example, after a new dental patient expressed her terror of needles, I almost pounced on her like I was trying to extinguish a kitchen fire! I explained that I would do everything in my power to make it better and detailed all the measures I would take including numbing gel, local anesthesia, and even relaxation techniques that she could try during the procedure. Explaining skillfully is an important ability (and is the next ISLEEP skill), and although the impulse to reassure with explanations may be well-meaning, explaining is not the same as empathy nor is it a substitute for empathy.

The last empathy substitute we will discuss is *sympathy*. While, at times, sympathy can be supportive, some research has found sympathy "unwelcomed and in some incidences despised by patients."[55] Why would it be so aversive? Like empathy, sympathy acknowledges the patient's suffering, and like empathy, the sympathizer feels emotion, for example, "I'm so sorry you're suffering." But unlike empathy (and this difference is subtle but significant), the sympathizer is not resonating with the patient's emotion. Rather they are more focused on their own feelings of pity or dismay. This emotional distance of the sympathizer may explain the aversion of patients in a study investigating preferences of terminally ill cancer patients: "Participants agreed that sympathy was the easiest of the three responses for observers to give away…an unwanted, pity-based response to a distressing situation, characterized by a lack of understanding and self-preservation of the observer."[55] In summary, "Sympathy and empathy, commonly confused with each other, are not the same. Sympathy is a statement of emotional concern while empathy is a reflection of emotional understanding"[56] and requires "approaching the patient's suffering in a vulnerable manner."[55]

Now that we know what empathy is NOT, we need to determine what exactly it is. And, more importantly, how does the HCP express empathy to a patient who is struggling? Let's return to the definition of empathy from Chapter 2 and its two main elements: "appreciation of the patient's emotions and expression of that awareness to the patient."[57] The first, "**appreciation** of the patient's emotions" (emphasis added), can by cultivated through several means as we saw in Chapter 2, including mindfulness practices, getting to know the patient's story, and mirroring words or nonverbal expressions. The second element of empathy, "**expression** of that awareness to the patient" (emphasis added),[57] will be the focus now.

Expressing Empathy With All ISLEEP Skills

Research shows that all six of the ISLEEP skills communicate empathy either explicitly or implicitly. Let's go back to the CARE measure (discussed in Introduce/Interconnect), a 10-item patient questionnaire that has been found valid and reliable in measuring "patient perception of relational empathy."[16] Interestingly, each of the ten questions of the CARE measure correspond to all of the six ISLEEP communication skills. For example, question #4, "How was the doctor at being interested in you as a whole person?" refers the skills of *introduce* and *interconnect*; question #2, "How was the doctor at letting you tell your story," refers to the ISLEEP skills of *soliciting* and *listening*; question #3, "How was the doctor at really listening, paying close attention to what you were saying," requires the ISLEEP skill of listening, and so on. See Appendix O for the CARE measure and corresponding ISLEEP skills (more about this in the Conclusion section). So, according to the CARE measure, skillful use of *all* ISLEEP skills can be a means to expressing empathy.

Verbal Expression of Empathy

By definition, an empathetic response includes two ingredients. It is "a response that demonstrates an accurate *understanding* and *acceptance* of the patient's feelings or concerns" (emphasis added).[24] Let's look at some examples.

Empathetic response = Understanding + Acceptance

Understanding: "*I see/hear/imagine your* _____ (emotion)."

+

Acceptance/validation: "*It makes sense you would feel* _____ (emotion)."

Note that the patient's reaction always makes sense from *their* perspective, although it may not from the perspective of the HCP. So, validating the patient's experience with words like "it makes sense" does not require that it make rational sense to you!

The story of Joyce, the terrified denture patient, is a great example of expressing empathy with words. In her first visit she shared her traumatic dental experience from childhood. In response, I said, "It makes total sense that you would be terrified after this experience. I really honor you for the courage it took to come here." She was visibly soothed on hearing these words, letting out a big exhale.

Experts report at times simply "repeating...some of the emotion-laden words we have heard,"[23] or *mirroring*, is a great way to convey empathy and understanding.[4] For example, soon you will see a video of a dental patient who is terrified of needles saying, "I'm so nervous." In this case, I could have simply mirrored the patient's words, "nervous... don't like needles," while at the same time expressing the same in my face and body.

When a patient does not label their feelings, the HCP might verbalize what they *think* the patient is feeling based on their nonverbal communication such as, "You seem a little upset."[24] However vague, the HCP must try to "clarify a patient's muddy expression of her experience" with their words.[58] For example, if a patient in a surgical consultation says, "My sister had the same procedure done and it was awful," an expression of empathy might be, "I imagine you might be afraid that you will have the same experience as your sister did," and then give the patient a chance to confirm and clarify what they are thinking and feeling.

Experiment With Verbal Empathy:
Imagine a patient is anxious about an upcoming procedure or complaining of pain during a procedure. Demonstrate verbal examples of the following types of responses:
1. Minimizing (includes shaming and punishing)
2. Explanations and Advice (what you will do, what they should do, etc.)
3. Sympathy (I'm so sorry/it's such a shame)
4. Empathy (understanding and acceptance—see above)

Pairs Experiment:
One person is the speaker and the other the listener. The speaker describes something bothering them in their life right now. The listener then demonstrates the four different types of responses listed above. Afterwards, reflect on your experience of each type of response as the speaker and the listener. Switch roles.

Nonverbal Expression of Empathy

Traditionally, empathy training for HCPs has focused on the words, but unfortunately, a focus on verbal communication ignores the hard-wired nature of the human brain. So, before you get caught up in the words you should say, consider how the brain processes interpersonal communications. In the words of leading empathy researcher, Dr. Helen Reiss:

> *The most subtle nonverbal approach and avoidance signals are detected in the amygdala more quickly than the prefrontal cortex is able to process verbal content. Not only are nonverbal cues processed faster but they have a greater impact on the perceiver than corresponding verbal statements (emphasis added).*[48]

Similar to the ways we discussed to express mindful listening nonverbally, there are several key nonverbal behaviors for expressing empathy, identified by Drs. Riess and Kraft-Todd. These are captured in an acronym, EMPATHY: *eye* contact, *muscles* of facial expression, *posture, affect,* and *tone* of voice (H and Y are more general: *hearing* the whole patient, and *your* response).[48]

Eye contact is an important way of expressing empathy, and one which has become increasingly challenging in this age of technology when the HCP's gaze is often pulled away from the patient. Second, *muscles* of facial expression convey the HCPS's emotional response to the patient, mirroring what the patient is feeling. Third, a *posture* that conveys empathy is one of "mutual respect and openness"[48] such as sitting at eye level with relaxed arms and hands. Finally, empathy is expressed in one's *tone* of voice—not "dominant" but "conveying warmth and anxiety about a patient's condition."[48]

Video 3.9 shows me and my colleague Dr. G in an unscripted reenactment of a real patient scenario. Notice all of the verbal and nonverbal ways Dr. G expresses empathy for the patient. Mirroring emotions, something Dr. G demonstrates well, has been rated by experts as the "most efficient" way to establish "a therapeutic, empathetic bond."[23] The HCP can mirror a patient's facial expressions and body language or even the emotion they are describing verbally but may not be visibly expressing. Dr. Ronda demonstrates this in Video 3.7 (shown in previous section on demonstrating mindful listening) with a subtle, fleeting facial expression mirroring the surprise and frustration of her patient about her aging father's unreasonable demands. See if you can find it.

Interestingly, mirroring not only *communicates* empathy, but it also helps *cultivate* empathy for the HCP (as discussed in Chapter 2). "If we can adopt the characteristics of others for just a few moments, we have a better idea of what is going on with the other. We understand better who the other person is, what they are about, and what they are feeling."[23] So, when a patient seems tense and you notice them knitting their brow, you could simply mirror their facial expression. By doing so, you can sense better what it feels like to "walk in their shoes," and at the same time, you are communicating empathy to them.

Note the circular relationship between mirroring and empathetic understanding depicted in Fig. 3.2; as the HCP mirrors, they understand better, which in turn helps the HCP express empathy better through mirroring. Mirroring is a way to both cultivate and express empathy.

Video 3.10 was filmed immediately before a dental extraction. The patient was a recent college graduate who was preparing to move from across the country for an opportunity through AmeriCorps to teach underprivileged children. She was excited about this new chapter of her life, but first she had to obtain dental clearance, which required her to undergo a tooth extraction and several restorations. (If her job didn't require dental clearance, she probably would not have sought treatment, because traumatic dental experiences in her childhood had left a fearful imprint). This patient expressed her anxiety very directly (which is uncommon). Note how the patient expresses her emotions verbally and nonverbally, and how the HCP expresses empathy through mirroring.

Patient: I'm so nervous!

Doctor: *Mirroring nonverbally*

Patient: I don't like needles. So, if I get tense, that's why.

Doctor: Okay. *Mirroring.*

So much is conveyed without words. Notice the patient's nonverbal communications, including eyes (looking away), face (smiling tensely), hands (wringing),

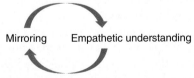

Fig. 3.2 Virtuous Cycle of Mirroring and Empathetic understanding.

tone of voice (high pitch/laughing). Notice which of these expressions are mirrored in the doctor's nonverbal communications.

Pairs Experiment with Mirroring:

One person is the speaker and the other the listener. For one to two minutes, the speaker describes an experience they had which evoked anger, sadness, fear, or happiness. The partner listens while counting backwards from 100.

Switch roles. This time the listener notices carefully the facial expressions and body language of the speaker and tries to mirror them.

Compare and contrast the two experiences from the perspective of both partners.

Timing Matters: Pacing and Pausing

Consider expressing empathy as a gradual, gentle process similar to the way one would approach a shy animal in the woods, gently coaxing it to come out into the open. Experts in medical communication identified four distinct stages: one in which the HCP "recognized emotion in the patient's voice or posture…a second question or comment said softly and gently, encouraged the patient to talk more," and finally "summarizing and expressing empathetic understanding."[59] In Video 3.9, Dr. G gently asked the patient four different times in different ways before the patient disclosed the worst of his trauma (you will see this video in its entirety in Chapter 5.) Challenging emotions are uncomfortable terrain therefore require a gentle approach.

Skillful timing of empathy also requires knowing when to pause. This is because when premature, empathy can "prevent the full disclosure of affect"; experts suggest, "Clinicians might delay their responses to empathetic opportunities…to allow the full story to emerge…to offer an appropriate and effective empathetic response."[42] Psychiatrist and philosopher Dr. Jodi Halpern has noted, "Pausing at moments of heightened anxiety" helps patients "disclose information. If physicians did not pause at such times, patients did not share vulnerable information, despite physicians asking the patients appropriate and accurate questions."[60] As a rule of thumb, wait a few seconds longer than you think the patient needs before responding, to allow space for feeling and sharing.

To Feel or Not to Feel?

Verbal or nonverbal, explicit or subtle, immediate or delayed—expressing empathy is complex! Is there anything that could serve as a compass to guide the delicate dance of expressing empathy for another's feelings? In a nutshell, feeling the feelings.

The question about whether or not feeling is required to express empathy has been controversial in medicine. Although the common definition of empathy involves feeling or "vicariously experiencing another's emotions by recognizing, understanding, and resonating with their emotional state,"[61] the medical use of the term has traditionally focused on the cognitive aspect of empathy at the exclusion of feeling. For example, a medical definition of empathy from a meeting of the Society of General Internal Medicine involves "the act of correctly acknowledging the emotional state of another *without experiencing* that state oneself" (emphasis added).[62] Medical educators define empathy as "a form of detached cognition."[60] This stance is likely motivated by the belief that clinician emotions might compromise mental clarity and objectivity.

Indeed, clarity of mind is important for any HCP, but unfortunately that is not enough. Patients want and need more than an accurate diagnosis or straight sutures. Research shows, "patients value empathy above all else,"[63] and the empathy we are talking about involves feeling. "Patients sense whether physicians are emotionally attuned…patients trust physicians who respond to their anxiety with their own responsive worry."[60]

Attuning to and resonating with the patient's emotions provide a compass for the complex process of expressing empathy both verbally and nonverbally. Fortunately, this ability to attune to and feel another's emotions is hardwired. Mirror neurons were discovered by an Italian team of researchers who reported these neurons "became active both when the monkey performed a given action and when it *observed* a similar action performed by the experimenter" (emphasis added).[64] Mirror neurons are activated not only when we observe another's actions but also when we observe their emotions. As researchers report, "The discovery of mirror neurons allows a comprehension of empathy as an immediate and compassionate partaking of a response, enabling an understanding of the other person's feeling."[65]

In conclusion, with a little time and attention, the HCP can tune into and feel the patient's emotions, thus allowing them to express empathy in a way that is meaningful and helpful. In the words of Dr. Halpern:

> *Attuning to patients does not always involve resonating with strong feelings…a subtle sense of where another person is emotionally…Emotional attunement guides the timing and the tone…when to ask questions, when to stay silent, and when to repeat important words.*[60]

Balancing Feeling With Thinking

While my experience dealing with anxious dental patients has shown me the value of tuning in to patients' emotions, too much focus on this can distract from the technical demands of a procedure. I once found myself trying so hard to empathize with a patient that I lost track of the sequence of my filling procedure (luckily my assistant was paying attention!). The mind can only contain so much.

This scenario illustrates the research findings that neural networks governing empathy and cognitive problem solving are anticorrelated. In other words, "increases in one network necessitate decreases in the other."[66] Therefore, HCPs, especially those of us who deal with complex technical procedures, must learn how to toggle between feeling and thinking modes. For difficult medical and dental procedures, one approach is to train support staff (who are not also needing to focus on the procedure) to look out for empathetic opportunities and encourage them to attend to the patient empathetically while the provider focuses on the technical task at hand. In addition, the HCP can set an intention to share empathy and compassion immediately before and after the procedure, then allow the mind to focus on the procedure for its duration.

Jump-Starting Empathy: Compassion Practice

For the times when empathy is not available for whatever reason—(e.g., the HCP is too stressed or too tired)—the HCP can always turn to compassion practice as a catalyst for empathy. Remember, compassion includes both empathy and a wish for another's well-being. By practicing compassion, the HCP activates the neural networks mediated by oxytocin and dopamine, which promotes their own well-being while finding empathy and the motivation to help others. The practice of loving kindness introduced in Chapter 2 cultivates compassion, and a simplified version of this practice can bookend any procedure or consultation as described below:

> **Practice With a Patient**
> A simplified form of compassion practice which can precede or follow a difficult procedure is simply wishing the person in your care to be free of suffering and to be well. (And when this wish is not available, simply set an intention to wish this.) You might also try bringing attention to the area of your heart. The simple setting of an intention can spark empathy and compassion for the person in your care. In addition, when we set an intention, even though we might forget the intention, often times it comes back to find us.

Finally, What Situations Call for Empathy?

Empathy does not have to be limited to the patient's illness or treatment. Experts assert an empathetic response is called for at "any expression of moderate to strong negative affect."[24] The emotions can be related to a procedure, any aspect of the office experience, or something totally unrelated. Let's close our discussion of empathy with a couple stories to illustrate.

A dental resident I was overseeing had just finished the second long appointment for a molar root canal. Unfortunately, he was unable to complete the treatment. When the patient heard that they would need yet another appointment they frowned and exclaimed, "another appointment!?" The resident and patient both walked out of the treatment room in a tense silence, leaving me wondering if the patient would return (and wanting to bite my fist!)

Unfortunately, the resident missed the cue for an empathetic response. If he had said something empathetic like, "I can imagine your disappointment over not completing this procedure…it's hard for you to make more time," he might have helped ease her frustration, avoided alienation, and cultivated connection.

Video 3.11 demonstrates empathy for a challenge unrelated to illness or treatment. Notice how the doctor expresses empathy for the patient's challenging drive to the clinic.

As a final note, empathy can also be expressed for positive experiences, too! The day that Joyce received her complete dentures was the first day she could smile confidently in 60 years. The dental assistant and I shared her happiness, smiling broadly and saying, "You must be so happy, you have waited all your life for this day!" Our empathy magnified her joy and deepened our connection.

TYING IT TOGETHER: INTRODUCE/ INTERCONNECT, SOLICIT, LISTEN, EMPATHIZE

Emotional scenarios are hard to capture on video because they tend to occur early in the relationship (and I don't like videorecording patients early on because I feel it is too invasive). In lieu of videos, short scenarios will be shared to demonstrate ISLEEP skills for difficult emotions. The following two similar scenarios—one medical and one dental—illustrate all of the ISLEEP skills covered so far. In addition to illustrating the skills covered so far, we will preview examples of the final two ISLEEP skills: *explain* and affirming *power* of the patient.

Scenario #1: The Dreaded Pap Smear

Introduction/Interconnect

The physician introduces herself to the patient, who is 40 years old and new to the practice. She ascertains that the patient likes to be called Liz and takes a moment to comment on the blizzard-like conditions of the past week in the area. Liz and the physician share their hardships getting through it.

Solicit

Physician: What brings you in today, Liz?

Liz: I know I need a pap smear, but I have been dreading it so much.

Physician: What do you think makes the thought of a pap smear so hard for you?

Listen

Liz: I have a history of a sexual assault *(begins to cry).* The exam I had afterwards in the emergency room was almost worse than the assault, and I've never been back.

Listen With Mindfulness

Physician: *(Feeling anxiety about what she should say first. She breathes a few times to allow space for this disclosure.)*

Liz: *(Trying to regain composure.)* That was a long time ago, and I'm grown up now, so I just need to get it done. I'm sorry.

Empathy: Nonverbal

Physician: (Takes a couple of breaths looking at Liz and nodding and expressing understanding.)

Empathize/validate

Physician: I can imagine how scary those experiences were for you. They are very traumatic events which have impacted your life. I can understand why you would dread having a pap smear.

Liz: Yes, thank you *(looks slightly relieved).*

Explain

Physician: I am so glad you came today and are interested in taking care of your health. I'm also grateful to you for sharing your past experiences to help me understand how you are feeling. We will discuss ways we can minimize your discomfort during a pap smear.

Affirm Power of the Patient

Physician: Also, I will proceed only when you are ready to do so, and you can ask me to stop any time if you feel uncomfortable in any way.

Scenario #2: Dental Phobia: A True Story

Ginger, a petite, blonde, middle-aged woman, sits tensely in the chair as the dentist walks in. This is her first visit to the clinic.

Introduce

Dentist: Hello, Ginger! I'm Dr. D. Welcome to the clinic. *(Sits down next to Ginger.)*

Interconnect

Dentist: I see you're coming all the way from Dover. How was your drive?

Ginger: Not too bad. *(wringing her hands.)*

Solicit

Dentist: What brings you to the clinic today?

Ginger: I haven't been to a dentist in 10 years. I am terrified, but I have to get this done. My mouth is a mess. I have to do something. There's no avoiding it.

Solicit

Dentist: What do you think has been keeping you away?

Listen

Dentist: *(Totally silent and still, smiling gently with her eyes resting on Ginger.)*

Ginger: Ten years ago, I had a root canal. I was having terrible pain during the procedure, but the dentist wouldn't stop. I kept telling him, "It hurts, I can't bear it," but he wouldn't listen. *(She looks down, and a tear trickles out of her eye.)*

Listening With Mindfulness and Empathy

Dentist: *(Feeling inner tightening and uncertainty about what to do next. Not wanting to offer premature reassurances, she waits, mirroring the patient's facial expressions of anxiety and nodding with understanding. Feeling the sensations of the breath she holds the space.)*

Ginger: I'm such a baby. You don't have time for this.

Empathy: Nonverbal and Verbal

Dentist: *(Continuing to look at Ginger, mirroring her upset facial expressions and nodding with understanding.)*

The experience you describe was traumatic for you. (*With a gentle, caring tone of voice*) It felt violating. It makes sense you would be afraid it will happen again!

Ginger: (*Her tears begin to flow*) Yes, yes! (*Sobbing quietly for a few moments before looking at the dentist with a shy smile. Her shoulders drop, and she lets out a big sigh of relief.*)

Explain

Dentist: I want to help you get your smile back and am willing to work within your comfort zone. We will make sure you are totally numb before any treatment. We will take a small step at a time. I will explain everything I am going to do and what it will feel like before doing anything.

Affirm Power of the Patient

Dentist: Also, you can stop me any time you need a break or feel uncomfortable.

Ginger: Thank you so much (*smiling, seeming reassured*).

As of the date of this writing, Ginger has completed a root canal, several restorations and extractions, and is ready to replace her missing teeth to restore her smile. Interestingly, she refuses to see any other dentist, even if she must wait weeks for appointments. While Ginger reports still feeling some anxiety before appointments, she tolerates her procedures well. She reports feeling safe.

The true scenario above demonstrates how the ISLEEP skills can help transform a person's health care experience from a traumatic one to a healing one with just a few words and a little time. It may feel discouraging or alarming to an HCP when a patient gets emotional. It may feel awkward to sit in silence with a patient when they are upset. Try it. You may find, as I have countless times, that you don't have to *do* anything. Simply by listening mindfully and empathizing with patients, they feel understood and gain trust. You may find that they refuse to see anyone else but you. You may find you feel less stressed and enjoy your work more.

Experiment: Solicit/Listen/Empathize

Try the following experiment with a partner, and then switch roles. Allow the speaker 1 to 2 minutes.

1. Solicit: ask a question that elicits negative or positive emotions such as:
   a. "What is bothering you in your life right now?"
   b. "What are you looking forward to?"
2. Listen and empathize nonverbally: Demonstrate your attention and empathy with body language such as eye contact, muscles of facial expression, posture, and tone of voice. Cultivate and express empathy by mirroring verbal and nonverbal expressions of emotion.

Note: Listener avoids interrupting with reassurances, explanations, advice, sympathy, or personal stories.

3. Empathize: express understanding, "I sense/see/hear your___" (emotion) and acceptance, "It makes sense you would feel_____."

Questions for Reflection

1. What was it like be heard and to listen in this way?
2. How was this experience different from how you normally listen/are listened to?
3. How do you think mindful listening and empathizing could impact your relationships both professionally and personally?

If you find it helpful, write down your reflections in a journal.

Preparatory Questions for ISLEEP Skill Explain

1. Before, during, and after hands-on procedures, what do you explain to patients to help them feel safe and respected?
2. Do you use different words to explain the same procedure to different people? If so, why? What are some of the words you use to help people understand the technical procedures you do?

ISLEEP: EXPLAIN

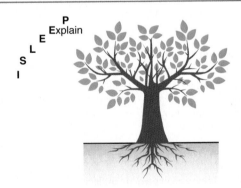

*When I was a child, ironically enough, I was very afraid of the dentist. I died a little inside every time my hygienist would scale my teeth. When I got older, I had a new hygienist who **explained** everything so well to me (emphasis added). She even showed me in the mirror the bits of calculus (tartar) on my*

mandibular anterior linguals (back of lower front teeth). She showed me what they looked like when she was done cleaning. When she noticed me pulling away as she was scaling, she offered some topical numbing gel. At that time, I didn't even know it existed! I will never forget her and the small acts of kindness and consideration she showed me. I remember her every day, with every one of my patients now.

Jessie M, RDH

Jessie's story captures the importance of the ISLEEP element **explain** to addressing fears and concerns. Explaining what a patient needs to know, in a way they understand, can avoid misunderstandings, disappointment, and litigation.[67] In a study of 45 depositions of suits brought against a large hospital in the United States, 26% of cases were the result of "delivering information poorly."[24] Explaining skillfully can also reduce anxiety[14] and even pain[68] (more in Chapter 5). The ability to explain skillfully correlates strongly with patient-centered care and patient satisfaction; research on communication in dentistry identified six main factors that determine patient satisfaction[69]; one of the six factors is called "sharing information," and five of six factors include questions pertaining to **explain**.

Especially when dealing with anxiety-provoking procedures, there are three essential areas to explain: "information about *what will happen* (procedural information), information about what *sensations* the individual will experience (sensory information), information about what the individual can do to *cope* with the situation (coping information)" (emphasis added).[28] This third item, explaining what a patient can do to cope, will be discussed more fully in Chapter 5 on managing procedural pain and anxiety. For now, let's briefly look at *what* to explain in each of the different phases of care. After that we will discuss *how* to explain—the choice of language.

What to Explain During Each Phase of Care
Explain During Consultations

Skillful explaining during the consultation is essential for informed consent and patient-centered care, and this includes explaining the risks and benefits of treatment options. Explaining well avoids misunderstandings and disappointments. For example, many times when I inform my dental patients they need a root canal retreatment, they usually assume the reason is because the first one was

done improperly or poorly, and they are disappointed. But it is a well-established fact that even when a root canal is done perfectly, there is always a slight chance that the tooth will need further treatment to remove all of the infection. Most likely, the patient didn't understand the risks (or forgot)—I (or whoever did the first root canal) may not have explained well.

A patient-centered approach to treatment planning called *shared decision-making* emphasizes choices and options. Visual aids such as issues cards, decision boards, and option grids help distinguish and clarify the options.[70]

Experiments:
1. Find visual aids to explain the different diseases and conditions that you deal with as well as the diagnostic and treatment options that you offer.
2. Explore how can you help patients understand their own conditions with a "show and tell" approach. For example, a dentist can use a simple hand mirror or intraoral camera to show the patient the condition of their mouth or dental fillings.

Explaining about procedures is especially important to the anxious patient. Explain your commitment to managing their anxiety. From a dental hygiene text, "Reassure the patient that his or her concerns are being taken seriously, that dealing with dental anxiety is an element of providing care, and that the hygienist is trained in anxiety management techniques."[38] Explain the nature of the procedure and the comfort measures you will offer.

Be aware that, for some patients, too much information can actually increase anxiety. One of my patients had a consultation with an oral surgery resident to prepare his mouth for denture fabrication with alveoloplasty (removal of boney overgrowths). The patient returned from the consultation alarmed by the resident's description of the procedure reporting, "He said he was going to flap my gum and file down the bone!" Although accurate, this is too much information for most patients. Usually, a general description of what the procedure will *accomplish* and its *benefits* is more helpful than detailed descriptions of the procedure itself. For example, in the scenario above, the doctor could simply explain, "The gums will be *shaped* so the denture will *fit better*." To help gauge how much information to share, dental fear experts suggest, "It may be useful to ask patients how much information they would like to have."[34]

Explain During Clinical Exams

Many times, after I have completed an oral exam, patients have commented, "I have never had such a thorough exam!" They most likely have had similar exams but were not aware because the provider did not explain *what* they were doing. Explaining during exams allows the patient to understand and appreciate a thorough examination (and reduce the number of complaints about being charged a fee when "nothing was done today"). I have found that explaining during physical exams also keeps me on task and helps me avoid missing something. Video 3.12 documents a complete extraoral and intraoral exam demonstrating the ISLEEP skill *explain*.

In addition to explaining what you are looking for during clinical examinations, it is also important to explain any *sensations* that may be felt during testing or manipulation of the body. Imagine being a patient for a procedure—perhaps having your blood drawn or your teeth cleaned—and having your body touched and manipulated without any explanation. To many of us, this can feel objectifying and unpleasant. In contrast, when a provider explains what they are doing and how it will feel, they convey respect and care. Video 3.13 demonstrates *explain* before palpation and percussion testing of the teeth (a way of identifying an offending tooth). This clip also demonstrates the P in ISLEEP, *power* of the patient, when the HCP asks permission: "Can I do a little tapping?" More on affirming patient power in the next section.

Explaining Immediately Before Procedures

Jessie's dental hygiene patients love her, and one of the reasons is her willingness and ability to *explain* well before she does anything to them.

> As a hygienist, most of my patients understand and know when they are there for a cleaning. But I do always clarify when bringing them back. I've also found helpful stating what I am about to do before doing it. For example, taking x-rays, which x-rays I am taking, when I'm about to polish, floss, and especially when I use the ultrasonic scaler. Many patients are unfamiliar with this type of scaler and can be afraid of it if I use it without warning. I've had many patients tell me that they appreciate me explaining what I'm doing. And it helps me stay on track too.
>
> **Jessie M, RDH**

Immediately before a procedure, review the procedure and the rationale with the patient. Review the risks and benefits. Review the expected duration of the procedure.[71] Most importantly, explain how you will address any specific concerns or fears that they have expressed about the upcoming procedure. For example, if the patient is afraid of needles, explain the comfort measures you will provide during the injection such as topical anesthesia. This is demonstrated in Video 3.14, which includes the ISLEEP skills *listen*, *empathize*, and *explain*. (We saw this video in the section on empathy. This time, focus on what the HCP explains to the patient.)

The benefits of explaining to the anxious patient immediately before and during procedures is illustrated by the following story about a dental hygiene patient:

> She came into the office after not having seen a dentist in years. She came in for a new patient exam and x-rays. She shared her concerns with me and cried for most of the appointment. However, I explained everything to her in detail and explained we could stop at any time without repercussion or judgment. Once her [full series of radiographs] was completed, I sat her back and picked up my probe. I showed her my instrument and explained its use. Through tears she thanked me and said no one had ever explained that to her before. It hit me right then the impact something as simple as that could have on a patient.
>
> **Kevin T, RDH**

For the anxious patient immediately before procedures, it is also helpful to **explain** the ways that the patient can cope with difficulties during procedures. The hygienist above explained to the patient that she could stop at any time. Also, explain any techniques, such as deep breathing, that patients may employ during the procedure. (See Chapter 5 for more interventions for procedural pain and anxiety.)

Explaining During Procedures

Most of the procedure-oriented HCPs' time is spent "hands on." This is a particularly vulnerable time for a patient, especially if they are unable to speak. Therefore, as with the clinical exam, *explain anything that will produce a sensation*. A study of pediatric dental patients found, "Children who received sensory information about the dental experience showed fewer disruptive behaviors, were more cooperative, were rated as less anxious and distressed, and had lower post-treatment pulse rates than children in a control group."[38] In the case of an uncomfortable sensation, one might think that telling a patient to expect discomfort would increase anxiety. On the contrary, dental fear experts report: "Being in a potentially threatening situation and never knowing when the actual negative event will occur keeps the person in a constant state of anticipatory anxiety"; in contrast, "If it is clear that all danger will be signaled, absence of the danger signal or warning can be taken as a 'safety signal.'"[34]

Explaining sensory information during a procedure includes any of the senses, including touch ("I'm going to gently pull your cheek"), smell ("You might smell alcohol now"), sound ("You'll hear the whistle of the dental handpiece now"), and sight ("Now I'll use a bright blue light to harden the filling material"). "Tailor to the patient's understanding, anxiety level and/or need for details"; you might simply ask, "Would you like continuous updates of what is going on, or would you prefer to relax your mind while I am working?"[52] In general, explaining during procedures decreases surprises and by doing so, increases trust and ease.

Finally, explaining upcoming uncomfortable sensations during procedures is even more helpful when coupled with ways to cope.[34] In Video 3.15, Nicholas, a severely phobic dental patient, describes what helped him cope with dental treatment despite his fear.

You tell me what's going to happen before you do it, what to expect, if anything. You prewarn me of pain... what I can do to alleviate it as you're working. I haven't had a problem. I feel very good.

(The breathing techniques that Nicholas alludes to will be discussed in more detail in Chapter 5.) Video 3.16 depicts an HCP **explaining** during a dental extraction on Nicholas.

> **Exercises:**
> 1. Imagine procedures that you commonly perform from start to finish. Make a list of all the sensations and all the senses a patient might experience including smells, tastes, sights, and sounds.
> 2. If you perform the procedures with a team, discuss with your team who would be the best person to explain these sensations and sensory stimuli to the patient during the procedures.
> 3. With a partner, simulate a common procedure you do in two different ways: first without any explanation and then explaining everything your "patient" will feel, smell, taste, see, and hear. Compare and contrast the two experiences.

Explaining Postoperatively

After the procedure is complete, explain what signs and symptoms to expect, such as sensitivity, swelling, or pain. Also, explain what the patient can do to care for themselves, and provide these instructions in writing if needed. As always, verbal and written instructions should be appropriate for the language and socioeconomic status of the patient. The next section focuses on the language we use to explain.

Table 3.3 summarizes what to explain during each phase of health care.

TABLE 3.3	Summary of Explain During Different Phases of Care		
ISLEEP Skill	**HANDS OFF** Consult/tx Plan	**HANDS OFF** Treatment Visit: Preop and Postop	**HANDS ON** Treatment Visit: Procedures and Clinical Exams
E. *Explain/ reassure*	• Treatment options • Risks/benefits • Check understanding NOTE: Avoid overly technical information about procedures (unless requested)	• Review procedure and rationale • Review risks and benefits • How provider will address patient concerns about procedure • How provider will address pain and anxiety • What patient can do for pain and anxiety • POST OP—what to expect and how to manage it	• What sensations will be felt (especially if uncomfortable) • EXAMS: What you are looking for • What the patient can do to minimize pain and anxiety

Note: The Appendices provide summaries of what to explain and sample language for each of the phases of care, including the consultation (Appendix D), pre- and post-operative phases (Appendix E), and the hands-on phase during procedures and clinical exams (Appendix F).

How to Explain: Choice of Language

Imagine being discharged from the hospital after surgery with these important postoperative instructions:

在與病人以口語或書面溝通時，使用病人能夠了解的通俗詞彙，是十分重要的.

This simulates the experience of many patients when the language is not appropriate for their needs! (Translation from Mandarin Chinese: "When communicating with patients either verbally or in writing, it is important to use language that is easy to understand.")

The HCP should use language that is "easily comprehended and match[es] the patient's requirements and expectations."[6] Any explaining should be culturally competent, defined by the American Hospital Association as "the ability of systems to provide care to patients with diverse values, beliefs and behaviors, including the tailoring of health care delivery to meet patients' *social, cultural, and linguistic needs*" (emphasis added).[72] This applies to both verbal and written communications.

Use of Medical Jargon

The comic strip "Garfield" once featured a dentist telling the patient, "You have acute gingivitis," to which the patient responded, "People tell me I have a cute smile too!"[73] The use of medical terminology can create several problems, as described by communication experts:

Jargon is a barrier to communication as it impairs the relationship and may result in the patient being afraid to ask questions that may appear stupid. Using jargon alters the power dynamic of the relationship: instead of the power being equal with the patient actively involved in the process, it becomes clinician-centered and not patient-centered.[4]

The patient in Video 3.17 (previously seen in Chapter 1) adores her neurosurgeon, who apparently is very skilled at the ISLEEP skill **explain**. When asked the open-ended question, "What do you like about your doctor," listen to what she says.

He takes time to tell me in detail everything he's going to do. He explains…he has someone come and explain it again…makes sure you understand. Some doctors give you all these big words. He'll tell you the big words but then explains what they mean.

Clearly, the ISLEEP element **explain** is core to this patient's definition of quality care.

One common obstacle to explaining effectively, especially for new clinicians, is having learned their profession only in technical terms. This technical/professional language must then be translated into lay language when speaking to a patient. There are three main considerations when translating medical terminology—*understandability, connotations, and alternative meanings*. First, when speaking to a patient, choose words that are common and *understandable*; some dental examples include translating "amalgam restoration" into "silver filling" and "periodontal disease" into "gum infection." Second, avoid lay terms that have a negative or inflammatory *connotation*. For example, the word "discomfort" would be preferable to "pain," "tip" to "needle," and "squirt" to "inject." Finally, be aware that some medical terms may have *alternative meanings* in mainstream culture. For example, "soft tissues" are a paper product to most people, and "recession" (as in recession of gums in the mouth) is a downward economic trend. In dentistry, the term "recall" to indicate a maintenance visit should itself be recalled, since it is synonymous with a defective product. In summary, use language that is understandable, non-inflammatory, and doesn't have negative or confusing alternative meanings to communicate with patients clearly and effectively.

Exercise

Create a list of commonly used medical terms in your specialty. Then create a list of corresponding lay terms using the guidelines described above. See Appendix G for medical and dental examples.

Preparatory Questions for ISLEEP Skill Power

1. Research shows that "pain experienced by a patient in control is not likely to lead to fear."[34] What are the ways that you give you patients control or the perception of control during challenging procedures?
2. What are some ways you honor the power of the patient in the consultation?

ISLEEP: POWER OF THE PATIENT

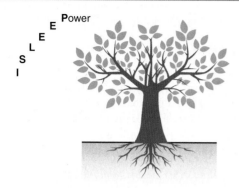

Let's listen to Joyce, a dental patient we have met before. After avoiding dentistry for decades because of fear and anxiety, she has just completed her treatment and received her complete dentures. In Video 3.18, she describes poignantly why she was so afraid and which aspects of her dental care enabled her to overcome her fear and complete her treatment. (Note that this video is slightly longer than previous ones.)

For Joyce, lack of a sense of control during one health care encounter as a child resulted in a lifetime of trauma. It tainted subsequent dental experiences, making dental care "like going to the gas chamber." Ultimately, it tainted every aspect of her life, including her career and social life. When asked what made it possible to overcome her fear and undergo treatment, she responds, "You gave me the **power**."

Imagine being a patient in the following scenario: you are situated under a bright light, unable to speak, unable to move, and anticipating discomfort or pain induced by the dental professionals who loom overhead. Considering the resemblance of this health care scenario to a spy interrogation, it is not surprising that patients would feel vulnerable, intimidated, and anxious! Many medical and dental procedures put patients in vulnerable situations that arouse anxiety and induce pain. This is particularly true of procedures that limit patients' ability to speak (dentistry) or their ability to move (magnetic resonance imaging [MRI], suturing wounds). The vulnerability of patients in many medical and dental procedures underscores the importance of affirming their power.

Much has been studied and written about patient power and perceived control in dentistry, which has relevance to any HCP, especially those who are procedure-oriented. Lack of a sense of control has been cited as one of the most anxiety-producing aspects of treatment.[34,74] Conversely, "According to the principle of 'perceived control,' if an individual believes he has some control over what is happening to him in an undesirable environment, he will experience less stress."[74] Most notably, "Pain experienced by a patient in control is not likely to lead to fear."[34] This last ISLEEP element, affirming **power** of the patient, addresses the need for control and perceived control to reduce anxiety and to increase trust and comfort for the patient.

Every step of a health care encounter—from checking the hospital wristband, to positioning the patient, to exiting the treatment room—is an opportunity to honor the patient's **power.** Remember, the patient doesn't *have to* do anything. They have the right to choose their own treatment options. They have the right to walk out at any time, even in the middle of a procedure or hospital stay. By remembering this important fact, the HCP is more likely to act in a patient-centered way.

> **Exercise** (although written for nurses, applies to all HCPs)
> *Nurses inevitably occupy a position of power in relation to their patients, whether conscious or unconscious. As the powerful person in this transaction, you have the means and the responsibility to do what you can to mitigate this difference. After reflecting on what barriers are presented by the physical environment, the different roles you occupy, your approach to caring processes and your understanding of how the patient might feel, think about what you can do to reduce these barriers.*[75]

How does the HCP affirm the **power** of the patient, especially during challenging procedures? Let's look at ways of affirming patient power while working "hands on" and then "hands off." Because patients are much more vulnerable and prone to feeling powerless in hands-on mode, we will spend most of our time here.

Affirming Patient Power While Hands On (Procedures)

Already, by practicing the previous ISLEEP skills, you have affirmed the **power** of the patient implicitly. For example, **soliciting** a patient's level of comfort during a procedure by asking, "Are you okay," affirms their **power** to express their discomfort and request comfort measures. Also, skillful **explaining** during a procedure, like,

"You're going to feel a cold sensation now," provides a sense of predictability that facilitates a sense of power and perceived control.[52]

Now, let's look at three general ways to more explicitly affirm the **power** of the patient. Video 3.19 provides examples of all three. (We met this patient in the section on empathy, when she shared her fear of dentistry.)

- Clip #1: Offering Options
  "Please stop me anytime if it's bothering you." (Option to stop treatment.)
- Clip #2: Asking Permission
  "Now I'm going to give the Novocaine. *If it's okay*, I'll bring the chair back a little more."
- Clip #3: Making Requests
  "When you're ready, *if you could please* open big and look straight up at the light."

While these three ways of honoring the power of the patient may seem obvious and simple, they make a world of difference to a patient who is anxious or afraid as Joyce described in her last video. Now let's unpack each of these three ways to affirm the patient's power while working hands on.

Requesting, Not Demanding

Making a request instead of a demand affirms the **power** of the patient. In the previous video, notice how subtly the HCP affirms the **power** of the patient by simply choosing language that is invitational ("When you're ready, if you could open") rather than demanding ("Open big"). Invitational language changes the tone of a statement from intimidating and demanding to empowering. Even when the HCP doesn't anticipate any objection, requests are a good practice.

In Video 3.20, Joyce describes the sense of safety that arises from gentle requests. Instead of demands, like, "Do this," Joyce prefers requests, like, "Will you do this for me," or "Can you do this for me?" She also shares her appreciation for a gentle tone of voice, which will be discussed more in Chapter 5 (nonverbal communication). Framing tasks as a request instead of a command or demand communicates to patients that they will not be forced to do anything and that they are in control.

Next, you will find an example of making a request during an intraoral exam (Video 3.21). Rather than manipulating the patient's head or commanding the patient to turn, the HCP affirms the **power** of the patient by making a request. Notice the invitational language, "*If you could*, turn towards me a little bit." Notice also how the request accompanies the movement without adding time to the procedure.

Asking Permission

Consent is more than a signature on a form, and written consent does not provide the HCP license to continue a procedure, no matter what. In this age of heightened awareness of sexual harassment and assault, we know that consent in intimate relations can be withdrawn at any time. The same is true in health care:

> *Nurses and other health professionals are required to obtain valid consent before starting any form of treatment or intervention. Even when they give consent, patients may withdraw it at any point, and professionals must generally respect patients' wishes, regardless of their own personal views.*[76]

When the HCP affirms the **power** of the patient by making requests and asking permission, they ensure they are proceeding with the patient's consent, moment to moment.

While *making requests* pertains to what the HCP wants the patient to do, *asking permission* pertains to something the HCP does for the patient. Even the simplest, most routine act, such as obtaining blood pressure, can be preceded by asking permission. Certified nurse midwife Martha B shares, "The patient must be asked: Can I check your blood pressure? Can I listen to your heart and lungs? No permission is assumed" (from a personal correspondence). Asking permission may seem obvious or simple, but it is essential to patient-centered care when working hands on to facilitate perceived control.[52] Again, dental anxiety experts have much to offer: "Asking permission is checking to see if the patient is ready to proceed. It enhances her control, and has the paradoxical effect of allowing quicker progress than if you tried to push."[34] Asking permission is also a way of showing respect.

Let's look at four examples of asking permission. In Video 3.22, the dentist wants to put protective goggles on the patient and then administer local anesthesia. The dentist asks, "We have some goggles to protect your eyes. *Is that alright?*" The dentist also asks, "Would you like to be numbed or try without?" This demonstrates offering options as a way of honoring the **power** of the patient, an approach that will be discussed more in the next section.

Video 3.23 demonstrates asking permission to insert a cotton roll in the mouth. "I'm going to tuck a cotton roll next to your cheek, *okay?*" In this case, the HCP asks permission—not because she anticipates an objection but as a gesture of respect and to honor the patient's power. Notice how asking permission can be woven into the flow of the procedure without adding extra time.

For a fearful patient like Nicholas (next video), jumping into something like percussion testing of his teeth could be very triggering. Here, the HCP asks the patient's permission to percuss the teeth as a way to facilitate perceived control and honor his power. In Video 3.13, the dentist asks permission by saying, "Just a gentle finger pressure, *okay?*" And then, "*Can I do a little tapping with my mirror?*"

The last example of asking permission pertains to procedures of a subjective nature, such as cosmetic reshaping of teeth. In these situations, asking permission can be a way to facilitate collaboration with a patient. One of my favorite patients, Albert, is a gentle giant who is always calm and gracious despite multiple serious medical problems. His favorite subject is his 6-year-old grandson, whom he is raising single-handedly. Whenever I ask about his grandson, Albert's eyes twinkle, and he smiles broadly. Video 3.24 shows me adjusting Albert's upper anterior teeth on his new complete denture. Notice how we are both engaged in the process of optimizing Albert's smile.

You may have noticed that I ask for the patient's permission several times as I work: "If you're okay with it…" then, "I'll do the same thing on the other side?" And, "Can I do it here, too?" Each time I ask permission, I am welcoming feedback and affirming his power. Each time he grants permission, he confirms his approval and satisfaction with my care.

Note for Special Populations

Some individuals benefit from a firm, directed approach, as opposed to asking permission and making requests. For example, a special needs patient or a neurotypical child may interpret a question such as "Could you open your mouth now" literally and respond with a "no!" Similarly, a high anxiety patient may respond "no" to the question, "Would it be ok if I looked in your mouth," due to their fear. For such patients, consider simple, specific, direct requests, such as, "Let's start with opening your mouth for three seconds." If the patient refuses, their "no" must be respected by backing away, waiting a minute, and then starting again. Start with small tasks and gradually build on them. (See more in Chapter 5, gradual exposure.) Table 3.4 contrasts the more common approach of affirming patient power with a more directed approach.

Offering Options

Making requests and asking permission, while affirming the **power** of the patient, also introduces the possibility of the patient refusing a request or not granting permission. What if the patient says no? Indeed, there have been several times when I have said to a dental patient, "I'm going to recline the chair now, is that okay," and the response has been, "No!" A routine action for the HCP, such as reclining the dental chair or placing a hospital wristband, can be problematic for a patient. For example, a person with a back injury or a history of sexual abuse may find it too painful to have the dental chair reclined; a person with a history of incarceration may find a hospital wristband emotionally triggering. Making requests and asking permission allow the HCP to uncover a patient's needs, express empathy, and *offer options* when possible. Maybe, the back-injured patient needs a pillow, or maybe they just need to go slowly. Patients with a history of trauma or abuse especially benefit greatly from the sense of control that comes from being offered options (more in Chapter 5).

Exercise:
Think of the procedures you do that arouse anxiety or induce pain. What are some possible options you could offer patients to grant them a sense of control? For example, they could choose which dental impression to do first (top or bottom teeth), which arm to use for vaccination, etc.

TABLE 3.4 Alternative Approaches for Special Populations

Affirming POWER	Neurotypical Adult	Special Needs, Pediatric, and High Anxiety Patients
Asking permission	*Is it OK for me to_____?*	*I'm going to_____.*
Making requests	*Could you please _____?*	*It's time to _____.*

Admittedly, there are times when a declined request would not be workable because of associated risks. For example, when I am preparing a patient's tooth for a filling, a "no" to the request to keep their mouth open introduces the risk of injury from a high-speed dental bur. In such cases, explain to the patient in advance the importance of keeping their mouth open (or whatever the critical instruction is) using invitational language, such as, "As much as possible for you, please stay open," instead of commands and ultimatums like, "You have to_____" or "You can't_____." Even more importantly, *offer options* for what to do in the event the patient cannot comply to the request, as we will discuss next.

Stop signals and breaks. The most basic option during a medical or dental procedure is the option to stop. A *stop signal* is a common way of giving patients a sense of control,[74] and researchers report this practice "has been shown to be effective in dental settings and a wide variety of other medical settings."[28] "Since many patients are unaware of this possibility or afraid of causing an inconvenience, every new patient should be introduced to an explicit, agreed nonverbal stop signal."[52] Even when offered this option, many patients with a history of abuse might not feel comfortable using it. For such patients, rehearsing the stop signal could encourage them to use it when necessary. Not surprisingly, patients' use of stop signals changes with time: "Early on patients may interrupt frequently but as trust increases interruptions decline."[38]

Another option the HCP can offer is the option to *take a break* during a procedure. As a dentist, I like to offer patients breaks often—even if there is no indication the patient wants one—simply to affirm their power: "Can you continue a little longer or do you need a break?" Offering the option to take a break could prevent a patient from struggling needlessly or, even worse, from injuring themselves if they end up having to stop at a critical time.

Offering options when discomfort or pain arises during procedures. The HCP's response to a patient's complaint of pain during a medical or dental procedure will make or break the relationship.

Scenario: Imagine you are an HCP running far behind schedule. As you perform a procedure for your patient, they suddenly flinch and moan in pain. You feel the internal tightening and the impulse to ignore and continue. You could try to decrease pain by numbing more, but this would take more time—time you don't have. Should you stop? Should you go on? While the decision to continue treating a patient in pain without offering options may save time in the short term, it comes at a great price. Throughout the years, I have heard so many patients report feeling violated, angry, and afraid when the HCP ignored them in these situations. They rate these providers very poorly. Unfortunately, many times the provider does not know the impact of their actions because the patient does not return. **The most important time to honor the power of the patient by offering options is when the patient complains of pain during a procedure**.

Research findings show the importance of responding to a patient's pain during procedures. First, doing so affects patient satisfaction as demonstrated by a large-scale dental study: "A patient's judgment of dentists' skills and quality of care are based on personal interactions with the dentist, the *level of comfort*, and post-treatment sensitivity" (emphasis added).[77] Second, not responding to pain contributes to procedural anxiety as reported by dental anxiety expert Dr. Corah. Conversely, the most important behavior linked to anxiety reduction is the provider's "dedication to prevent pain."[78]

So, when a patient expresses discomfort during a procedure, whenever possible, try to offer options, even if it is just the option to take a break. When a patient declines this option and permits the provider to proceed, they are also permitting the possibility of discomfort again. This is a very different experience from that of a provider marching on without giving the patient any choice. Dental fear experts assert, "Pain experienced by a patient in control is not likely to lead to fear."[34] When offered options, patients can endure procedures, even uncomfortable ones, and still maintain a sense of safety and trust.

What about procedures in which pain or discomfort is unavoidable? One example of unavoidable discomfort is the pain of an injection of local anesthesia as a means to avoid procedural pain. For such cases, other ISLEEP skills are useful to solicit the nature of the patient's discomfort, empathize, and explain the value of discomfort now to enhance comfort later. Another example of unavoidable pain involves situations when pharmacologic means of sedation, analgesia, or anesthesia would interfere with detection of the root cause.[79] For such situations, is it possible to decrease a patient's procedural pain or increase their pain tolerance non-pharmacologically? Indeed, it is! Chapter 5 is dedicated to the complex and subjective nature of pain perception and includes many non-pharmacologic tools for managing procedural pain and anxiety.

Note: See Appendix F for sample dialogue for power of the patient while hands on.

Affirming Patient Power While Hands Off (Consultations)

The concept of informed consent [extends] beyond that of simple information transfer towards honoring informed preferences...At its core shared decision-making rests on accepting that individual self-determination is a desirable goal and that clinicians need to support patients to achieve this goal wherever feasible.[70]

Several times in my career as a dentist, I have overheard a dental assistant tell a patient before obtaining a full series of radiographs, "You have to get an FMX." Each time, I cringed. First of all, what is an "FMX" to most patients? As we discussed in the ISLEEP skill *explain*, using a lay term, such as "a full set of x-rays," is clearer communication. More importantly, the patient doesn't *have to* do anything, and most patients don't like being told what to do (with the exception of some older patients and those of lower socioeconomic level, who "seem generally to prefer a directive style of consultation"[16]). "Patients have indicated they prefer a collaborative role for decision-making."[6] This is expressed clearly by a patient in a study of patient preferences as she describes her doctor: "She shares her knowledge and suggests options, but she doesn't speak in absolutes or dictate my actions. It seems more like we are partners."[80] How does the HCP convey this sense of partnership?

For affirming a patient's power in the consultation, the previously discussed ISLEEP skills are essential. For example, by **soliciting and listening** to a patient's concerns, wants, and needs and **empathizing** with them, the HCP affirms the patient's power implicitly,

as well as by **explaining** treatment options and the risks and benefits of each option in language the patient can understand.

Here is a true medical story shared by Martha B, CNM, describing how an HCP affirms a patient's power in a consultation:

A neighbor with a history of medical trauma told me of trying to return to medical care after a while of staying away. She had a couple of false starts from physician encounters that were too directive and describes being printed out a list of all the medical screening tests she was now delinquent in. The approach she described as effective for her was a physician who sat and looked at her and listened and did not insist on any exams or tests in that first encounter. The physician left the patient with a sense of hope. She describes the physician as saying, "We're going to help you get your groove back," and then scheduled another appointment very soon so the beginning thread of possibility they had established would not be lost; the relationship could continue and they could work on issues little by little over time. The patient felt that the physician heard her, cared for her and wanted the best quality of life for her.

The physician in this scenario did not dictate what should be done or when, even though the patient was long overdue. Instead, they focused on listening and affirming power by simply giving space. By doing so, this HCP was able to budge a boulder of resistance created by a patient's traumatic past.

When presenting treatment options, the approach that research has found best is to "present treatment plan using a suggestive tone instead of an imposing one."[33] I wish I had understood this earlier in my career. In the beginning, I routinely commanded patients to get a cleaning before any fillings could be done. My intention was to "do the right thing" and to maintain the standard of care instilled in me during school. Over time, I have found that patients are much more likely to follow my guidance when I don't tell them what to do but rather honor their **power** by *sharing recommendations and suggestions* and *explaining why.* Now I say to patients, "I recommend a cleaning first, so I can provide better quality fillings for

TABLE 3.5	**Summary of Affirming Power During Different Phases of Care**		
ISLEEP Skill	**HANDS OFF** **Consult/tx Plan**	**HANDS OFF** **Treatment Visit:** **Preop and Postop**	**HANDS ON** **Procedures and Clinical Exams**
P. *Power of the patient*	Ask permission to give info Pt chooses tx based on their preferences, needs, and values *NOTE: Recommendations and suggestions (not commands)*	Agree on a stop signal (esp. for pain or anxiety)	• Ask permission • Make requests • Offer options (esp. when uncomfortable)

you." The following 10-second video clip (Video 3.25) demonstrates affirming the **power of the patient** after an intraoral examination.

Of course, there are times when a patient's unwillingness to do or not do a test or procedure might preclude an HCP's ability to care for them. How does the HCP respectfully encourage a patient to do unwanted but necessary tests or procedures? How does the HCP set limits respectfully when a patient requests testing or treatment that is unethical? The next chapter explores how to apply ISLEEP skills and mindfulness to these and other common clinical challenges.

Table 3.5 summarizes the skill of affirming patient power in the different phases of care.

> Note: Appendices D, E, and F provide sample language for POWER, including the consultation (Appendix D), before and after procedures (Appendix E), and hands-on mode (Appendix F).

Table 3.6 contrasts the language of affirming power with the opposite, both hands on and hands off.

Pairs Experiment in Explain and Power:
Think of procedures and tasks that you regularly provide to patients that you can simulate with a partner. Let's explore the difference between doing a procedure TO the patient versus FOR the patient.

One person plays the role of the patient, and the other plays the provider. The HCP simulates performing these procedures in two different ways.

1. No explanation is given, and the patient is powerless: tasks are done TO patients (without asking permission), patients are commanded to do tasks (without making requests), and no options are given (such as the option to take a break).
2. Now try performing a procedure demonstrating the ISLEEP skills *explain* (what you will do, why, and what the patient will feel) and affirm *power* (make requests, ask permission, give options).

Switch roles. Compare and contrast the two experiences.

(If time is limited, skip over the skills introduce/interconnect, solicit, listen, and empathize. Otherwise, you can practice these skills as well.)

TABLE 3.6	**Contrasting Language of Affirming Power Versus No Power**	
	Hands Off	**Hands On**

No power	Commands:
	   "You have to…"
		Demands
		   "Open wide."

Affirming power	Recommendations:
	   "I suggest…"
		Making requests:
		   "Could you open wide?"

Reflection Questions
Although the ISLEEP skills are tightly intertwined and overlapping, the differentiation of the six skill categories allows for identification of an HCP's strengths and weaknesses and allows for growth and development in these areas.

1. Which ISLEEP skills are you best at?
2. Which skills would you like to improve on and how?

TABLE 3.7   **Summary Chart of ISLEEP in Different Modes of Health Care**

ISLEEP Skill	HANDS OFF Consultation	HANDS OFF Treatment Visit: *Preop and Postop*	HANDS ON Clinical Exam and Procedure
I. *Introduce/ Interconnect*	(See Table 3.1)	(See Table 3.1)	Continue interconnecting during procedure breaks (i.e., waiting for anesthesia)
S. *Solicit*	• Chief complaint • Symptoms • Concerns/fears • Needs, wants, values • Beliefs about condition/tx options • Experience of the condition/tx • Questions	Preop: • Questions • Fears/concerns • Requests for comfort measures Postop: • Questions • Feedback on experience	Comfort level (physical and emotional) Details about discomfort
L. *Listen*	(See Table 3.1)	(See Table 3.1)	Tuning in to nonverbal cues about discomfort, pain, anxiety
E. *Empathize/ Validate*	(See Table 3.1)	(See Table 3.1)	(When patient expresses discomfort)
E. *Explain/ Reassure*	• Treatment options • Risks/benefit • Use visuals • Check understanding of info *NOTE: Avoid overly technical information about procedures (unless requested)*	Preop: • Review procedure and rationale • Review risks and benefits • How will address the fears • What patient can do to alleviate pain and anxiety Postop: • What to expect and how to cope • After-hours support	EXAM: what looking for (i.e., decay, defective restorations) EXAM and PROCEDURES: What sensations will be felt (especially if uncomfortable) What the patient can do to help with pain and anxiety • Breathing techniques • Mindfulness • Distraction
P. *Power* of the patient	Patient chooses tx based on their preferences, needs, and values *NOTE: Recommendations and suggestions (not commands)*	Agree on a stop signal (esp. for pain or anxiety)	• Ask permission • Make requests • Give options • Gradual exposure

Table 3.7 summarizes all of the ISLEEP skills in each phase of care and can also be found in Appendix H.

A final note about ISLEEP: The boundaries between the six different ISLEEP skills are not always well-defined. For example, an HCP might affirm a patient's *power* by asking them questions (*solicit*), such as "Are you ready to decide" or "Do you want more time?"[70] They might interconnect by soliciting personal information like, "How is your family?" They might explain options as a way to affirm a patient's power. Table 3.8 highlights some interrelationships between the six skills. One relationship which is not captured by the table is what I call the "triple crown"—*soliciting* permission to *explain* information as a way to affirm *power*. Clearly the skills are highly intertwined!

TABLE 3.8 Interrelationship Between ISLEEP Skills

Skill	Introduce/ Interconnect	Solicit	Listen	Empathize	Explain	Power
Introduce/ Interconnect	_____	Solicit information about the person				
Solicit		_____				
Listen			_____			
Empathize				_____		
Explain		Solicit what patient already knows (before explaining) and what they understood (after explaining)			_____	
Power	Getting acquainted with the person affirms their presence as a human, not just a body or a tooth problem	Solicit preferences And readiness to proceed with decisions or during procedure	Listen to affirm power	Empathize to affirm power	Explain options to affirm power during consultation and procedures	_____

REFERENCES

1. Cocksedge S, George B, Renwick S, et al. Touch in primary care consultations: qualitative investigation of doctors' and patients' perceptions. *Br J Gen Pract*. 2013;63:e283–e290.
2. Orsini CA, Jerez OM. Establishing a good dentist-patient relationship: skills defined from the dental faculty perspective. *J Dent Educ*. 2014;78:1405–1415.
3. Huntington B, Kuhn N. Communication gaffes: a root cause of malpractice claims. *Proc (Bayl Univ Med Cent)*. 2003;16:157–161.
4. Curtin S, McConnell M. Teaching dental students how to deliver bad news: S-P-I-K-E-S model. *J Dent Educ*. 2012;76:360–365.
5. McKenzie CT. Instructor and dental student perceptions of clinical communication skills via structured assessments. *J Dent Educ*. 2016;80:563–568.
6. Wener ME, Schönwetter DJ, Mazurat N. Developing new dental communication skills assessment tools by including patients and other stakeholders. *J Dent Educ*. 2011;75:1527–1541.
7. Ayn C, Robinson L, Nason A, et al. Determining recommendations for improvement of communication skills training in dental education: a scoping review. *J Dent Educ*. 2017;81:479–488.
8. Lanning SK, Ranson SL, Willett RM. Communication skills instruction utilizing interdisciplinary peer teachers:

program development and student perceptions. *J Dent Educ*. 2008;72:172–182.
9. Miller GE. The assessment of clinical skills/competence/performance. *Acad Med*. 1990;65:S63–S67.
10. Omar H, Khan SA, Toh CG. Structured student-generated videos for first-year students at a dental school in Malaysia. *J Dent Educ*. 2013;77:640–764.
11. Quinn S, Herron D, Menzies R, et al. The Video Interaction Guidance approach applied to teaching communication skills in dentistry. *Eur J Dent Educ*. 2016;20:94–101.
12. Stamenkovic DM, Rancic NK, Latas MB, et al. Preoperative anxiety and implications on postoperative recovery: what can we do to change our history. *Minerva Anestesiol*. 2018;84:1307–1317.
13. Carnegie D. *How to Win Friends and Influence People*. New York: Pocket Books; 1936.
14. Ayer WA. *Psychology and Dentistry: Mental Health Aspects of Patient Care*. New York: Haworth Press; 2005.
15. Diering SL. *Love Your Patients! Improving Patient Satisfaction With Essential Behaviors That Enrich the Lives of Patients and Professionals*. Nevada City: Blue Dolphin; 2004.
16. Mercer SW, Maxwell M, Heaney D, et al. The consultation and relational empathy (CARE) measure: development and preliminary validation and reliability of an empathy-based consultation process measure. *Fam Pract*. 2004;21:699–705.

17. Babar MG, Hasan SS, Yong WM, et al. Patients' perceptions of dental students' empathic, person-centered care in a dental school clinic in Malaysia. *J Dent Educ.* 2017; 81:404–412.

18. D'Arro C. Mindful dentist. *Int J Whole Person Care.* 2018;5:29–37.

19. Tweedy D. *Black Man in a White Coat.* New York: Picador; 2015.

20. Langewitz W, Denz M, Keller A, et al. Spontaneous talking time at start of consultation in outpatient clinic: cohort study. *BMJ.* 2002;325:682–683.

21. Marvel MK, Epstein RM, Flowers K, et al. Soliciting the patient's agenda: have we improved? *JAMA.* 1999;281:283–287.

22. Leebov W, Rotering C. *The Language of Caring Guide for Physicians: Communication Essentials for Patient-Centered Care.* 2nd ed. USA: Language of Caring LLC; 2014.

23. Virshup BB, Oppenberg AA, Coleman MM. Strategic risk management: reducing malpractice claims through more effective patient-doctor communication. *Am J Med Qual.* 1999;14:153–159.

24. Frankel RM. Emotion and the physician-patient relationship. *Motiv Emot.* 1995;19:163–173.

25. Dailey YM, Humphris GM, Lennon MA. Reducing patients' state anxiety in general dental practice: a randomized controlled trial. *J Dent Res.* 2002;81:319–322.

26. Appukuttan DP. Strategies to manage patients with dental anxiety and dental phobia: literature review. *Clin Cosmet Investig Dent.* 2016;8:35–50.

27. Heaton LJ, Carlson CR, Smith TA, et al. Predicting anxiety during dental treatment using patients' self-reports: less is more. *J Am Dent Assoc.* 2007;138:188–195.

28. Newton T, Asimakopoulou K, Daly B, et al. The management of dental anxiety: time for a sense of proportion? *Br Dent J.* 2012;213:271–274.

29. Hornung CA, Massagli M. Primary-care physicians' affective orientation toward their patients. *J Health Soc Behav.* 1979;20:61–76.

30. Riley JL III, Gordan VV, Hudak-Boss SE, et al. Concordance between patient satisfaction and the dentist's view: findings from The National Dental Practice-Based Research Network. *J Am Dent Assoc.* 2014;145:355–362.

31. Levinson W, Gorawara-Bhat R, Lamb J. A study of patient clues and physician responses in primary care and surgical settings. *JAMA.* 2000;284:1021–1027.

32. Mostofsky DI, Fortune F. *Behavioral Dentistry.* Ames: Wiley Blackwell; 2014.

33. Orsini CA, Jerez OM. Establishing a good dentist-patient relationship: skills defined from the dental faculty perspective. *J Dent Educ.* 2014;78:1405–1415.

34. Milgrom P, Weinstein P, Heaton LJ. *Treating Fearful Dental Patients: A Patient Management Handbook.* 3rd ed. Seattle: Dental Behavioral Resources; 2009.

35. Schuster PM. *Communication: The Key to the Therapeutic Relationship.* Philadelphia: F.A. Davis; 2000.

36. Awdish R. *Shock: My Journey from Death to Recovery and the Redemptive Power of Hope.* New York: St. Martin's Press; 2017.

37. Raja S, Shah R, Hamad J, et al. Patients' perceptions of dehumanization in dental school settings: implications for clinic management and curriculum planning. *J Dent Educ.* 2015;79:1201–1207.

38. King D. Anxiety control. In: Daniel S, Harfst S, eds. *Dental Hygiene; Concepts; Cases, Competencies.* St. Louis: Mosby; 2002:576–584.

39. Krupat E, Frankel R, Stein T, et al. The Four Habits Coding Scheme: validation of an instrument to assess clinicians' communication behavior. *Patient Educ Couns.* 2006;62:38–45.

40. Stein T, Krupat E, Frankel RM. *Talking with Patients Using the Four Habits Model.* Kaiser Permanente; 2010 [Online]. Available at: http://www.careinnovations.org/wp-content/uploads/2016/03/four-habits-monograph_new-agenda.pdf. Accessed May 5, 2020.

41. Suchman AL, Markakis K, Beckman HB, et al. A model of empathic communication in the medical interview. *JAMA.* 1997;277:678–682.

42. Schwartz B, Bohay R. Can patients help teach professionalism and empathy to dental students? Adding patient videos to a lecture course. *J Dent Educ.* 2012;76:174–184.

43. Covey SR. *The 7 Habits of Highly Effective People: Powerful Lessons in Personal Change.* New York: Free Press; 2004.

44. *Quote by Rumi: "The Quieter You Become, The More You Are Able To Hear"* [Online] Available at: https://www.goodreads.com/quotes/6822193-the-quieter-you-become-the-more-you-are-able-to.

45. Peck MS. *The Road Less Traveled: A New Psychology of Love, Traditional Values, and Spiritual Growth.* New York: Simon and Schuster; 1978.

46. Haidet P. Jazz and the "art" of medicine: improvisation in the medical encounter. *Ann Fam Med.* 2007;5: 164–169.

47. Carroll M. *Awake at Work: 35 Practical Buddhist Principles for Discovering Clarity and Balance in the Midst of Work's Chaos.* Boston: Shambhala; 2006.

48. Riess H, Kraft-Todd G. E.M.P.A.T.H.Y.: a tool to enhance nonverbal communication between clinicians and their patients. *Acad Med.* 2014;89:1108–1112.

49. Riess H. *The Power of Empathy: Helen Riess at TEDxMiddlebury—YouTube.* TEDx TALKS; 2013 [Online]. Available at: https://www.youtube.com/watch?v=baHrcC8B4WM. Accessed May 5, 2021.

50. Riess H, Kelley JM, Bailey RW, et al. Empathy training for resident physicians: a randomized controlled trial of

a neuroscience-informed curriculum. *J Gen Intern Med.* 2012;27:1280–1286.

51. Morse DS, Edwardsen EA, Gordon HS. Missed opportunities for interval empathy in lung cancer communication. *Arch Intern Med.* 2008;168:1853–1858.

52. Torper J, Ansteinsson V, Lundeby T. Moving the four habits model into dentistry. Development of a dental consultation model: do dentists need an additional habit? *Eur J Dent Educ.* 2019;23:220–229.

53. Yarascavitch C, Regehr G, Hodges B, et al. Changes in dental student empathy during training. *J Dent Educ.* 2009;73:509–517.

54. Birnie KA, Chambers CT, Taddio A, et al., HELP in Kids & Adults Team. Psychological interventions for vaccine injections in children and adolescents: systematic review of randomized and quasi-randomized controlled trials. *Clin J Pain.* 2015;31:S72–S89.

55. Sinclair S, Beamer K, Hack TF, et al. Sympathy, empathy, and compassion: a grounded theory study of palliative care patients' understandings, experiences, and preferences. *Palliat Med.* 2017;31:437–447.

56. Hirsch EM. The role of empathy in medicine: a medical student's perspective. *Virtual Mentor.* 2007;9:423–427.

57. Haslam N. Humanizing medical practice: the role of empathy. *Med J Aust.* 2007;187:381–382.

58. Dohrenwend AM. Defining empathy to better teach, measure, and understand its impact. *Acad Med.* 2018; 93:1754–1756.

59. Branch WT, Malik TK. Using "windows of opportunities" in brief interviews to understand patients' concerns. *JAMA.* 1993;269:1667–1668.

60. Halpern J. What is clinical empathy? *J Gen Intern Med.* 2003;18:670–674.

61. Luberto CM, Shinday N, Song R, et al. A systematic review and meta-analysis of the effects of meditation on empathy, compassion, and prosocial behaviors. *Mindfulness (N Y).* 2018;9:708–724.

62. Markakis K, Frankel R, Beckman H, et al. Teaching empathy: it can be done. Working paper presented at the Annual Meeting of the Society of General Internal Medicine, San Francisco, CA, April 29–May1, 1999.

63. Vergnes JN, Apelian N, Bedos C. What about narrative dentistry? *J Am Dent Assoc.* 2015;146:398–401.

64. Gallese V, Fadiga L, Fogassi L, et al. Action recognition in the premotor cortex. *Brain.* 1996;119:593–609.

65. Häusser LF. Empathy and mirror neurons. A view on contemporary neuropsychological empathy research. *Prax Kinderpsychol Kinderpsychiatr.* 2012;61:322–335.

66. Haque OS, Waytz A. Dehumanization in medicine: causes, solutions, and functions. *Perspect Psychol Sci.* 2012;7:176–186.

67. Hickson GB, Federspiel CF, Pichert JW, et al. Patient complaints and malpractice risk. *JAMA.* 2002;287: 2951–2957.

68. Czarnecki ML, Turner HN, Collins PM, et al. Procedural pain management: a position statement with clinical practice recommendations. *Pain Manag Nurs.* 2011;12:95–111.

69. Schönwetter DJ, Wener ME, Mazurat N. Determining the validity and reliability of clinical communication assessment tools for dental patients and students. *J Dent Educ.* 2012;76:1276–1290.

70. Elwyn G, Frosch D, Thomson R, et al. Shared decision making: a model for clinical practice. *J Gen Intern Med.* 2012;27:1361–1367.

71. Studer Group. *AIDET Patient Communication.* Available at: https://www.studergroup.com/aidet.

72. *"Becoming a Culturally Competent Health Care Organization."* American Hospital Association; 2021 [Online]. Available at: https://www.aha.org/ahahret-guides/2013-06-18-becoming-culturally-competent-health-care-organization. Accessed September 10, 2021.

73. *"A Cute Gingivitis Postcard."* Garfield Paws [Online]. Available at: https://www.smartpractice.com/Apps/WebObjects/SmartPractice.woa/wa/style?id=SQPC1991&cid=506779&m=SPD. Accessed May 7, 2020.

74. Singh H, Meshram G, Warhadpande M, et al. Effect of "Perceived control" in management of anxious patients undergoing endodontic therapy by use of an electronic communication system. *J Conserv Dent.* 2012;15:51–55.

75. Corless L, Buckley A, Mee S. Power inequality between patients and nurses. *Nurs Times.* 2016;112:20–21.

76. *"What does consent mean in clinical practice?"* Nursing Times; 2013 [Online]. Available at: https://www.nursing-times.net/clinical-archive/patient-safety/what-does-consent-mean-in-clinical-practice-01-11-2013/. Accessed September 14, 2021.

77. Riley JL III, Gordan VV, Rindal DB, et al., Dental Practice-Based Research Network Collaborative Group. Components of patient satisfaction with a dental restorative visit: results from the Dental Practice-Based Research Network. *J Am Dent Assoc.* 2012;143:1002–1010.

78. Corah NL, O'Shea RM, Bissell GD, et al. The dentist-patient relationship: perceived dentist behaviors that reduce patient anxiety and increase satisfaction. *J Am Dent Assoc.* 1988;116:73–76.

79. Adler T. What is a nurse's role in pain management? *Nurse Choice.* 2019;2 [Online]. Available at: https://www.nursechoice.com/blog/profiles-and-features/what-is-a-nurses-role-in-patient-pain-management/. Accessed September 14, 2021.

80. Stevens PE Lesbians' health-related experiences of care and noncare. *West J Nurs Res.* 1994;16:639–659.

4

Applying Mindfulness and ISLEEP Skills to Clinical Challenges

Most health care professionals (HCPs) enter the field with the intention to alleviate suffering and to help others. Those who enter the field for fast money will quickly realize there are much easier ways to earn a living! The life of the HCP is full of challenges. In an ideal world, patients accept and adhere to recommendations and are satisfied with their care. In an ideal world, medical and dental procedures are successful. Yet, the road is rarely straight. HCPs encounter procedures that deviate from the textbook, patients who refuse necessary procedures, and patients who are dissatisfied with their care.

During such clinical challenges, there are two people who need attention and care: the patient and the HCP. Chapter 2 equipped us with practices for cultivating EASE: equanimity, attentiveness, self-awareness, and empathy. Chapter 3 described the fundamental communication skills—ISLEEP—needed for patient-centered care. In this chapter, we have the chance to integrate and apply all these skills (and some new ones) to real-life clinical challenges for our own and our patients' well-being. Just like it is important to put the oxygen mask on yourself before you help others in an airplane, it is also important to know how to manage your own challenges in order to be able to escort patients through theirs. Soon, we will cover several common health care challenges, but first, prepare yourself for a little self-help talk tailored to the HCP. This chapter will equip you with time-tested, evidence-based tools that will empower you to navigate clinical challenges at work with steadiness and confidence.

CARING FOR THE CAREGIVER IN CHALLENGING CLINICAL SITUATIONS

Clinical challenges can arouse a range of difficult emotions, such as anxiety, frustration, and anger for both patients and HCPs. Mindfulness can be very helpful in these situations, as the following true story illustrates.

A review of my schedule triggered a sudden wave of panic:

Sarah White: Bridge Delivery, Teeth #13–15

A cascade of images and thoughts come tumbling down—I flash back to Sarah enduring weeks of dental work complicated by her small mouth and gag reflex. I worry about Sarah's upcoming vacation and her expectation that her bridge will be done before she leaves tomorrow. If the new bridge does not fit, Sarah will be disappointed and maybe even angry at me.

The time comes to try on the new bridge. First, we remove the temporary bridge, clean the abutments (supporting teeth), then try on the new, permanent bridge. The color looks great. The contact with neighboring teeth, fine. Oh no—my worst fear. The margin is open on #13. Maybe it's not going down all the way? Or worse yet, maybe it is defective and must be remade! I apply pressure with my fingers and check again. Still open. I catch myself not breathing, cueing me to my panic. "Sarah, could you please excuse me while I check on something for a moment? Thank you!" I make eye contact with my assistant, who nods with understanding.

As I step into the neighboring treatment room, I intentionally connect with my breath. Tuning into my body, I notice my neck braced and my chest constricted. I stay with the sensations for just few seconds, allowing them to be there, without trying to change them or make them go away. Within just a couple breaths I start to feel calmer. Thoughts come into my awareness like bubbles surfacing in a pond, "It's not going to fit, she will be angry, I am a bad dentist." I continue to breathe, holding on to the breath as an anchor. I feel a release in the tension in my neck.

Suddenly, an idea spontaneously arises. I remember a similar situation in my first job for which my employer/mentor had taught me a remedy. (Have the patient bite down on a soft wooden stick on the bridge for a few minutes.) I returned to Sarah to try this technique. Problem solved! We completed the procedure just in time for her vacation. I was relieved, and Sarah was pleased and grateful.

In this true story, mindfulness helped me to regain calm and focus after being triggered into panic during a clinical challenge. Even more, by regaining a calm state, I was able to find a solution to the problem. To better understand how mindfulness works, it is important to understand what triggers stress.

The Real Source of Stress (Not What You Think) and How Mindfulness Helps

It is a common belief that stress is caused entirely by the events and conditions of our lives. For the HCP, the event might be something like a failed medical procedure or a dissatisfied patient. Prepare yourself for a radical statement: the events and conditions of our lives are not the main source of our stress. If certain events were inherently stressful, then they would arouse the same negative reaction for everyone. To illustrate this point, consider the example of two people waiting for the bus, which is running late. One person becomes angry while the other is delighted (they are reconnecting with an old friend they just encountered). If the delayed bus were the direct cause of the angry passenger's stress, then both passengers should be equally upset. So, what made the delay stressful for the angry passenger yet pleasant for the other?

What triggers negative stress more than events and conditions are our thoughts *about* the events and conditions. The term "thoughts" includes thoughts of the future ("Now that the bus is late, I will be late for work, and my day will be ruined"), thoughts of the past ("I should have taken the earlier bus"), and expectations/beliefs

("Buses should never be late"). In the mindfulness tradition, there is a teaching about two arrows—the first arrow represents the actual event or condition we are experiencing, and the second arrow represents our thoughts *about* the events.[1,2] Meditation teacher and author Sharon Salzberg calls the second arrow our "add-ons."[3] For example, when there is a pain in the knee, the pain is the first arrow. This is often followed by the add-ons of future thoughts ("Oh no, I'm going to need surgery!" or "I'll never be able to run again!") or past thoughts ("I shouldn't have run so much.") or judgments (It's my fault I have this pain."). While we can't avoid the first arrow, there is a way to avoid the stress of the second arrows— the add-ons—which make the pain and the stress worse.

> **Note:** In Chapter 5, we will discuss the influence of thoughts on pain and anxiety and ways to support patients during procedures with mindfulness practices and other techniques.

One common approach to the add-ons is trying to get rid of them. Unfortunately, this doesn't usually help. To illustrate, Dr. Craig Hassad, physician and mindfulness educator, invited us in a seminar to try the following experiment.

> **Experiment:**
> Notice a sound in the environment. Now try to make it go away. Notice what happens.

Most people find that not only is it impossible for them to stop noticing the sound, but also that the more you try, the more noticeable and annoying the sound becomes. Similarly, trying to get rid of or to fight against our thoughts, beliefs, and expectations about the events and conditions of our lives only makes it worse. In the words of Swiss psychiatrist Carl Jung, "What you resist not only persists, but will *grow* in size."[4] So how do we let go of the add-ons that trigger stress?

Mindfulness Practice: Exercising the Letting Go Muscle

Mindfulness offers a way out of stress reactivity by helping us notice and let go of all the add-ons. The Chinese philosopher Lao Tsu captures the essence of mindfulness in his quote, "If you are depressed you are living in the past. If you are anxious you are living in the future. If you are at peace you are living in the present."[5] Regular, formal mindfulness practice makes it possible to remember to come back to the present instead of spinning in a vortex of thoughts, beliefs, and expectations about the future and the past. The default mode of the mind, however, involves constantly looking for threats to our safety and happiness. This functions to keep us safe, but it also provides an abundance of second arrows and stress. According to the teaching of the two arrows, we can let go of the second arrows and the stress they generate by *noticing* and *allowing* the **first** arrow—what's present right now, especially in the **body**. This is the essence of mindfulness, and it can be practiced both formally and informally.

Mindfulness "on the cushion": formal practice. Recall the three basic instructions for awareness of the breath meditation from Chapter 2: find a good seat, focus on the breath, notice when the mind has wandered, and return to the breath.

This simple (but not easy!), formal mindfulness practice trains the mind to avoid stress in two main ways. First, as we try to focus on the breath (or another real-time anchor such as body sensations or sounds), we learn to notice when the mind is lost in the add-ons—the thoughts *about* the events that can trigger stress. A thought is simply a mental event which may or may not be true. Recognizing a thought as just a thought is already a huge step, because normally many triggering thoughts fly under the radar, rendering us like a puppet on a string, reacting unconsciously. So just by *noticing* thoughts, we are already short-circuiting the default mode that causes stress.

Further, each time we notice the mind has wandered into thoughts and we choose to return to the breath, we are doing what Sharon Salzberg calls "exercising the letting go muscle."[6] With practice, the ability to notice and let go of thoughts, false beliefs, and expectations increases as does our resilience during challenging times. Some of my teachers have described the effect of mindfulness as "increasing the gap between the itch and the scratch." Over time, like a trickling stream creates a deep rock canyon, mindfulness practice can penetrate even the most solid, deep-rooted thoughts.

> **Note:** Not all add-ons are useless mental events to be set aside. For example, if you smell smoke while meditating and the thought arises, "My house is on fire," that may be an important thought to act on! If you have an urgent thought like, "I must remember to tell the patient about that treatment option," that can be earmarked mentally or even jotted down during meditation to act on later. Mindfulness helps us regain the

power to choose which thoughts to put aside and which to act on.

Mindfulness "off the cushion": informal practices. Mindfulness can help calm and focus us in the heat of a clinical challenge, and this effect increases the more you practice "on the cushion." When you are in the heat of the moment, try to come back to a neutral, grounding, present-moment anchor—either the breath sensations, body sensations (contact of feet with floor, hands), or sounds. In the previous story of my patient Sarah, I used my breath sensations as an anchor to the present. Every storm has an eye of stillness and by connecting to the breath, we connect to that still place that is always available. The nature of the mind is that it can only attend to so much. So, by focusing on the present moment, we take away the focus on the add-ons—the thoughts of the future and the past that fuel stress reactivity—and by doing so, the power of the add-ons naturally deflates.

Once you steady yourself with the breath, you can expand your awareness to include any sensations in the body that are present. In the previous story, I noticed tightness in my chest and neck. Leaning into the uncomfortable body sensations in the moment, although it can be uncomfortable temporarily, further deflates the power of the triggering thoughts ("This procedure is taking me too long," or "The patient is going to hate me.") and by doing so, diminishes stress.

Interesting fact: while we can *think thoughts* in the past and future, we can only *feel sensations* in the present. This is why awareness of the real-time sensations of the *breath, body,* and *sound* is the gateway to the present and key to staying steady. Awareness of the present coupled with an attitude of acceptance is mindfulness. Mindfulness allows us to experience everything from "the wider container of awareness."[7] Just like a drop of color will dye a large container of water more than a small one, a stressful event will have less effect on a mind that is aware with an attitude of acceptance. The wider perspective of mindfulness allows us to "transform our solid emotional reactions into something more porous. It's not that they disappear (although they might) but that we hold them much more lightly."[7]

"Even this" meditation: exercising the letting go muscle. The language we use can help us let go of thoughts that trigger stress. Meditating with awareness of the breath and the words *"even this"* (Video 4.1) encourages letting go of even the most difficult thoughts

and emotions—two types in particular. First are the emotionally charged thoughts that consume and dominate, such as the ones that come from a dire medical diagnosis in yourself or a loved one: "Something terrible is going to happen, someone could die." The second type of sticky thoughts are the self-critical thoughts of the moment: the subtle, insidious, commentary thoughts like, "I can't do this practice," or "I don't like this meditation," or "I wish this meditation were shorter." For whatever thoughts or judgments you notice, say to yourself silently, "*Even this* thought I can set aside for just one breath." Each time you do this, you are exercising the letting go muscle, and, in time, it gets stronger!

Let's try. Start by settling into the sensations of the body as it contacts the floor or chair. Then allow the attention to rest increasingly on the breath. Once the mind has settled a bit, open the awareness and notice whatever arises in the mind and body. Whatever you find, silently say "*Even this,*" as in "*Even this,* I can let be for now. *Even this,* I can say hello to and set down."

As always, feel free to modify the practice in the way that feels right to you—the position of your body (sitting, standing, lying down), your eyes (open or closed), your choice of anchor (breath, body, sounds), and if ever you feel like you are getting out of your window of tolerance, stop the meditation and resume when you are ready.

At times, a thought or emotion or sensation won't let go and calls for attention. In these cases, letting go may first require giving the experience some closer attention and care. For these experiences, the next practice, called RAIN, can be very helpful.

Practice: RAIN. Let's revisit the mindfulness practice of RAIN (Fig. 4.1) from the end of Chapter 2 as a way of dealing with clinical challenges in the moment. This practice blends mindful awareness with self-compassion.

R: Recognize

Ask yourself: What's bothering me right now? It might be an emotion like anxiety, fear, frustration. It might be an uncomfortable sensation or pain in the body. If it's not clear, then simply acknowledge, "I'm having a hard time right now."

A: Allow

Give the experience of the moment space. Instead of resisting or trying to make it go away, welcome it in. You might say to yourself silently and gently, "Hello _____ (e.g., frustration, tension in head, etc.), I see you."

Recognize what is going on;

Allow the experience to be there, as it is;

Investigate with interest and care;

Nurture with self-compassion.

Fig. 4.1 A Mindfulness and Self-compassion. Practice: RAIN.

I: Investigate

At times, recognizing and allowing may be enough to settle and focus. You can also go on to investigating the different aspects of the experience in the moment, including the body sensations, thoughts, and beliefs. Meditation teacher Tara Brach recommends to "bring your primary attention to the *felt-sense in the body*" (emphasis added).[8] Tune in to the direct sensations in the body—the location, the intensity, the quality (sharp/dull, deep/superficial, temperature, etc.).

N: Nurture with Self-compassion

Offer yourself the words that you would say to your best friend or a child in this situation. Perhaps, "I know you're having a hard time; I'm here for you." Here are some suggestions from the Mindful Self-compassion Program: "If you wish, placing a hand over the part of your body that feels uncomfortable, and just feeling the *warmth* and gentle *touch* of your hand. Perhaps imagining warmth and kindness *flowing* through your hand into your body" (emphasis added).[9] Kind words and touch are offered to yourself not to change or fix anything (which might set up an expectation and make things worse) but simply to comfort and soothe.

The Language of Letting Go and Focusing Practice

We saw how thoughts trigger stress, and linguisticians know that the language we use shapes our thoughts. Language can either keep us stuck in stress-triggering thoughts, or it can facilitate awareness and letting go. When we are not mindful, the default mode is identification, and our language reflect this. Identification is associated with "I/me/mine" language such as "*I am* angry" or "My patient is making *me* angry." On the other hand, certain language can be very helpful to *let go* of identification and thereby unhook us from the grips of negative emotions.

For example, a hospital nurse has done everything in their power to satisfy a patient's excessive demands, but the patient still complains, repeatedly pressing the call button. In this case, the nurse might say to themselves, "I am so angry," which frames the experience as something they *are*, reinforcing identification and stress. Compare this to the language, "Anger *is here*" or "*Something in me* is angry." Most people sense more spaciousness in the latter two phrases. The anger is not all of what I am but rather just a passing experience —a part of me that I can observe from a wider perspective.

Linguistics expert and leading focusing teacher Ann Weiser Cornell explains, when we can say, "I'm sensing something in me is angry," it allows the anger to "get a hearing, have some company, be able to make steps. Because someone is there, the 'I' keeping it company."[10] In other words, there is a mindful awareness. The words "I'm sensing something in me is angry (or whatever negative emotion)" also allows room for something else to be acknowledged, perhaps something in me that is opposed to the anger (such as guilt about the anger); many times, this is key to getting unhooked—allowing all parts to be heard and understood.

There is a powerful psychotherapeutic technique called *Focusing* that facilitates letting go of negative emotions. Focusing features two elements "the language of presence" coupled with awareness of the body sensations or the "felt-sense." Cornell shares several ways to use language to promote presence. For example, instead of "I am sad," she recommends the following possibilities: "Part of me is sad," "I have sadness," "Something in me is sad," "There is a sad place in me."[10] In her words, "The language of Presence…although it takes more words to say gives the Focuser support in finding a solid place to stand in relation to what they're feeling and a way to *be with* rather than *be in* their inner experiencing."[10] In addition to language, mindfulness of the body is key to Focusing practice. Detailed attention to the body sensations allows the sensations and their associated emotions to bloom and fade naturally without having to fix, analyze, or push anything away.

I had a first-hand experience of the benefits of Focusing—using language of presence and attending to the felt-sense in the body—in the final weeks before submitting the draft of this book to the publisher.

After years of researching and writing and rewriting and videotaping and editing and re-editing, I was just weeks away from the deadline for this book, and I started to get headaches—sharp, squeezing pain distracting me from writing. I pushed through for a few weeks until I hit a wall of exhaustion. I just couldn't do any more, and I was so worried I would miss the deadline and the chance to share with you the tools in this book. Then, I tried Focusing. Lying in bed in the morning after a good night's sleep, I grounded in my body, feeling the sensations of contacting the pillow and the mattress and my breathing. I tuned into a pressure in my upper chest and the thought, "I'm sick and tired of this book, I can't take it anymore, I am burned-out." Then I tried to reframe it in the language of letting go: "Something in me is feeling tired and burned-out and doesn't want to write anymore." As soon as I had turned to this part, suddenly another sensation emerged calling for attention, this one in my forehead—another part of me, a scared part… "Something in me is scared of the part that's burned out, because it believes if I don't keep going, I will miss the deadline." It was as if the scared part didn't want me to get sidetracked attending to the burned-out part! Feeling into the forehead and naming it silently, "scared squeezing."

Now that both conflicting parts of me had been acknowledged, I focused on the stronger one—the part that was scared. My forehead started tightening even more, and I realized it was the start of a good cry. I let the tears flow and stayed with it, feeling the pain. After just a few moments, it eased and then let go. Soon, I was sitting at my computer happily writing to you again, just a little tired but no more headache and at peace.

By simply tuning into the sensations in my body, I discovered the second arrow—the scared part of me that was making the fatigue so much worse. By using the language of letting go, I unhooked from the perception that the emotion was who I am and instead could see the "something in me," something I can keep company and that will pass, as everything eventually does. Even more, the language of letting go helps define who "I" am as a "compassionate witness…the one who can turn towards anything."[10] I realized the headache was a call for attention all along. There was no need for analysis. There was no need for medication. Once I could bear witness to it, see it fully so it could feel understood, it served its purpose and let me go.

While practices like "even this" meditation, RAIN, and Focusing are very helpful in loosening the grip of many thoughts that generate stress, certain thoughts are particularly challenging for many HCPs to let go of and call for something more. Let's look at these more closely and some approaches that can help.

The Role of Expectations and Self-criticism in Generating Stress

> **Reflection:**
> 1. *When was the last time you said to yourself, "Today, I did enough," or "I did a good job?"*
> 2. *When you feel you have not done enough or not done a good job, ask yourself "What would be enough? What would be a good job?"*

Several times when I have felt disappointed with myself and asked myself what would be enough, I arrive at an expectation that is humanly impossible. For example, when I had to do a dental filling on a restless special needs patient and was disappointed for taking so long, I realized I was expecting myself to do all fillings quickly and perfectly no matter what the circumstances.

Expectations are a particularly sticky kind of thoughts—expectations about the way things should be, the way others should be, and (the stickiest of all) what I, myself, should be and should do. Expectations are often accompanied by the word "should." If your car doesn't start one morning and you become angry, this reflects an expectation that your car *should* start every day. If you are burned out and disappointed with your less-than-stellar patient care, this might reveal an expectation that you *should* perform perfectly all the time. Author and lecturer Brené Brown states, "Disappointment is unmet expectations, and the more significant the expectations, the more significant the disappointment."[11]

HCPs are known to be high achievers with high expectations of themselves; these set up the HCP for disappointment. Researchers have noted that dentistry "tends to attract people who often have unrealistic expectations and unnecessarily high standards of performance,"[12] and similar trends have been noted among medical professionals,[13] as the following true story captures:

My colleague, Dr. G, is a mother of five; the owner of a private dental practice employing about ten employees; and a high-quality, high-tech, compassionate dentist. If that weren't enough, she manages and offers dental care at a non-profit dental clinic that she founded, which is dedicated to special needs patients. The Covid-19 pandemic turned both of her dental practices upside-down as she and all HCPs scrambled to find ways to keep themselves and everyone safe at work. During the height of the pandemic, more than once she confided in me something that she felt bad about. She told me she has been struggling with feeling "grumpy" with others lately.

It saddened me that despite how hard she was working and the incredible stress she was shouldering that she—like so many other HCPs—would still expect herself to be unruffled, pleasant, perfect.

Exercise:
1. Recall a time when someone you cared about was struggling with a failure or a mistake they had made and how you responded to them. Write down the words you shared, and describe your tone of voice.
2. Now, recall a time when you were struggling with a failure or a bad outcome at school or at work. Write down how you treated yourself.
3. Notice any differences between your approach to your friend and to yourself.

Admittedly, high expectations are necessary to gain admission to a professional training program, survive the rigors of training, and cope with the challenges of the health care profession. Unfortunately, excessively high expectations can be problematic both on and off the meditation cushion.

One of the consequences of extremely high or unrealistic expectations is that when they are not met, they can result in harsh self-criticism. While self-criticism can motivate one to work hard, achieve a lot, and avoid mistakes, it is also very corrosive. (A colleague of mine calls self-criticism "dirty fuel" because it keeps us going short term but damages us long term and is therefore unsustainable.) Christopher Germer and Kristin Neff, leading researchers and teachers of mindful self-compassion, describe self-criticism as "the stress response turned inward," explaining, "Since we are both the attacker and the attacked when we are being self-critical, the sympathetic nervous system can become especially strongly activated."[9] Harsh self-criticism is not only stressful but also a threat to mental health. Paul Gilbert,

British clinical psychologist and founder of compassion focused therapy, found, "The self-persecuting function of self-criticism was especially linked to self-harm, depression, and anxiety."[14]

Caring for the Inner Critic

The experience of self-criticism is marked by two features that make it particularly impenetrable and entrapping. First, while most emotions are accompanied by sensations in the body—something you can literally feel, like butterflies in the stomach (anxiety) or heaviness in the chest (sadness)—inner criticism usually shows up as just a voice, and it feels like THE VOICE OF TRUTH. Lacking a felt sense in the body, the experience of self-criticism is much harder to notice and therefore much harder to let go of.

The trickiest part of self-criticism is that it is an expression of an emotion disguised as another—what feels like something big, authoritative, and scary is scared itself; what looks like an accusation is a veiled fear. This has been the universal finding of Ann Weiser Cornell while working with people worldwide over the past several decades. She likens the inner critic to a nervous mother. When your mom says, "You're going to die of pneumonia!" as you run outside in the winter with no coat on, what she means is, "I'm *afraid* you will catch a cold. I *want* you to be healthy." Like the nervous mom, the part of us that criticizes is voicing the very thing it fears will happen. The inner critic is a part of you that wants to protect, but it can't do anything except try to control you by giving orders. So, when something in me was saying, "You're so screwed. You're going to miss your book deadline," it was trying to say, "I'm *afraid* you're going to miss your deadline!"

The knowledge that there is a fear underlying the inner critic makes it possible to find a way out of its clutches by simply using the skills you already have—the language of letting go and the ISLEEP skills. First, the language of Presence helps to disidentify, to get some space around the part of you that is criticizing while you remain the mindful presence of it all. For example, I can shift my language from, "I am such a loser dentist," to, "*I'm sensing something in me that says* I am such a loser dentist." (The italicized words are from Ann Weiser Cornell).[10] This language reframes "me" as the Presence that can "turn toward the criticizing part, and toward any other part, with interested curiosity."[10]

Now, that there is a presence that can *be with* the inner critic (instead of *being in* the criticism), we can relate to it as we would a friend who is afraid of something. It may take a little imagination and suspension of disbelief. Start by saying hello to the part that is criticizing, ask how it's feeling, listen to what it fears, offer it empathy, all while honoring its power, respecting its boundaries, and moving at its pace. Does this sound familiar? Introduce, solicit, listen, empathize, power—the ISLEEP skills—are all that is needed to relate to this scared part of ourselves— the inner critic!

This part that is disguised as something powerful, big, authoritarian, and scary just wants your attention; that's all. And, once it feels heard and understood, it lets us go. Ann Weiser Cornell has taught this approach—Inner Relationship Focusing—all over the globe for decades, and we can frame her instructions (in Table 4.1) with the ISLEEP skills to help us remember.

Once we can separate from the part of us that is criticizing and give it the space and attention it needs to feel safe, it will reveal its fears. According to Cornell, this type of listening calls for a willingness to stay "at the edge of not-yet-knowing" to listen for the answers to emerge. While the criticizing part "doesn't like to admit that it's afraid," often it is "willing to admit that it is worried or concerned."[10] And once the fears are known and held in kind awareness, they relax, transform, release. This is the magic of Presence.

Knowledge of what the inner critic does *not want* (what is feared) easily gives rise to what is *wanted*, which is even more helpful. Focusing on what is wanted is less stressful than focusing on the fear and, best of all, it can energize us to move forward in a more positive way.

Exercise: ISLEEP for the Inner Critic

Find a time and place when you can be still and uninterrupted, and recall a time when you were experiencing self-criticism. See if you can note it with language of Focusing, such as, "Something in me is saying I am_____/I am going to_____ (negative trait/ outcome)." Spend a few moments being with this part of you, using the ISLEEP skills as shown in Table 4.1 to understand what this part of you is afraid of and what it wants for you. Stay with the sensations in your body as they emerge, bloom, and fade.

Experiment: Mindfulness of Self-judgement (Thoughts Like Sounds)

See if you can catch yourself the next time something doesn't go your way at work. Try to notice your thoughts, as if they were detected by a microphone and amplified by speakers. Notice the *content* of the thought stream—the words that arise in your mind. Notice if the content is understanding like, "This is not what I

TABLE 4.1　**ISLEEP for the Inner Critic**	
ISLEEP Skill	**Inner Relationship Focusing for the Inner Critic**
Introduce	Say hello to the part that is criticizing
Solicit (three core questions)	1. "I'm wondering if you might be worried or concerned." 2. "I'm wondering what you might be not wanting to happen to me." 3. "What do you want for me?" or "What positive feeling or state are you wanting to help me experience?"
Listen	1. "I hear that you are _____." 2. "I really hear that you are not wanting me to be _____."
Empathy	"No wonder you're feeling worried if what you're wanting is for me not to be _____."
Explain (implicit)	I am not here to change you in any way but just to show I care by listening and keeping you company. You are not alone. I hear you.
Power (implicit)	Allow the felt-sense to emerge *in its own time.* Allow the criticizing part and its felt-sense to change *if it wants* to and *when it is ready.*

Cornell AW. *The Radical Acceptance of Everything: Living a Focusing Life.* Berkely: Calluna; 2005.
The quotes in the table are directly from Cornell.

had hoped for my patient's procedure," or if it is a judgment like, "I am such a bad nurse." Notice also the *tone* of the internal dialogue; is it friendly or harsh?

Try to receive the thoughts like you would receive sounds in the environment while connecting to an anchor (the breath, sounds, or body sensations). Notice any shift in the experience as you observe with mindfulness—in the body, thoughts, emotions. Journal your experience, if that is helpful to you.

Shame and Its Antidote

One of the side effects of harsh criticism is shame, "A highly unpleasant self-conscious emotion arising from the sense of there being something dishonorable, immodest, or indecorous in one's own conduct or circumstances."[15] Shame can arise from self-criticism and also from others', as illustrated in the next story.

I remember as a dental student spending eight long hours toiling over a denture set up—setting my patient's denture teeth in wax to prepare for a "wax try-in". When I finally submitted my case to the professor, he yelled at me in front of my classmates. "This is awful, start over!" He threw my work across the table. I felt anger and frustration, but most of all, shame.

(Fortunately, this teacher was not representative of my teachers in dental school, most of whom were very kind and supportive.) Interestingly, shame can arise even in the face of success, a phenomenon called "impostor syndrome," in which people "attribute their accomplishments to luck rather than to ability and fear that others will unmask them as a fraud."[16]

Shame is a corrosive emotion that is "now beginning to be appreciated as having a *unique and significant* association with mental illness" (emphasis added),[17] as confirmed by several studies.[18] A study of the experience of shame in medical students found shame can lead to "withdrawal, isolation, psychological distress, altered professional identity formation, and identity dissonance," and found an overarching theme of "the destabilizing nature of shame."[19] Shame is such a problem in medical education that leaders are looking for solutions; Will Bynum, a physician, educator, and researcher, offers several suggestions on how to avoid shame in the face of medical errors: "acknowledging the presence of shame and guilt in the learner; by avoiding humiliation, and by leveraging effective feedback."[20] Let's look at a remedy we can try on our own.

Self-compassion: an Antidote to Harsh Self-criticism and Shame

Be kind to your sleeping heart. Let it out into the vast fields of Light, and let it breathe.

Hafez[21]

Fortunately, there is a powerful remedy for shame, one that calms and soothes the HCP while also motivating them to help others. This antidote to self-criticism is its opposite—self-compassion. In contrast to shame and self-criticism, which trigger the sympathetic nervous system, compassion engages two calming and soothing systems: the parasympathetic nervous system and the mammalian caregiving system.[22] As with self-criticism, when we offer ourselves compassion, we are both the giver and the receiver—only this time, instead of doubly harmful, it is doubly beneficial. And the benefits of self-compassion extend beyond ourselves because self-compassion is closely linked to compassion for others.[23]

If you are like me and many other HCPs, the mere mention of self-compassion can be aversive. (For me it triggered hives.) We are so conditioned to push ourselves and be hard on ourselves that it becomes a habitual pattern and a way of life. You might think, "How can there be time or space for such softness when I don't even have time to sleep, eat, or go to the bathroom?" (I had an image of myself as a champion weightlifter trying to stop to smell the roses while lifting a potentially back-breaking weight.) In addition, for many of us high achievers, there is a fear that "if we don't judge ourselves harshly, then we'll become lazy, incompetent or unsuccessful."[24] Yet, a growing body of evidence is proving the contrary.

The research of psychologist Kristin Neff provides answers to the following questions: "What qualities do people with self-compassion have in common," and "What are the benefits of self-compassion especially for shame." Her research yielded a working definition of self-compassion that has been validated by research and includes three main components: "being kind and understanding toward oneself in instances of pain or failure…perceiving one's experiences as part of the larger human experience…and holding painful thoughts and feelings in mindful awareness."[25]

If we compare these three hallmarks of self-compassion with the features of shame, we can appreciate how self-compassion is a perfect antidote.[9] See Table 4.2 for a comparison of shame and self-compassion with examples.

TABLE 4.2   Comparison of Shame and Self-compassion

Shame	Self-compassion
Identification *I am bad.*	Mindfulness *I feel bad.*
Isolation *Everyone knows I'm bad.*	Common Humanity *Everyone makes mistakes*
Self-criticism *How could you be so stupid/bad?*	Self-compassion *This is hard for you. You will get through.*

Neff K, Germer C. *Teaching the Mindful Self-compassion Program: A Guide for Professionals.* New York: Guilford; 2019.

Shame is one of the most entrapping emotions, and the reason for this is that it is very difficult to be mindful with shame. Christopher Germer, psychologist and cofounder of Mindful Self-compassion Program, shares this interesting insight: "Shame has a way of wiping out the very observer who is needed to be mindful of our situation."[26] Because of this, mindfulness is the foundation of self-compassion and the way out. At the moment of contact with kindness, when you can say, "This is a moment of suffering," you have already started to hoist yourself out of the mire of shame.

Informal self-compassion practice: self-compassion break. A lot of self-care methods, like exercising, enjoying nature, and watching a movie, *are* helpful but can't be done at work (unless you are trying to get fired!). Informal practices, like this self-compassion break, can be done on the spot. This practice includes three steps: mindfulness, acknowledging common humanity, and self-compassion.

Practice:
You might try these steps using Kristin Neff's reminder phrases or words of your own choosing:
1. *This is a moment of suffering.* (Mindfulness)
2. *Suffering is a part of life.* (Common humanity)
3. *May I be kind to myself.* (Self-compassion)[27]

The third element of this practice, self-compassion, can also be expressed with *touch.* Research has found that touch, when it communicates compassion, induces physiologic changes that are soothing and calming.[28] (More on expressive touch in Chapter 5.) So, you might try gently placing your hand on your heart or belly if that feels comfortable to you. Notice the feel of the *contact* and the *warmth* of your hand and imagine *kindness* flowing into your body.

To illustrate, here is an example of a nurse navigating a clinical challenge with the self-compassion break:

Kendra is a critical care nurse who hasn't slept in two nights due to her work schedule and caring for her baby. She accidentally administers the wrong medication to a patient. Table 4.3 contrasts how this scenario would play out with self-criticism versus self-compassion.

TABLE 4.3   Comparison of Shame and Self-compassion: Nurse Scenario

Self-criticism Fueling Shame	Self-compassion Cultivating Resilience and Remorse
No mindfulness/identification: "I *am* a bad nurse, a bad person." **No mindfulness of triad:** Lost in emotions, negative thoughts and impulses (eating a box of donuts)	**Mindfulness/non-identification:** "I *did* something I regret." **Mindfulness of triad of experience:** *Body:* Feeling tension in forehead, chest tight *Thoughts:* Aware of future-oriented thoughts—"the patient will be harmed, I will be ruined." *Emotions:* "Worry is here, shame is here." Worry/shame feel like this in the body."
Isolation Loneliness, withdrawal	**Common humanity** "Others have made mistakes too."
Self-judgement (harsh words and tone) "I am the worst nurse in the world. I should have never gone into nursing."	**Self-kindness** (kind words, tone, and touch) "You are having a hard time, you are exhausted. I am here for you." "You will find the way to address the harm done and prevent it from happening again." Placing hand on belly, feeling the contact and warmth soothing and comforting.

Notes About Self-compassion Practice

Self-compassion is a practice of goodwill, not good feelings.[29]

The importance of setting healthy expectations, as discussed earlier, applies to our expectations of self-compassion practice, too! Kristen Neff warns, "If we use self-compassion practice to try to make our pain go away…things will likely get worse."[29] My own mindful self-compassion teacher, Mila de Koning, co-author of the book, *Heart for the Doctor*, offers the analogy of comforting a crying baby: we wouldn't hold, rock, and stroke a baby, and then, if it doesn't stop crying immediately, set the baby down and walk away angrily. We offer compassion to ourselves as we do for the baby, simply to care and to comfort, without expecting or requiring any particular outcome on any particular schedule—unconditionally.

At times, practicing self-compassion may arouse negative thoughts, emotions, or sensations. If so, you may be experiencing the contrast between how you normally approach yourself and the self-compassion that you are now offering. Maybe a sense of unworthiness is coming into relief. If so, you may try to explore this negative reaction by practicing RAIN as described earlier.

The Compassionate Counterpart to Shame

A common myth is that a focus on self-compassion will translate into not taking responsibility or making amends when we make a mistake, but research is proving the contrary. In fact, self-compassion is associated with *higher* motivation to making amends and with avoiding repeating mistakes.[30] Another set of studies showed "Self-compassion spurs positive adjustment in the face of regrets."[31]

Self-compassion promotes the healthier counterpart to shame. When things go wrong or we make a mistake at work and we practice self-compassion, we feel *remorse*. Both forms of self-evaluation—shame and remorse—are well-described by meditation teacher and author Sharon Salzberg. In the first type, "Our thoughts focus on our worthlessness: 'I'm the worst person in the world. Only I do these terrible things,'" and as a result, we feel depleted.[32] (Note that this version of self-criticism is referred to as *shame* in medical literature, but Salzberg calls it guilt.) With shame, the focus is on oneself and one's own pain and, as a result, we don't see the facts clearly and don't see what others may need. On the other hand, with *remorse*, she explains,

"We realize that we have at some point done something or said something unskillful that caused pain, and we feel the pain of that recognition. But crucially, remorse frees us to let go of the past. It leaves us with some energy to move on, resolved not to repeat our mistakes."[32]

Note to educators: Medical literature uses the term *shame* to refer to the toxic form of self-criticism and *guilt* for a more constructive type. Unfortunately, this positive use of the term guilt conflicts with the lay definition as "feelings of deserving blame especially for imagined offenses or from a sense of inadequacy"[33]—clearly not a positive emotion! Because of the incongruity between the professional and lay uses of the term guilt, I recommend the use of the term remorse instead of guilt to designate the healthier form of self-criticism.

Formal practice: forgiveness. The intention of this practice is to cultivate self-compassion when you feel you have done wrong, whether it is true or not. The object here is not to fabricate a particular feeling, so don't worry if you don't feel anything "warm and fuzzy." Simply set an intention to forgive. As described by Sharon Salzberg, forgiveness practice is done in three parts: asking forgiveness of others, offering forgiveness to others, and offering forgiveness to yourself.[32]

Start by sitting comfortably, with your eyes closed, if that is comfortable for you. Allow your attention to settle gradually on the anchor of your choice—the sensations of the breath, body sensations, or sounds. Once your attention has settled, silently invoke the first intention, "*I ask forgiveness of anyone I have harmed intentionally or unintentionally.*" Notice who or what comes to mind, if anyone. Stay with this intention. After a few minutes, move to the second part, offering to others what we have just received: "*I offer forgiveness to anyone who has intentionally or unintentionally harmed me.*"

In the last part, the most important part for dealing with self-criticism and shame, we practice forgiveness for ourselves. In Salzberg's words, "*If there are ways you have harmed yourself, or not loved yourself, or not lived up to your own expectations, this is the time to let go of unkindness toward yourself because of what you have done.*"[32] For the third part, consider, especially, the aspects of yourself that you tend to judge. For example, I tend to judge myself for being too slow at work and running behind schedule. If nothing comes up, stay a few moments and something will likely bubble up, when given the chance. In time, the self-compassion generated by watering the seeds of forgiveness will show up, often at times when you least expect. When that happens, note it and smile. Video 4.2 offers a guided forgiveness meditation.

> **Exercise:**
> Motivating yourself with self-compassion. The following exercise is inspired by the Mindful Self-compassion Curriculum.[9]
> Recall something you are struggling to change such as a health-related behavior (losing weight), or a skill needed at work (staying on schedule) that you are struggling with and that you give yourself a hard time about. Write a letter in one or more of the following ways:
> 1. From your compassionate self to your struggling self
> 2. From a good friend to yourself
> 3. From yourself to a person you care about with this issue.
> By relating to yourself in this way, you will soon find a new tenderness blooming.

Other Benefits of Self-compassion: Relieving Caregiver Stress and Promoting Well-being
Self-compassion for Caregiver Stress

Self-compassion is not just for self-criticism or shame; it is essential to navigating the inevitable challenges of caring for others in need. At the time of this writing, an unprecedented percentage of HCPs are suffering from burnout—no surprise given a global pandemic. The term compassion fatigue, used so often, is a misnomer as we know that compassion is beneficial (see Chapter 2). The real problem is too much *empathy* and *not enough compassion*—especially for the caregiver, themself. Kristin Neff reports, "When we give ourselves compassion, we create a protective buffer, allowing us to understand and feel for the suffering person without being drained by his or her suffering."[34]

Research is finding mounting evidence of benefits of self-compassion for caregivers. Some of the benefits of self-compassion particular to HCPs include less self-reported stress and sleep disturbance and better mental health[35,36] as well as increased satisfaction with the caregiver role.[37] The program for mindful self-compassion as adapted for HCPs was the subject of a research study that found the course may be "an effective way to increase self-compassion, enhance well-being, and reduce burnout for health care professionals."[38] An interesting study of parents of children with autism found benefits with implications for all caregivers, "Even though child symptom severity is often the strongest predictor of negative adjustment for parents,

self-compassion universally predicted parental well-being over and above the effects of child symptom severity" (emphasis added).[39] This underscores the importance of the ability of caregivers to care for themselves.

Compassion activates the soothing network in the body—the mammalian caregiving system mediated by oxytocin, as we saw in Chapter 2. This effect can be helpful to the HCP and the patient alike. The following practice offers a way to tap into the benefits of compassion in the middle of a patient encounter.

Informal practice: compassion at work (giving and receiving compassion). I am pretty good at self-care when I am alone, but when I am with a patient or anyone who is suffering, my tendency is to focus entirely on the other at the exclusion of myself. Many days it feels like I stop breathing when I walk in the door of my office and don't resume breathing until the workday is over! The practice of giving and receiving compassion is a way of caring for yourself as you work with patients, even in the heat of a clinical challenge. This practice comes from the Mindful Self-compassion Program curriculum[9] and can be done on the spot or as a formal meditation (imagining a challenging person). As with many informal/on-the-spot practices, it helps to practice them when you are not in the heat of the moment. As one of my teachers once said, the best time to weave your parachute is not when you are jumping off the plane!

> **Practice:**
> In the moment of difficulty, tune in to the sensations of your breath and body—especially the sensations of the stress you feel. Then, on the inhale, receive and absorb compassion for yourself. On the exhale, send compassion to the patient. Some suggested words you might say silently to yourself: (on the inhale) "one for me," and (on the exhale), "one for you." Alternatively, "in for me," and, "out for you."

If the need is great for yourself, you can focus on the inhale and receiving compassion ("one for me") until you are ready to give again, at which time you can offer more to the other again ("one for you"). Video 4.3a offers a description of the practice followed by a guided practice in Video 4.3b.

What I enjoy most about this practice is that it offers me at least 50% of my care or more if needed, which is more than the habitual 0%! By doing so it allows me to calm and soothe myself at the same time as I care for a person who is struggling. With practice, it can become a healthy habit that makes patient care less depleting, more rewarding, and more sustainable. In the words of Germer and Neff, "When we feel emotionally overwhelmed in the consultation room, the easiest way to activate the care state is by giving care to ourselves, and once we feel calmed and soothed, we are in the right state of mind and can extend care to our clients."[9]

Self-compassion for General Well-being

In addition to reducing negative experiences like shame and stress, self-compassion is also associated with decreased mental health disorders and increased positive states. A meta-analysis of 14 studies, all using Neff's self-compassion scale, found "a large effect size for the relationship between compassion and psychopathology," and that "Compassion is an important explanatory variable in understanding mental health and resilience."[40] Interestingly, the benefits of self-compassion are reflected in physiologic changes in the body. For example, self-compassion has been associated with changes in alpha amylase and interleukin-6, reflecting decreased sympathetic nervous system activity.[41] Self-compassion also increases positive states.[42] Corresponding positive physiologic changes have been noted, including increases in parasympathetic activity reflected by vagally mediated heart rate variability.[43]

Formal practice: "making rounds on yourself" (body scan with self-compassion). How do you know when you are stressed? Maybe you have a signature reaction like overeating or driving too fast that signals your stress reactivity. Before the reaction comes an impulse, and before the impulse, there is *something*. If we notice that something, we can catch the whole cascade before it unravels. That something is a sensation in the body. In fact, every negative emotion is accompanied by an uncomfortable body sensation.[7] Our language captures this phenomenon with many expressions, such as "my heart in my throat," "a pain in the neck," "broken-hearted," and "butterflies in my stomach."

Just like the caterpillar recoils when it feels an unpleasant sensation, we, too, have a hard-wired instinct to react to pain. Thanks to mindfulness, we have many more options than a caterpillar! As we practice mindfulness, we begin to notice the tightness in the chest that accompanies frustration and the impulse to interrupt a patient, and we have the freedom to choose a skillful response, like listening until the end of their story. Mindfulness is even helpful for overcoming the impulses that underlie addictive behaviors. Neuroscientist and addictions expert Judson Brewer reports, "Cravings are simply made up of body sensations," and, if we can notice and get curious about them, we can

"feel the joy of letting go."[44] In summary, mindfulness of the body sensations that lie upstream of our reactions offers us the option to avoid mindless *reaction* and to *respond* in ways that are helpful to our patients and ourselves.

Mindfulness is more than just paying close attention to the present moment. (Even a hit man pays close attention…to their target!) Remember the two wings of mindfulness—the *what* and the *how*. The "what" is the paying attention to the present moment, and the "how" is the attitude we bring to the moment. Jon Kabat-Zinn, the father of the mindfulness movement in health care, defines mindfulness as "the awareness that emerges through paying attention, on purpose, in the present moment, and *non-judgmentally* to the unfolding of experience moment by moment" (emphasis added).[45] Non-judgment calls for self-compassion. Whatever arises, simply notice what's here with the attitude you would bring to your best friend or cherished pet. And when judgement does arise, try not to judge the judging!

The foundational mindfulness practice of the body scan as instructed in Chapter 2 focused on the "what" by paying close attention to the present-moment sensations in the body; this focus is necessary and helpful to develop and strengthen the awareness of the body, since so many of us are stuck in our heads. Now we add a focus on the "how," the attitude we bring to what we notice, weaving together both awareness of the body and self-compassion.

This practice requires a little imagination to consider each body part as a separate being with its own thoughts and emotions, a being that we can relate to with compassion. It may feel silly at first, but I encourage you to follow along with the guidance in the video below; it is a profound way of cultivating self-compassion and well-being. I encourage practicing lying down to promote resting and releasing, but you can also practice seated. As always, you can modify the pace and the words in whatever way feels comfortable and comforting to you. Start on one end of the body, like the feet, and gradually travel to the other end. Video 4.4 will guide you through a body scan with self-compassion.

Practice:
For each body part, practice the following:
1. *Greeting* each body part with gratitude. "Hello_____ (feet, legs, etc). Thank you for what you have done and endured for me."
2. *Wish* each body part a sense of ease. Inviting each part to imagine being completely at ease. (Compassion)

3. *Tuning into the sensations* present in that part of the body without any agenda to fix, analyze, or get rid of anything. (Mindful awareness)
4. *Offer care* for that body part for what it is feeling right now. (Self-compassion) The care can be expressed with words or with touch. For example, "I see you, I am here for you, keeping you company no matter what are feeling right now, you are not alone." If it feels right, gently touch the area, feel the contact and the warmth, and imagine care flowing into the body.

Formal practice: awareness of the breath with emphasis on self-compassion. As with the last practice, this one (Video 4.5) also invites us to focus on both the "what" (the breath and everything else) as well as the "how" (the attitude of compassion).

Practice:
As you sit with the sensations of the breath, notice whatever arises and name it silently: for example, anxiety, restlessness, boredom, peace. Whatever arises, set an intention not to slap, swat, or judge. Instead, try silently saying to yourself, "Hello, _____ (restlessness/boredom/anxiety). Wishing care for this _____ (restlessness/boredom/anxiety/etc.)."
Then, return to the breath.

Self-criticism can show up in meditation practice as thoughts of not meditating well or not meditating enough. When you notice thoughts *about* your practice that start with some form of "I should _____ (be more focused)," or, "I should not _____ (wander/feel restless)," silently say something like, "Wishing care for this self-criticism." Then, when you are ready, return to the anchor—breath, body sensations, or sounds. Notice any shifts in your experience as you assume a gentler attitude. Discomfort may bloom or fade or both. Allow it all, and meet everything with an attitude of curiosity and patience.

Conclusion: Mindfulness and Self-compassion for Clinical Challenges

Together, mindfulness and self-compassion help to loosen the grip of shame and other aversive emotions that may arise for the HCP during clinical challenges. With *mindfulness*, we can note the experience silently, "shame is here," "restlessness is here," "tension is here," while staying with the anchor of attention, such as the breath. We can allow space for everything and hold every-

TABLE 4.4 Summary of Formal and Informal Mindfulness and Self-compassion Practices

Practice	Formal	Informal (on the Spot)
1) Rain	X	X
2) Mindfulness of self-critical thoughts (thoughts like sounds)		X
3) Self-compassion break	X	X
4) Forgiveness	X	
5) Compassion with equanimity (giving and receiving compassion)	X	X
6) Body scan with emphasis on self-compassion	X	
7) Awareness of breath with emphasis on self-compassion	X	

thing in a wider field of non-judging, patient awareness. In this way, mindfulness transforms a difficult experience from one that permeates and consumes to just a passing phenomenon. Through the lens of mindfulness, the experience naturally shifts from identification ("I **am** shameful/angry/disappointed") to disidentification ("shame/anger/disappointment **is here**").

Mindfulness is the foundation for self-compassion. With self-compassion the internal voice shifts from, "I should _____," to "I choose to _____"; from, "I should have," to "next time I will aim to _____." In the words of Marshall Rosenberg, you can "avoid 'shoulding' yourself!"[46] The effects of mindfulness and self-compassion together act like a balm for a wound, healing the corrosive effects of harsh self-criticism, shame, and stress that challenge many HCPs.

Table 4.4 summarizes the formal and informal (on-the-spot) practices that will help cultivate both mindfulness and self-compassion for the HCP.

CARING FOR THE PATIENT DURING CLINICAL CHALLENGES: APPLYING ISLEEP AND MINDFULNESS

Now we move from the care of the HCP to the care of the patient in clinical challenges. The focus here will be on applying the ISLEEP skills to the following situations: *physical touch, the "difficult patient" (refusal of care, requests for unethical care), adverse outcomes, delivering bad news,* and *health counseling.* The challenge of procedural pain and anxiety is not included here as it will be the subject of Chapter 5. Examples of mindfulness and self-compassion for the HCP will also be included.

Attempts to describe communication skills with written words only are inevitably incomplete because they omit the non verbal communications—tone of voice, facial expressions, and posture—which we know are so important. Nonverbal communication will be discussed more in Chapter 5 as it pertains to pain and anxiety. This discussion of patient care using ISLEEP skills is offered as a framework for what to say to navigate tough clinical challenges. Scripts of dialogues will be provided to illustrate ISLEEP skills in specific clinical scenarios. As dentistry is my area of expertise and is an area of health care that most HCPs are familiar with (as a patient), dental examples will predominate. You may notice repeating patterns as you go through the various dialogues, and hopefully this will help reinforce how to apply these evidence-based communication skills. Finally, although touch is fundamentally different from the other clinical challenges, it is included here and featured first because of its central role in the delivery of health care, because it is a complicated phenomenon, and because it gets so little attention during most HCPs' training.

Preparatory Questions for Reflection about Touch

1. Recall instances, positive or negative, when you were the recipient of functional touch during a medical or dental procedure (e.g., a dental cleaning, venipuncture for a blood test). What did you like or dislike about the ways that HCPs touched your body?

2. In your opinion, what distinguishes the way an HCP should touch a patient's body from the way a car mechanic touches a car as they work?

Physical Touch in Health Care

Touch is fundamental to both diagnosis and treatment in medicine and dentistry, so it can quickly become routine to the HCP, making it possible to overlook the gravity of working in close proximity and touching a person's body. Many health care procedures involve entering patients' "intimate zone," the closest of the four

zones of personal space defined by American anthropologist, Edward Hall.[47] In addition, many health care providers routinely touch parts of the body that are inherently intimate, such as the face, mouth, and genitals.

In the absence of an explicit curriculum on health care touch, education is via modeling their mentors (the "hidden curriculum"), and the most common approach modeled is a detached and clinical one. This approach may be motivated by the need to focus on the technical aspects of care. It may also be driven by concerns about violating boundaries. Yet, as we shall see, a purely clinical approach to touching intimate parts of the body can be objectifying and therefore violating. The big question is: how does an HCP balance a patient's need for respect of boundaries while also expressing care for the whole person, not just their body?

First, let's clarify some nomenclature for touch in health care. There are two main types of touch described in the literature. "Expressive touch" is touch that aims to comfort; this will be discussed in Chapter 5 as a means to alleviate pain and anxiety. "Functional touch" is touch that is task-oriented. A specific kind of functional touch called "intimate touch" designates "task-oriented touch to areas of patients' bodies that might produce feelings of discomfort, anxiety, fear, or might be misinterpreted as having a sexual purpose."[48] Intimate touch applies not only to genitals but to any area that is emotionally charged for a given patient. For example, when one considers the integral role of the mouth in many basic human functions—nourishment, communication, maternal-child bonding, and physical intimacy—it becomes clear that the mouth is laden with emotional associations, and therefore it qualifies as intimate touch for many patients. For patients with a history of abuse, touch in any area of the body can be particularly sensitive as touch "may be prone to retriggering memories of trauma, depending on the nature of the trauma."[49]

For any patient, there lies "potential for harm if intimate touch is provided inappropriately…" such as "increased stress and anxiety, damaged therapeutic relationships and even allegations of sexual assault."[50] Despite the gravity of touching inappropriately, very little guidance exists on how to touch in health care, leaving clinicians to learn by "trial and error on the job, an inconsistent method that is not in line with evidence-based practices."[48] Research on touch suggests "touch in the health care profession is a conflicted and ill-defined practice."[51] Fortunately, mindfulness and the ISLEEP communication model provide much needed guidance on touch. First, let's see how mindfulness helps navigate the experience of touch in health care.

Mindfulness for Touch

While the concepts of functional and expressive touch are helpful academically, in practice, the distinction does not exist. Researchers have noted, "a single encounter may comprise several types of touch."[48] This blurry distinction between functional and expressive touch is highlighted by one model of touch depicting a continuum between functional, on one end, and expressive, on the other.[52] A dualistic model of touch is misleading because it denies the fact that *all touch is expressive.*

> *Touch…bears within it expressive content. Whether I probe an injury…stroke a cheek, or punch someone with a fist, these are actions which embody gestural significance, be it investigative, amorous, or hostile in nature. The body manifests meaningful intentionality that may or may not be fully conscious and articulable.*[53]

Not only is all touch expressive, but research has also shown that humans are very perceptive of the intention behind another's touch. One study on touch perception asked study subjects to guess the emotion conveyed through touch (out of a possible 12 emotions). Touch was provided from behind a barrier, which allowed only the hand and arm of the toucher to pass through, and the duration of touch was only 1 second. While the chance of determining the correct emotion conveyed in the touch was only about 8%, subjects guessed accurately over 50% of the time![54] These findings have profound implications for HCPs.

If all touch is expressive of something, what is expressed when an HCP engages in functional touch? Purely functional touch, or touch which is "not primarily communicative or empathic but analytical," has been called "objectifying touch."[53] While purely functional or objectifying touch can be valuable at times "to avoid inappropriate intimacy which can violate boundaries," it can be damaging as it also bears "the power to exacerbate, rather than heal, the disintegrations of illness."[53] Imagine the experience of having lost your front tooth in an accident and having a parade of clinicians and trainees probe and poke in your mouth without acknowledging your experience of the accident or of being touched at this vulnerable time. As one

researcher expresses so well, "objectifying touch can exaggerate the patient's sense of having a distressingly flawed object for a body."[53]

It is important to recognize that *all touch in health care is expressive* and holds the potential to convey care and thereby heal—or harm. "Touch, even when it performs essential clinical tasks, can be interpreted as an expression of compassion, empathy, and presence."[51] Functional/procedural touch can convey both care and respect, when the HCP is *mindful.*

If we return to the definition of mindfulness, "The awareness that emerges through paying attention, on purpose, in the present moment, and non-judgmentally,"[45] we remember there are two parts: the what and the how:

$$\text{Mindfulness} = \frac{\text{awareness of the present}}{\text{(what)}} + \frac{\text{an intention of care/respect}}{\text{(how)}} \quad \textbf{1}$$

Similarly, **mindful procedural touch** includes these two elements. For example, as I retract a patient's cheek during an intraoral examination, awareness of the present might include the temperature and smoothness of the cheek and the tension of the cheek muscles (what). At the same time, I connect with an intention of care and respect (how).

Mindful procedural touch avoids something that patients have reported as aversive, "being handling carelessly,"[55] as well as the risk of injuries (such as a dentist cutting the corner of the patient's mouth). Most importantly, mindfulness allows all touch—even functional touch—to convey both care and respect.

Note: Mindful procedural touch is not an ideal to strive for at all times. As we discussed earlier, the mind can only attend to so much. Because of this, there are times, as in the case of challenging, complex technical procedures, that might require the HCP to focus all their attention on the procedure itself—purely functional touch—to avoid harming the patient. But many instances of touch in health care do not require such hyper focus and provide an opportunity for mindful touch. Examples include the moments of contact while doing simpler tasks, such as placing a blood pressures cuff or placing a bib on a dental patient. The HCP must always use their judgement moment by moment to gauge where their attention is needed most.

We have seen how mindful touch can benefit the patient, and in Chapter 5, we will explore even more benefits of touch for procedural anxiety and pain. What about the provider—are there benefits of mindful touch to the HCP?

Mindful Procedural Touch: Good for the HCP, too

Every time a professional touches a patient, they are themselves touched.[51]

I have been pleasantly surprised by my experiences while exploring mindful procedural touch. When I notice the sensations of touch during dental procedures (e.g., warmth, softness, and slipperiness of a patient's cheek) and connect with an intention of caring for the patient, many times I feel an instantaneous sense of calming, soothing, connection, and uplifting of my mood. Such experiences led me to search for an explanation.

We know that compassion—without any touch involved—confers physiological benefits to the giver. As discussed in Chapter 2, compassion is associated with the neurotransmitter oxytocin (which creates feelings of calm, soothing, and connection) as well as the neurotransmitter dopamine (which mediates the experience of pleasure). When we add the act of touching to compassion, we may be magnifying these known physiologic benefits of compassion. Dacher Keltner, psychologist and director of the Greater Good Science Center affirms that "the act of touching is physiologically rewarding for the toucher," and research is beginning to uncover the mechanisms for this effect.[56]

Experiments

(A) Mindful Touch for Self

As you go about your personal hygiene routine—brushing your teeth, showering, and combing your hair—notice your habitual way of touching your body. Is it mindful or mindless? As you touch, try to notice the sensations of touch and any other senses like smell, taste, etc. Also, try to connect with an intention of care for yourself.

Questions for Reflection

How do you compare the experience of mindful versus unmindful touching?

How does this experiment inform the way you touch a patient during a procedure?

(B) Mindful Procedural Touch Experiment (Pairs)

Round 1 (mindless): One person plays the patient, the other the HCP. The provider first performs a simple work-related task (e.g., extraoral exam, BP reading, etc,) while counting backwards from 100. This is a way of simulating mindless touch or purely functional touch.

Round 2 (mindful procedural touch): Repeat the activity this time focusing on the present moment sensations and connecting with an intention of care and respect.

Switch roles and repeat both rounds.

Questions for Reflection

How would you compare the two experiences?

How does this experiment inform the way you touch a patient as you work?

(C) Mindful Procedural Touch With a Patient

Choose a simple task that allows you to experiment with your focus of attention such as:

- Placing blood pressure cuff on patient
- Tying a tourniquet on patient arm for phlebotomy
- Placing dental bib on patient
- Placing hand on the patient's shoulder as you guide a patient into treatment position (such as reclining the dental chair)

Whenever you can, even for just a few seconds at a time, notice the sensations as you touch a patient's body, such as warmth, contact of the hand, the texture of the patient's clothing. Connect with an intention of care and respect. Notice what that feels like and how it affects your attitude toward the patient.

ISLEEP for Procedural Touch

Touch is a highly subjective experience, and research on touch in health care has found "patients may have a different understanding than that of clinicians, whereby clinicians' behaviors demonstrate respect."[50] Several possible reasons for such differences have been proposed, including the following: (1) "Clinicians find intimate care so routine…that they do not approach intimate care in a mindful manner." (2) "Clinicians assume acquiescence from patients toward intimate touch as a component of the patient role." (3) "Clinicians have unrealistic expectations of patients to trust that the clinician's intentions are good and that clinicians' proficiencies with touch are unquestioned."[50]

The many differences in perspective about touch between patients and providers underline the importance of mindfulness as well as understanding *patient perspectives* on touch. "Congruent with a patient-centered paradigm, the perceptions, experiences, and preferences of the patient take precedence over the clinician concerns and become the primary driver of recommendations and guidelines on how the clinician should provide intimate touch in the context of clinical care."[50]

Research findings on patient preferences about touch in health care emphasize the importance of all six ISLEEP skills. For example, the value of *soliciting* was expressed clearly by one patient in a study of patients with a history of sexual abuse: "That would be great for a dentist to ask 'Do you have a problem with people touching you?' as a matter of fact, all doctors could ask you that."[57] A qualitative, systematic review study of literature from 1970 to 2016 aimed to "identify and synthesize findings on the perceptions, experiences, and preferences of patients receiving a clinicians' touch during intimate care procedures." This study also aimed to "identify evidence on patients' recommendations for clinicians for providing intimate touch in a manner that communicates professionalism and respect for patient dignity."[50] The requests and recommendations of these patients can be easily categorized in terms of the ISLEEP skills: introduce/interconnect, solicit, listen, empathize, explain, and power of the patient. This suggests that by applying each of these six skills to procedural or functional touch, the HCP will increase the chances of conveying respect and care. What follows are the thoughts and words of patients in the review study, pertaining to each of the ISLEEP skills.

Experiments:

1. Before reading the patient's recommendations relating to each ISLEEP skill, imagine possible ways to demonstrate each skill as you touch a patient during procedures.
2. Photocopy the following bullet points, cut out each point, and scramble them. Then try to identify which ISLEEP skill each point demonstrates.

Introduce/Interconnect
- "The most in-depth discussion among participants centered on their desire for rapport... if the care involved intimate touch." "Tell me your name...make a human connection."[48]
- "Positivity was conveyed about providers who had storied knowledge of their clients, that is, a recognition of the multidimensionality....as well as an understanding of the specific circumstances particular individuals faced."[55]
- Patients welcome some self-disclosure by the provider of touch, such as hobbies and interests to make the provider more human.[48]

Solicit
- Providers of touch "should solicit feedback from patients while providing care."[48]
- "Operationalization of clinician respect is likely to be highly variable among different care contexts and patients, hence the need for meaningful communication and solicitation of patient feedback."[50]
- "Asking for feedback if you sense discomfort."[48]

Listen (with ears and eyes)
- Patients want providers "to listen to their concerns and answer their questions" as a way to "increase their comfort with intimate touch."[48]
- Patients want providers of touch to "monitor verbal and non verbal cues from patients in evaluating the effectiveness of their touch.[52]
- "...since it is the patient who is in the greatest position of vulnerability while receiving touch from a clinician, it is the responsibility of the clinician to be attentive to the responses of the patient during the touch encounter and make behavioral and procedural adjustments as necessary."[50]

Empathy/Compassion
- "Competence alone was not enough...clinical expertise must be built upon an ethic of compassion and generosity... negative experiences were related to providers who dismissed women's complaints."[55]

Explain
- "Explain what you're going to do before you do it."[48]
- "Participants...said communication was of the utmost importance and must occur before the intimate touch could take place." "Don't touch me without telling me."[48]
- "Participants wanted kind words and assurances... that they'll do what they can to ensure comfort."[48]

Power
- Patients expect that the HCP "seek permission before initiating intimate touch and they want to be involved in deciding when and how it's given."[48]
- "Patients were emphatic in their rejection of an assumed perspective that they must simply acquiesce to any physical contact deemed necessary by the clinician."[50]
- Researchers recommend HCPs to "halt the intimate touch...if you sense discomfort."[48]
- Patients report the unaffirming experience when a provider "spoke in abrupt commands."[55]
- "They discussed clinical situations in which they'd felt powerless and devalued by not being given the chance to express their preferences concerning

intimate touch…They were emphatic that if intimate touch was needed, they'd want control over the procedure."[48]

Reflection on Touch in Health Care:
1. When you are a patient, what ISLEEP skills are most important to you during functional touch?
2. What ISLEEP skills do you think are most important to your patients for touch?

The "Difficult" Patient

They might be in pain, scared, and suffering. They might be angry, frustrated, disenfranchised. They might be worrying about bills…They might be addicts. They might have made terrible choices. They might be easy to judge. They might not have the skills to be kind while in pain; they might never in their lives had kindness shown to them. They might have been abused or violated by someone they trusted. They might be many things. But one thing is true: they are doing their best. The patient, even the accusatory and fearful patient, is doing their best.

Dr. Rana Awdish, Author of In Shock: My Journey from Death to Recovery and the Redemptive Power of Hope[58]

Medical and dental training inculcates the "right" way—the standard of care. For example, in dental school I was taught to remove disease (place all fillings) before replacing missing teeth (dentures, an implants, etc.), and the reverse order would be heresy. Unfortunately, patients' priorities don't always align with this order—in fact, in my experience they seldom do! For example, I have met many patients with multiple, abscessed teeth, yet their chief complaint is the desire to whiten their teeth.

So, the HCP has the challenge of a delicate balancing act. On one hand, they must uphold the standard of care established by the profession. At the same time, they must provide patient-centered care: care that "is respectful of and responsive to individual patient preferences, needs, and values," and ensures that "patient values guide all clinical decisions."[59] How should the HCP proceed when a patient's values and preferences conflict with standards of care?

When a patient requests something (or refuses something) that would violate the standard of care, many times HCPs label them as "difficult," and struggle ensues. In some cases, patients' wishes may reflect ignorance. Other times, their values may simply differ from the provider's. Whatever the case, the HCP must balance the duty to do no harm and do good while respecting the patient's autonomy, and at times these aims are conflicting. For example, not doing harm may require taking radiographs, but respecting a patient's autonomy may require not forcing a patient to take radiographs they don't want.

Let's look at a couple situations in which patients' wishes conflict with the principle to do no harm, exploring how mindfulness, self-compassion, and ISLEEP skills can help find a way forward.

Patient Refusal of Necessary Testing or Treatment

Think of a common procedure in your specialty that patients often refuse. In such situations, some HCPs may be tempted to assume a paternalistic approach like, "You have to _____," like the dental assistant telling a patient, "You have to get an FMX (full mouth series of radiographs)." This approach can easily arouse resistance, resentment, or conflict. Table 4.5 illustrates how to apply the ISLEEP skills, mindfulness practice, and self-compassion for the scenario of the dental patient refusing radiographs. This is by no means intended to be a script but simply one of countless possible ways to apply the skills.

Experiment 1:
By covering the right column, you can practice verbalizing each skill on your own.

Experiment 2:
By covering the left column, you can try to identify which skill is at play.

Experiment in Pairs:
Hide the right column. One person plays the patient, the other the HCP.

No matter what a patient's objection is, express **empathy**. Even if it doesn't make sense to you, *it makes sense to the patient*. Empathy softens resistance. Further, by **explaining** information relevant to the patient's objections, the HCP has a chance to reassure and move forward while staying connected. If the patient still declines, and this would create an unethical situation, the patient's autonomy can still be honored by politely offering the option to seek a second opinion (ISLEEP skill *power of the patient*), for example, "I encourage you to seek another opinion and would be happy to refer you to a trusted colleague."

TABLE 4.5   ISLEEP for Refusal of Care: Dental Radiographs

ISLEEP Skill, Mindfulness Practice, and Patient Response	Sample Dialogue
Explain (what is needed and why, in language the patient can understand)	*"Since most of the tooth structure is under the gums, many dental problems can only be seen on x-rays."*
Power (recommend not command)	*"So, we <u>recommend</u> a full set of x-rays."*
Patient refuses without sharing the reason	Patient refuses without sharing the reason
Solicit	*"Can you share with me your concern?"*
Mindfulness **Self-Compassion**	*Doctor feels their own breath and body sensations (e.g., tension, constriction)* *Breathing in Compassion for self, out for patient (Compassion at Work practice)*
Patient cites worry about radiation	Patient cites worry about radiation
Empathize/validate	*"It makes sense that you would be concerned about radiation. Radiation can pose health risks at high doses."*
Explain	*"Fortunately, modern dental x-rays provide very low exposure. In fact, you may be exposed to more radiation when you fly in an airplane.* *We must also consider this: there are risks of NOT taking x-rays, such as missed diagnosis and untreated disease. In your case, the risk of not taking x-rays is much greater than the risks of taking them."*
Solicit (Patient feedback on explanation)	*"How does that sound to you?"*
Patient Consents	Patient Consents
Power (ask permission to begin)	*"Ready to begin?"*

Experiment:

For the remainder of this chapter, think of examples of each different type of clinical challenge in your health care niche. Write your own script or role-play the challenge with a partner in two ways:

1. Try the scenario in a paternalistic, doctor-dominated way, without ISLEEP skills (e.g., imagine how you would want to act when you are tired, grumpy, or in a hurry. Have fun!).
2. Try the same scenario in a patient-centered way, using the ISLEEP skills.

Requests for Suboptimal Care

In addition to refusing necessary care, patients may at times request care that is not on par with the standard of care. A common example of a request for suboptimal care is that of a patient requesting antibiotics for a viral upper respiratory infection. In the scenario in Table 4.6, the HCP has determined that the patient's symptoms do not represent a bacterial infection and advises symptomatic care (without antibiotics). The patient is angry and states they always need antibiotics to recover.

Through the years, I have had many dental patients request suboptimal care. A common example is the request for restorations (fillings) before a prophylaxis (cleaning). This can pose a problem when the gums are inflamed because inflamed gums bleed easily, which can compromise the bond of the filling to the tooth. Here is an example of how to navigate this situation with ISLEEP skills.

Tom has been a patient for many years. He presents on a Monday morning with tooth #9 (upper front tooth) severely fractured from a sports injury. Examination reveals the tooth is restorable with a large filling and a crown. Unfortunately, Tom hasn't had a cleaning in a year and his gums bleed easily. Not an ideal situation, but a filling could be done.

Experiment with Table 4.6 and Table 4.7 as before:

Experiment 1:

By covering the right column, you can practice verbalizing each skill on your own.

Experiment 2:

By covering the left column, you can try to identify the ISLEEP skill.

TABLE 4.6 Patient Requests Suboptimal Care: Medical Scenario

ISLEEP Skill, Mindfulness Practice, and Patient Response	Sample Dialogue
Patient requests antibiotic	Patient requests antibiotic
Empathize/validate	*I can understand wanting to get better quickly and wanting to take a medicine that might clear up your infection.* *(Note that the statement "it makes sense" refers to the patient's beliefs. Validating a patient's beliefs does not require that it make sense to the HCP.)*
Explain	*All medications have risks and therefore we don't want to use them unless the benefits are greater than the risks. The risks of taking antibiotics include allergic reactions, adverse drug reactions, and drug interactions. Right now, there is NO benefit to you taking antibiotics because antibiotics only work for infections that are caused by bacteria, and your infection is caused by a virus.*
Power (recommend not command)	*Here is what I recommend to help you heal quickly....(symptomatic care strategies)*
Solicit (questions/concerns/feelings)	*Do you have any questions or concerns about what I have shared?*
Patient accepts recommendations	Patient accepts recommendations

TABLE 4.7 Patient Requests Suboptimal Care: Dental Scenario

ISLEEP Skill, Mindfulness Practice, and Patient Response	Sample Dialogue
Patient requests restoration today due to appearance of tooth, exam done	Patient requests restoration today due to appearance of tooth, exam done
Empathy	*"I can understand your wish to fix a broken front tooth as soon as possible!*
Power (recommend, not command)	*I would recommend that you have a cleaning first...*
Explain (reason for recommendation)	*so we can do the best quality filling."*
Patient asks for restoration without cleaning today	Patient asks for restoration without cleaning today
Solicit (reasons for not accepting recommendation)	*"What are the advantages to you of doing the filling before the cleaning?"*
Patient cites time constraints	Patient cites time constraints
Empathy	*I hear your need to stay on schedule on a work day—your time is limited.*
Explain (specific reasons for the recommendation)	*Unfortunately, your tooth is not clean and the gums bleed easily so the filling may not last. This means the filling may need to be redone after the cleaning, which would cost more time and money.*
Solicit (reaction to explanation)	*Are you willing to take that chance?*
Patient accepts risks of filling before cleaning	Patient accepts risks of filling before cleaning

> **Experiment 3 (Pairs):**
> Hide the right column. One plays the patient, the other the HCP.

In this case, it was a reasonable option to restore the tooth without cleaning first, even though it was a deviation from ideal care. Patient wishes were honored without compromising care unreasonably. By explaining the risks of restoring the tooth without first doing a prophylaxis (cleaning), patient expectations of possible outcomes were managed. For sample dialogue, see Table 4.7.

Requests for Unethical Care

> **Reflection:**
> Think of a common patient request for something you cannot do or something patients commonly refuse which you cannot do without. How do you avoid setting ultimatums, which can create conflict, yet maintain standard of care?

Let's revisit the last scenario, only this time, a dental restoration without a cleaning would be unethical.

Scenario:
Patty has not seen a dentist in 2 years. Limited exam reveals her gingiva (gums) are severely inflamed and she has heavy calculus (tartar buildup). She asks for two white fillings to be done today.

In Patty's case, restorations would most likely fail (due to the inability to control bleeding and due to calculus buildup). A paternalistic approach might involve an ultimatum without any explanation: "You have to have a cleaning before the fillings can be done." Ultimatums can result in alienation. Let's apply mindfulness, self-compassion practice, and ISLEEP skills to navigate this scenario in Table 4.8.

Notice how the ISLEEP skills help uncover the objections and obstacles to treatment and find a way forward in collaboration with the patient—like a dance. By **soliciting** skillfully, the HCP may uncover social determinants of health, such as financial or transportation issues, that the health care team might help surmount. Most importantly, when the HCP **solicits** and **listens** to a patient's story, it allows the HCP a means of shifting from a stance of judgment or frustration to one of **empathy** and compassion. And when the patient feels heard and understood, it builds trust and a therapeutic relationship.

What if the patient still refuses?

If the patient persists with an unethical request or declines essential tests or treatment, the professional must set limits respectfully. Always present recommendations in terms of the patient's best interests and a commitment to quality care, for example, "Unfortunately, *I will not be able to do a quality filling for you* until the teeth are cleaned and the gums have healed." If the patient persists, you might say, "*You are welcome to seek another opinion.*" By offering the option to seek a second opinion, the HCP affirms the power of the patient.

> **Informal Compassion Practices for Difficult Patients:**
> 1. Imagine the patient as a frightened child. This may help to soften your approach and increase patience.
> 2. Remind yourself that if you were exposed to the same life challenges and influences as the patient, you might think and act similarly.
> 3. Forgiveness practice: acknowledge the stress this patient arouses in you and set an intention to forgive them. (See formal forgiveness practice at the beginning of Chapter 4.)

Adverse Outcomes

Early in my career, I enjoyed a lot of "geographic success." This term, coined in jest by my residency director, is defined as the false perception of success that arises from not practicing long enough in the same location! Any HCP, no matter how skilled, who stays long enough in one location learns that things go wrong. For example, in dentistry, restorations can fall out, new dentures can be loose, and patients' teeth can break during an extraction. When things go wrong, what happens next can either compromise the relationship with the patient or, conversely, strengthen it as demonstrated by the following story.

I met Dr. M while he was a general dentistry resident, and I clearly remember his kind presence and excellent chairside manner. Recently, one of his patients posted this five-star review online (printed exactly as written):

I highly recommend Dr m, I had previously went to Dr m to replace a cracked filling, then i went to him for a checkup. He found that it was difficult to get dental floss past that tooth that he had filled , and said that he wasn't happy with the filling , so he offered to redo that filling ,at no additional cost , so i had him redo that filling , and i'm very happy that i did cause i can now get dental floss past that tooth, thank you very much Dr m.[60]

TABLE 4.8   Patient Requests Unethical Care: Dental Scenario

ISLEEP Skill, Mindfulness, Patient Reaction	Sample Dialogue
Patient asks to have fillings done today	Patient asks to have fillings done today
Empathize	*"I understand your wish to have the fillings done today."*
Explain (need for hygiene)	*"Because of the tartar buildup on your teeth and the bleeding gums, any fillings I would do right now would not seal, and the leakage of bacteria under the fillings would cause harm to your teeth."*
Power (recommend hygiene not demand)	*"So, I recommend first a cleaning, time for the gums to heal, and then the fillings."*
Solicit (reaction to explanation and recommendation)	*"How does that sound to you? What questions do you have?"*
Listen with mindfulness	Staying still. Making eye contact.
	Feeling the breath and body sensations.
Patient expresses frustration. Wants fillings today (doesn't share why)	Patient expresses frustration. Wants fillings today (doesn't share why)
Solicit (social determinants)	*"What are the advantages, from your perspective, of having the fillings done first instead of the cleaning?"*
Listen with mindfulness	HCP connects with the breath and uncomfortable or strong body sensations.
Self-compassion	Breathing in compassion for self, out for the patient (Compassion at Work practice)
Patient starts crying (describes difficulties as a single mom of a special needs child)	Patient starts crying (describes difficulties as a single mom of a special needs child)
Listen with mindfulness	Not interrupting, making eye contact, nodding with understanding and acceptance.
Empathize/validate	*"So many moms struggle to care for their little ones, and their own health gets pushed to the bottom of the list. This is a hard time for you!"*
Patient stops crying. Begins to look reassured and relaxed	Patient stops crying. Begins to look reassured and relaxed
Solicit	*"How would you like to proceed?"*
Affirm Power (implied by soliciting preference)	
Listen with mindfulness	HCP continues to sit still, making eye contact with the patient, smiling
Patient states times that would be possible for a cleaning. She looks calm and receptive.	Patient states times that would be possible for a cleaning. She looks calm and receptive.

Many HCPs assume that an adverse event, such as a faulty dental filling, would inevitably result in an angry or disappointed patient. Yet, as this glowing review demonstrates, an adverse outcome doesn't have to tarnish the provider-patient relationship. In fact, when handled skillfully, an adverse outcome can actually *enhance* trust and loyalty. I believe this patient's review of her dentist was higher than if the restoration had been perfect the first time. His transparency demonstrated his honesty, and the offer to replace it at no cost demonstrated his commitment to quality care.

Patient satisfaction with their care is largely determined by their expectations, and as we discussed earlier, *all disappointments reflect an unmet expectation.* Because of this, the way an HCP helps set patient expectations and manages unmet expectations can have even more impact on patient satisfaction than the treatment outcome. In the above example, the patient expected the filling not to have a problem and was therefore disappointed when it failed. But, when Dr. M replaced the patient's faulty filling at no cost, he exceeded her expectations, resulting in a rave review despite an adverse event.

Before treatment, the HCP can help set healthy expectations by "front-loading," providing appropriate and ample information about possible outcomes. The ISLEEP skill, *explain*, is paramount to managing expectations upstream. Once the adverse event has occurred, other ISLEEP skills can help navigate the choppy waters of unmet expectations, mitigate disappointment, and avoid litigation.

> **Experiment:**
> Call to mind a scenario in which a product or procedure you provided a patient was defective or failed. Imagine how you would navigate this scenario with ISLEEP skills.

Let's practice applying ISLEEP skills to two clinical scenarios: a faulty product and a failed procedure.

The Faulty Product

Recently, I delivered a new complete maxillary (upper) denture to a patient, Eileen. Preoperative examination led me to expect good retention in the final denture, so I hadn't forewarned her about the possibility of looseness. To my dismay, the denture was so loose, the patient was unable to wear it without large amounts of denture adhesive. The patient was disappointed, and so was I. Table 4.9 provides a sample dialogue.

> **Solo Experiment:**
> As before, the ISLEEP skill will be listed on the left and the sample dialogue on the right. You can experiment with covering the left column to practice identifying the ISLEEP skill or covering the right column to imagine what words would demonstrate each skill listed on the left.

> **Pairs Experiment:**
> One person plays the patient and the other the provider. Cover the right column and create your own dialogue.

Note that the dentist refers to the disappointment as "ours" and the options as "ours" to emphasize that the HCP and the patient are on the same team—that the disappoint-

TABLE 4.9   The Faulty Product

ISLEEP Skill, Mindfulness, Patient Reaction	Sample Dialogue
Patient reports new denture very loose after trying for 1 week	Patient reports new denture very loose after trying for 1 week
Empathize/validate	*"I am sorry that your denture is so loose. It makes sense that you would be disappointed, and I am too."*
Power of the patient (options)	*"Here are our options:* 1. *Do nothing and see if it improves on its own.* 2. *Try an adjustment.* 3. *Send back to lab to reline."*

ment and the options are shared, although ultimately, the patient gets to choose. In the case of Eileen, she chose to try adjusting the denture and then, after some time, to reline the denture. Despite this adverse outcome, our relationship was maintained and, in my sense, strengthened.

The Faulty Procedure (Need for Redo)

Dr. Jones, a general dentist, has just obtained an impression for a crown on a lower back tooth for Sarah, a petite, young woman. The procedure was very difficult for Sarah, due to the location and limited space for the suction, handpiece, and mirror. She gagged many times during the procedure. On inspection of the impression, Dr. Jones announces with frustration, "We have to take another impression" and walks away to check another patient while the assistant sets up for another impression. Sarah is visibly disappointed and fights back tears, wondering how she will survive another impression.

Remember, every disappointment reflects an unmet expectation. In this case, the dentist didn't prepare the patient for the possibility of having to retake the impression, so it came as an unpleasant surprise and a big disappointment, especially since the first impression was so challenging. Before a difficult procedure, the ISLEEP skill *explain* can help prepare the patient for the possibility of a retake or redo. A simple preparatory statement can help set appropriate expectations: *"Most of the time we can capture the tooth on the first impression, but sometimes we need more than one."* When the patient knows this, and the first attempt is successful, the patient will be extra appreciative. If the first impression is not successful, the advanced warning will help avoid or at least mitigate disappointment.

At times of adverse outcomes, mindfulness and self-compassion are key to keeping calm. When I notice myself getting upset, I may excuse myself for a moment to regain balance. *"Please excuse me, I need to inspect this impression more closely in the other room."* In the other room, I can inspect the impression...and also my breathing! The sensations of the breath are always available as an anchor for the attention when navigating choppy waters. Feel and allow the sensations to be there for a breath or two. Notice any other sensations in the body, perhaps a constriction or bracing against the reality of the moment. You might also try noticing the believed thoughts—if a microphone could amplify the thoughts in your head...what would you hear? My thoughts have a theme in these cases: *"I'm stupid, and I'm a bad dentist."* Allow the thoughts to be on the sidelines, without suppressing, or adding more and staying with the breath.

In addition to mindfulness, self-compassion helps. Practicing self-compassion on the spot could include a reminder that everyone makes mistakes and has unfortunate outcomes. Offer a kind word to yourself silently with a caring tone of voice. Offer yourself a caring touch, feeling the contact and warmth of your hand. Because of our hard-wiring, our own touch can induce the release of oxytocin to calm and soothe in a difficult moment.

Now, let's revisit the failed dental crown impression, but this time applying mindfulness, self-compassion practices, and ISLEEP skills. Table 4.10 offers a sample dialogue.

TABLE 4.10 The Faulty Procedure (Need for Redo)

ISLEEP Skill, Mindfulness	Sample Dialogue
Dentist has left the treatment room to confirm the impression needs to be redone.	Dentist has left the treatment room to confirm the impression needs to be redone.
Mindfulness	HCP feels their breath and body sensations. Notice and allow any judgments about self or patient.
Self-Compassion	(Doctor to self silently while gently placing hand on chest) "Everyone makes mistakes. This is hard, but I will get through."
Doctor returns to patient	Doctor returns to patient
Empathy (for challenges already faced)	*I know that was challenging for you. You worked so hard to get through that and I appreciate it!*
Explain (need to retake impression and why) **Power** (recommend not demand)	*Unfortunately, the impression does not capture everything needed by the lab to make the best quality crown for you.* *So, I recommend taking another impression.*
Patient appears visibly upset	Patient appears visibly upset
Solicit	*You look upset. Can you share what you're feeling right now?*
Patient reports feeling tired.	Patient reports feeling tired.
Empathy	*I can imagine you are tired. You have been sitting a long time!*
Solicit	*What would be helpful for you? Maybe you would like to take a break or use the bathroom?*
Patient agrees to a bathroom break. She returns looking more at ease.	Patient agrees to a bathroom break. She returns looking more at ease.
Explain	*I believe we can finish in the next few minutes, and once we obtain the impression of the tooth, the lab will be able to make a high-quality crown for you.*
Power (offer options)	*We can do another impression today or, if you need to stop now, we can schedule another appointment.*
Patient agreeable to working more today.	Patient agreeable to working more today.
Power (permission)	*Are you ready to get started?*
Patient agrees	Patient agrees

> **Reflection:**
> Compare the paternalistic approach described first ("We *have to* take another impression") with the dialogue in Table 4.10.

In situations where we need to redo a part of a procedure, many HCPs are tempted to coerce the patient to redo it immediately even when it would be possible to stop at this point. Reluctance to offer the patient the option to take a break or schedule another appointment may be due to cost or time concerns. Yet not offering the patient options can be violating, especially if the patient is experiencing pain or anxiety (more on this in Chapter 5). Many patients have reported trauma resulting from being pressured by an HCP.

By taking just a few moments to *solicit* and *listen* to patient's needs; *empathize*; *explain*; and affirm *power*, the experience above was quickly reframed from potentially traumatic to a tolerable discomfort. The entire dialogue above took about 30 seconds (not including the bathroom break). When given the option to say "Yes, I will," most patients will consent to trying again—they want to get the job done too! In the rare cases where the patient does *not* consent, the provider avoids violating the patient and, by doing so, can maintain the patient's trust.

Delivering Bad News

Delivering bad news is an inevitable part of health care. In my work as a dentist, a common example would be informing a patient that their tooth requires extensive treatment or is not restorable at all. These situations are hard for the patient *and* the HCP. "The bearer of bad news often experiences strong emotions such as anxiety, a burden of responsibility for the news, and fear of negative evaluation."[61] Formal practices of mindfulness and self-compassion help the HCP to remember to be mindful and compassionate with themselves in the heat of the moment—feel the breath, feel the body sensations, reconnect with an intention of care for yourself and for the patient.

The way an HCP delivers bad news is important because it "can have a significant impact on the patient's perception of the problem, the relationship with the clinician, and satisfaction."[62] As we saw before, patient expectations have a profound influence on the impact of the bad news. "The impact on the patient is proportional to the gap between the patient's expectations and the reality of the situation."[62] The professional can help minimize this gap by employing ISLEEP skills. Let's look at three examples of delivering bad news in order of increasing gravity.

Minor Bad News: Interruptions and Delays

Modern health care is fraught with interruptions, and technology is probably the main source of interruptions of interactions between providers and patients. Too many interruptions can undermine the provider-patient connection, especially when not handled skillfully, and the ISLEEP skills can help manage interruptions in a way that maintains and even strengthens connection.

When the interruption is related to the patient's care, the HCP can provide reassurance and maintain connection with the ISLEEP skill *explain*. For example, before turning to the computer I might tell a dental patient, *"I'm going to check your x-rays first, and then we'll check your tooth,"* or *"I'm going to enter some notes into your chart while we wait for numbness to set in."* When the interruption is *not* related to the patient's care, other ISLEEP skills are helpful. In the next scenario, the dentist must interrupt a patient's procedure to check on a dental hygiene patient (more common than I wish!). The dialogue in Table 4.11 demonstrates how, in just a few seconds, the ISLEEP skills can help the HCP transform a potential annoyance to an opportunity to express care and respect.

Moderate Bad News: Moderate Disease

Even when the bad news is not their fault, many HCPs feel responsible and feel guilty, and this can create a lot of stress for themselves. Previously, dental hygienist Jessica described the anxiety she feels when delivering the bad news about a patient's gum disease, saying it is especially stressful "when the patient is angry, in a bad mood, or questions my knowledge." Bad news is stressful for patients too, especially when the HCP doesn't explain adequately, uses medical jargon, or tells them what they "have to do."

Again, mindfulness and self-compassion can support the HCP as they deliver bad news. Mindfulness allows the experience to be held in a wider space, thus diluting its negative charge. Before starting the conversation, feel the breath, noticing any sensations of constriction, holding, or restraining, and allow them space. Self-compassion in the moment, such as breathing in

TABLE 4.11 Minor Bad News

ISLEEP Skill	Sample Dialogue
Explain (what and possibly why, if that would be helpful)	*I need to step out for just a moment to check on a patient.*
Empathize (assume possible disappointment even if not expressed by patient)	*I'm sorry for the interruption.*
Solicit needs or wants (doctor)	*Are you comfortable? Is there anything you need while you wait?*
Patient declines offer	Patient declines offer
Power—offer options (assistant)	*(assistant) Would you like to stay in this position or sit up while you wait?*
Patient opts to sit up and expresses gratitude	Patient opts to sit up and expresses gratitude

compassion for yourself (*compassion at work* practice) can soothe and calm.

The next scenario (Table 4.12) demonstrates ISLEEP skills for delivering the bad news of periodontal disease (gum disease). Let's fast-forward past *introducing/interconnecting, soliciting* the patient's chief complaint, *listening,* and *empathizing.* Also, *power* of the patient was honored by asking permission to obtain radiographs and perform the clinical exam. Based on the findings, the dentist has determined the need for periodontal treatment (scaling and root planing) in lieu of a routine cleaning.

At this point, the ISLEEP skill *explain* is key. Explaining with visual aids helps the patient learn about different stages or types of disease and different treatment options. You may also explain using the patient's own images/radiographs or clinical presentation (e.g., dentist using a mirror or intraoral camera). In this way, the patient has a chance to connect their own condition with a

TABLE 4.12 Moderate Bad News

ISLEEP Skill/Patient Reaction	Sample Dialogue
Explain—using visuals to describe condition and treatment options	**Explain**—using visuals to describe condition and treatment options
Power (recommend treatment, don't tell what to do)	*I recommend treating your gum disease with scaling and root planing, which is similar to a routine cleaning, only deeper and with local anesthesia to numb your gums so you will be comfortable.*
Solicit (using open-ended questions)	*What questions do you have? What concerns do you have?*
Listen	Sitting at eye level, still and silent. Body language expresses attention and care (nodding, eye contact). Not interrupting.
Patient expresses fear of pain	Patient expresses fear of pain
Empathize/validate	*I hear your concern. It makes sense you would be anxious, thinking the procedure could be uncomfortable.*
Explain (how will address concern, using layterms)	*We will take several measures to make sure you're comfortable including use of a numbing gel and other numbing medicine.*
Power (options)	*Also, you can stop for a break any time, especially if you are ever uncomfortable.*
Solicit and listen	*How does that sound to you? What other questions or concerns do you have?*
Patient expresses frustration about the extra cost.	Patient expresses frustration about the extra cost.
Empathize	*You expected a routine cleaning, so it makes sense you would be surprised and maybe even disappointed it would cost more than expected.*

Continued

TABLE 4.12   Moderate Bad News—cont'd

ISLEEP Skill/Patient Reaction	Sample Dialogue
Explain	Remember this is not just a cleaning but actually a treatment for an infection in your gums that, if left untreated, could result in losing your teeth. The treatment coordinator can discuss the specifics of fees and scheduling options when we are done.
Solicit	How does that sound? What other concerns?
Patient consents to proceed.	Patient consents to proceed.

particular disease or stage of disease. Through the years, I have met many patients who, given the right information, could diagnose their own stage of periodontal disease, thus taking the burden of the bad news off me! It also allows the patient to experience the diagnosis more objectively and less as a judgment or an imposition.

As discussed in Chapter 3, *explain* includes: recommended treatment options; benefits of treatment; risks of treatment, risks of non-treatment.

Remember to describe treatment using lay language (e.g., "removing tartar buildup," instead of "scaling and root planing") and non-inflammatory terms (e.g., "numbing the gums," instead of "injecting local anesthesia"). This is especially important when delivering bad news as it can affect a patient's receptivity to the news. Many providers stop here, thinking the job is done and the patient should accept the recommendation, given adequate information. But we have only set the stage for patient-centered care.

The HCP is able to uncover potential objections and obstacles to treatment and to address them by employing the ISLEEP skills soliciting, listening, and empathizing. For example, the patient may have a concern about discomfort during the proposed procedure. *Soliciting* these concerns allows the HCP the chance to *empathize and explain* what comfort measures will be offered during a procedure—a prime concern for most patients. If the patient was expecting a simpler diagnosis or treatment, the HCP might solicit the patient's disappointment, frustration, or skepticism.

Notice that until there is a sense of resolution of the patient concerns, the HCP can circle back to *soliciting* to continue uncovering objections, questions, emotions, and concerns. By demonstrating skillful *listening, empathizing,* and affirming the patient's *power* (e.g., making recommendations instead of commanding, offering options), the HCP helps the patient identify, process, and resolve their concerns.

Severe Bad News

Many HCPs deal with serious diagnoses sometimes involving life and death issues. While my own profession seldom involves such grave scenarios, there *are* situations that bear emotional weight, such as the loss of a front tooth due to disease or injury. Experts on dental fear suggest to "let the patient know what is 'ok' about [their] health first and present the problems in a non-overwhelming way."[63] Also, try to preface bad news "with a warning statement to prepare the patient emotionally" and to avoid alarming the patient with too much information.[62] Most importantly, resist the impulse to interrupt or break a silence, especially after sharing bad news, as this may be an expression of a "need to rescue" or to "make it right or better."[62]

Let's look at two different ways to deliver bad news—with and without ISLEEP skills.

Scenario: Loss of a Front Tooth (Without ISLEEP)
Gabrielle is a 50-year-old female with a large cavity in her front tooth. Currently, she denies any symptoms. Her last visit to the clinic was 3 years ago.

"What can I do for you, today?" Dr. Smith asks.

"I'm hoping you can fill this tooth for me, Doctor. It looks awful," Gabrielle reports, pointing to her upper front tooth.

After a limited examination and review of a radiograph, the dentist reports matter-of-factly, "I'm sorry. The tooth is not restorable, and it has to be extracted." He goes on to explain, "It can be replaced in three different ways." Gabrielle begins to cry but suppresses her tears out of shame—shame about her teeth and shame that she is getting emotional in front of the doctor and the assistant, who are looking down on her, literally and figuratively. She imagines going to work with no front tooth. She imagines her boyfriend's reaction to her. She hears Dr. Smith explaining several different tooth replacement options.

She nods politely through watery eyes, but the words don't register; she is too upset. She tells him she needs to think about it and let him know. Dr. Smith looks at his assistant from behind the patient, shrugs his shoulders, and moves on to the next patient.

Let's replay the same scenario—this time applying the ISLEEP skills as illustrated in Table 4.13.

Reflection:

1. What thoughts and emotions arise as you read this scenario?
2. How would you compare the impact of this scenario to the previous one—to the patient, to the HCP?
3. What are common scenarios in your specialty in which you must deliver bad news that evokes strong patient emotions? Write a dialogue or role-play the scenario applying the ISLEEP skills.

You may have noticed a cyclical pattern of ISLEEP skills, as in Table 4.12. Several times during this interaction, the provider *solicits* the patient's questions, feelings, or concerns. Each time the patient expresses an emotion or question, the provider has the opportunity to *listen* mindfully and express *empathy*. This cycle of *solicit-listen-empathize* can repeat until the patient has reached some degree of resolution. Often, especially in patients with high anxiety or a history of trauma, the most important and sensitive concerns don't surface immediately, and you will see a video example of this in Chapter 5.

In reality, this scenario would be much more subtle and nuanced. There might be nonverbal expressions of empathy. There might be pauses to hold the space for the emotions that arise. Remember the healing power of simply bearing witness to someone's pain. Remember what distinguishes a healer from a technician is the ability and willingness to listen with no agenda other than

TABLE 4.13 **Severe Bad News**	
ISLEEP Skills, Patient Reaction	**Sample Dialogue**
Introduce **Interconnect**	Hi Gabrielle, I'm Dr. Smith. Welcome back. Good to see you. How is your family?
Patient reports husband's job loss and financial woes	Patient reports husband's job loss and financial wo[...]
Empathy and compassion	I'm sorry to hear you are having these problems! I hope you are able to find the resources you need to get through this tough time!
Introduce (agenda for the visit)	Today, our goal is to see what the issue is and help you get comfortable until we can treat the problem in the way that you chose.
Solicit 1 (chief complaint)	So, can you tell me what brings you in today? How can I help you?
Listen mindfully	Doctor sits at eye level, without interrupting. Feeling their own the breath and connecting with an intention of care.
Patient reports hole in upper front tooth. She denies any symptoms, but she is embarrassed about her appearance.	Patient reports hole in upper front tooth. She denies any symptoms, but she is embarrassed about her appearance.
Empathy	So, you feel self-conscious about your appearance. I can appreciate wanting to have a smile you feel good about!
Power (ask permission) **Explain** (what will you do next view x-ray and perform exam)	If it's OK, I'll take a look at your x-ray and then your tooth so we can see what options would be best for you.
Patient consents	Patient consents
Explain (exam findings—share good news before the bad news)	The good news is that there are several ways to improve your smile. The bad news is that the tooth is severely infected and not savable. The only way to heal the infection is by removing the tooth.

Continued

TABLE 4.13   Severe Bad News—cont'd

ISLEEP Skills, Patient Reaction	Sample Dialogue
Solicit 2	How do you feel about this?
Listen mindfully	Making eye contact, breathing, allowing a few moments of space without trying to fix or rescue. Notices the patient looks teary-eyed.
Self-compassion	Doctor breathes in compassion for self, out for the patient. (Compassion at Work practice)
Patient STARTS TO CRY—expresses shame about appearance and about being emotional right now.	Patient STARTS TO CRY— expresses shame about appearance and about being emotional right now.
Empathize/validate	I can imagine how upsetting it is to lose your front tooth. This is big deal for you!
Explain (short-term solution to avoid being toothless—transitional partial)	What we can do right away is make a temporary, removable tooth that can be inserted the same day as the extraction. That way you never have to go without a tooth.
Solicit 3	How does that sound to you?
Patient expresses reassurance	Patient expresses reassurance
Power (offer option of more information)	Would you like some information on long-term solutions or is that enough information for now?
Patient consents	Patient consents
Explain	Describes two permanent options (bridge and implant) with visual aids including general descriptions, risks, and benefits. (Avoids procedural details and terminology which could confuse or alarm the patient.)
Solicit 4 (questions and concerns)	What questions or concerns do you have about what I've shared?
Patient EXPRESSES GRATITUDE, wants time to think about long-term options but consents to temporary removable tooth (transitional partial) and extraction.	Patient EXPRESSES GRATITUDE, wants time to think about long-term options but consents to temporary removable tooth (transitional partial) and extraction.
Power: Ask about readiness for next step (financial arrangements and scheduling next appointment)	Are you ready to talk to the coordinator about costs and scheduling?
Patient CONSENTS—looks reassured and calm now.	Patient CONSENTS—looks reassured and calm now.

to understand. With mindfulness, self-compassion, and the ISLEEP skills, even reactions to the most difficult bad news can be heard, held, and healed.

Health Promotion and Counseling

Every HCP knows patients whose diseases are caused by unhealthy lifestyle choices such as smoking, unhealthy eating, and alcohol use. I, myself, have known several dental patients who generate cavities faster than I can restore them and yet show up for their dental appointment with a bottle of soda in hand! People with a history of trauma are especially prone to "smoking, drinking, and high intake of sugary food and drink."[49]

HCPs are charged with addressing the behaviors that cause disease and promoting healthy lifestyle choices. The traditional approach of telling patients what to do, such as, "*Smoking is harmful to your health, you should quit*" or "*You have to brush and floss*," rarely inspires patients to change their behaviors. In fact, "There is evidence to suggest that traditional approaches to health education based on information giving and expert advice are largely ineffective, with success rates of only 5% to 10%."[64] It seems human nature resists being told what to do.[65] Researchers report, "Educating patients in dental and medical settings is frequently an exercise in overt persuasion...direct persuasion pushes the patient into a defensive position."[66] How can the HCP help patients change the behaviors that contribute to their health problems, and can the ISLEEP model help?

An evidence-based, patient-centered approach to behavior change, which employs all the skills of ISLEEP, is called motivational interviewing (MI). Originally designed to address problem drinking in the 1980s, this approach gained popularity in the 1990s for its effectiveness in managing chronic illnesses related to health behaviors.[65] A review of studies on MI found evidence of benefits for "reducing binge drinking, frequency and quantity of alcohol consumption, substance abuse in people with dependency or addiction, and increasing physical activity participation."[67] Systematic reviews of MI in dentistry found evidence of the efficacy of this approach for oral health behaviors as well.[68,69]

MI "uses collaborative and empathetic interactions to develop a client's internal and autonomous motivation to change."[64] At the heart of MI is the ISLEEP element, *power of the patient:* "The ethos of MI is to ask permission before providing unsolicited information…It is important to seek permission so the patient does not perceive [providing information] as 'telling them what to do.'"[70]

Soliciting is another core ISLEEP skill for MI, and there are many recommended issues to solicit. Because of the human inclination "to believe what we hear ourselves say," the patient themself needs to be the person "voicing the arguments for change."[65] Unfortunately, many times HCPs inadvertently elicit the patient's arguments NOT to change by giving unsolicited advice to change a behavior. Instead, the HCP must *solicit* the patient's own reasons for behavior changes. The acronym DARN represents the core issues to solicit for MI: it stands for the patient's own *desire* for change, *ability* to change, *reasons* for change, and *need* for the behavior change.[65] The provider also solicits the *importance* of the change to the patient, the *confidence level* in their ability to change, and the *pros and cons* of the behavior change in the eyes of the patient (see Appendix I for examples). So much to solicit!

A clever way of soliciting in MI involves the use of *rulers.* For example, "on a scale of 1 to 10, how important is it to you to quit smoking right now?" If the patient answers with a 5, asking the patient "Why 5 and not 2?" would help solicit the patient's personal reasons for wanting to change. By hearing their own reasons for changing behavior in their own voice, patients are more likely to change.

Listening is another ISLEEP skill that is essential to MI, and it involves mirroring or reflecting back the patients' words. First, listening includes reflecting back the patient's own words of *resistance* to change. For example, for the patient who doesn't want to take the time to brush their teeth, the HCP might reflect back, "It takes more time and effort to brush than you have." This serves to validate the patient's point of view, helps reduce resistance, and paradoxically inspires them to voice reasons to change, like, "I know I need to brush, or my girlfriend will notice my bad breath." Second, and most importantly, it involves reflecting back any *"change talk"* such as, "You want to quit smoking to set a good example for your kids." According to MI, emphasizing the patient's own reasons for change will motivate behavior change more than anything else.

Empathy in MI manifests by avoiding shame and scare tactics and, rather, expressing understanding and acceptance. For example, "It's hard to change routines, especially given all the stressors you are dealing with right now." Next, any *explaining* in MI is guided by the patient's interest and readiness for information. Before giving information, ask what the patient already knows and their willingness to listen. Further, MI experts suggest explaining the options for behavior change in terms of what *others* have done. For example, *"Some patients with a lot of tooth decay reduce sugar intake; others brush and floss more or use special fluoride products."* This indirect approach to explaining healthy behaviors minimizes resistance to change. Finally, the *power of the patient* is affirmed by asking permission to talk about issues and allowing patients the space to choose their own course of action, on their own timeline. For example, "What do you think you'll do? What would be a first step for you?"

Table 4.14 summarizes MI in the framework of ISLEEP skills. See Appendix I for sample dialogue to accompany the questions and actions in the table.

By employing the ISLEEP skills, the HCP promotes healthy behavior changes that endure. The information referenced above is from the book entitled, *Motivational Interviewing in Health Care: Helping Patients Change Behavior,* by Rollnick, Miller, and Butler.

Fig. 4.2 summarizes the practices, traits, skills, and the many acronyms we have explored. While this chapter focused primarily on challenges arising in the consultation, the next chapter addresses the challenge of managing pain and anxiety associated with medical and dental procedures.

TABLE 4.14 Summary of ISLEEP Skills for Motivational Interviewing	
ISLEEP Skill	**Changing Health-Related Behaviors: Motivational Interviewing[65]**
I. *Introduce/Interconnect*	

S. *Solicit*	• "DARN"
	  Desires
	  Ability to change
	  Reasons to change
	  Need for change
	• Rulers
	• Importance and confidence
	• Pros and cons of the behavior
	• What next?

L. *Listen*	Reflect resistance to change Reflect change talk (reasons for change)
E. *Empathize/validate*	NOTE: Avoid scare tactics and shame
E. *Explain/reassure*	Allow patient to ask for info Talk about what others do
P. *Power* of the patient	Ask permission to give info Offer choices Allow space to choose behavior changes and timeline

Rollnick S, Miller WR, Butler C. *Motivational Interviewing in Health Care: Helping Patients Change Behavior.* New York: Guilford Press; 2008.

The Patient-centered HCP

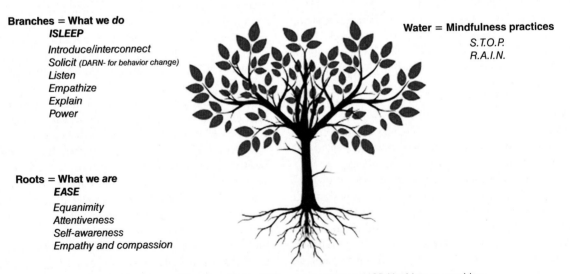

Branches = What we *do*
   ISLEEP

   Introduce/interconnect
   Solicit (DARN- for behavior change)
   Listen
   Empathize
   Explain
   Power

Water = Mindfulness practices
   S.T.O.P.
   R.A.I.N.

Roots = What we *are*
   EASE

   Equanimity
   Attentiveness
   Self-awareness
   Empathy and compassion

Fig. 4.2 Summary of Practices, Traits, Skills, and Acronyms. *HCP,* Health care provider.

REFERENCES

1. Sallattha S. *The Arrow*. Available at: https://www.dhammatalks.org/suttas/SN/SN36_6.html. Accessed January 6, 2022.
2. Samuel S. *Feeling Pandemic Guilt? Buddhism's "Second Arrow" Teaching Might Help*. Vox. Available at: https://www.vox.com/future-perfect/2020/5/1/21242047/coronavirus-pandemic-guilt-buddhism. Accessed December 19, 2021.
3. Salzberg S. *Real Happiness: The Power of Meditation: A 28-Day Program*. New York: Workman; 2011.
4. Seltzer L. *You Only Get More of What You Resist—Why?* Psychology Today; 2016. Available at: https://www.psychologytoday.com/us/blog/evolution-the-self/201606/you-only-get-more-what-you-resist-why. Accessed December 19, 2021.
5. Lao Tzu Quotes. Available at: https://www.goodreads.com/author/quotes/2622245.Lao_Tzu. Accessed September 21, 2020.
6. Salzberg S. *Week One of the 2019 Challenge*. 2019. Available at: https://www.sharonsalzberg.com/week-one-of-the-2019-challenge/. Accessed December 25, 2021.
7. Bayda E. *Being Zen: Bringing Meditation to Life*. Boston: Shambhala; 2002.
8. Brach T. *RAIN: A Practice of Radical Compassion*. 2020. Available at: https://www.tarabrach.com/rain-practice-radical-compassion/. Accessed December 25, 2021.
9. Neff K, Germer C. *Teaching the Mindful Self-compassion Program: A Guide for Professionals*. New York: Guilford; 2019.
10. Cornell AW. *The Radical Acceptance of Everything: Living a Focusing Life*. Berkely: Calluna; 2005.
11. Brown B. *Rising Strong: How the Ability to Reset Transforms the Way We Live, Love, Parent, and Lead*. New York: Spiegel and Grau; 2015.
12. Rada RE, Johnson-Leong C. Stress, burnout, anxiety and depression among dentists. *J Am Dent Assoc*. 2004;135:788–794.
13. Thomas M, Bigatti S. Perfectionism, impostor phenomenon, and mental health in medicine: a literature review. *Int J Med Educ*. 2020;11:201–213.
14. Gilbert P, McEwan K, Irons C, et al. Self-harm in a mixed clinical population: the roles of self-criticism, shame, and social rank. *Br J Clin Psychol*. 2010;49(Pt 4):563–576.
15. *APA Dictionary of Psychology*. Shame. Available at: https://dictionary.apa.org/shame. Accessed December 21, 2021.
16. Weir K. *Feel Like a Fraud?* APA. Available at: https://www.apa.org/gradpsych/2013/11/fraud. Accessed November 11, 2020.
17. Johnson EA, O'Brien KA. Self-compassion soothes the savage ego-threat system: effects on negative affect, shame, rumination, and depressive symptoms. *J Social Clin Psychol*. 2013;32:939–963.
18. Vizin G, Unoka Z. The role of shame in development of the mental disorders II. Measurement of shame and relationship. *Psychiatr Hung*. 2015;30(3):278–296.
19. Bynum WE IV, Teunissen PW, Varpio L. In the "Shadow of Shame": a phenomenological exploration of the nature of shame experiences in medical students. *Acad Med*. 2021;96:S23–S30.
20. Bynum WE IV, Goodie JL. Shame, guilt, and the medical learner: ignored connections and why we should care. *Med Educ*. 2014;48:1045–1054.
21. Hafez. *Be Kind to Your Sleeping Heart*. Take it out in...; n.d. Available at: https://www.goodreads.com/quotes/579308-be-kind-to-your-sleeping-heart-take-it-out-in. Accessed October 19, 2020.
22. Gilbert P. *The Compassionate Mind: A New Approach to Life's Challenges*. London: Constable and Robinson; 2009.
23. Gilbert P. *Compassion: Conceptualizations, Research, and Use in Psychotherapy*. New York: Routledge; 2005.
24. Scope. *The Benefits of Self-Forgiveness*. Available at: https://scopeblog.stanford.edu/2019/08/02/the-benefits-of-self-forgiveness/. Accessed September 21, 2020.
25. Neff KD. The development and validation of a scale to measure self-compassion. *Self Ident*. 2003;2:223–250.
26. Germer C. *To Recover from failure, Try Some Self-Compassion*. Harvard Business Review; 2017. Available at: https://hbr.org/2017/01/to-recover-from-failure-try-some-self-compassion. Accessed November 5, 2021.
27. Neff KD. *Exercise 2: Self-Compassion Break*. Available at: https://self-compassion.org/exercise-2-self-compassion-break/. Accessed November 16, 2020.
28. National Public Radio. *Human Connections Start with a Friendly Touch*. Available at: https://www.npr.org/templates/story/story.php?storyId=128795325. Accessed December 16, 2021.
29. Neff K. *Tips for Practice—Self-Compassion*. Available at: https://self-compassion.org/tips-for-practice/. Accessed December 12, 2021.
30. Breines JG, Chen S. Self-compassion increases self-improvement motivation. *Pers Soc Psychol Bull*. 2012;38:1133–1143.
31. Zhang JW, Chen S. Self-compassion promotes personal improvement from regret experiences via acceptance. *Pers Soc Psychol Bull*. 2016;42:244–258.
32. Salzberg S. *Loving-Kindness: The Revolutionary Art of Happiness*. Boston: Shambhala; 1997.
33. Merriam-Webster. *Guilt*. Available at: https://www.merriam-webster.com/dictionary/guilt. Accessed December 12, 2021.

34. Neff K. *The 5 Myths of Self-Compassion*. Psychotherapy Networker. Available at: https://www.psychotherapynetworker.org/magazine/article/4/the-5-myths-of-self-compassion. Accessed November 14, 2021.

35. Kemper KJ, Schwartz A, Wilson PM, et al. Burnout in pediatric residents: three years of national survey data. *Pediatrics*. 2020;145:e20191030.

36. Kemper KJ, McClafferty H, Wilson PM, et al. Do mindfulness and self-compassion predict burnout in pediatric residents? *Acad Med*. 2019;94:876–884.

37. Raab K. Mindfulness, self-compassion, and empathy among health care professionals: a review of the literature. *J Health Care Chaplain*. 2014;20:95–108.

38. Neff KD, Knox MC, Long P, et al. Caring for others without losing yourself: an adaptation of the Mindful Self-Compassion Program for Healthcare Communities. *J Clin Psychol*. 2020;76:1543–1562.

39. Neff KD, Faso DJ. Self-compassion and well-being in parents of children with autism. *Mindfulness*. 2014;6:938–947.

40. MacBeth A, Gumley A. Exploring compassion: a meta-analysis of the association between self-compassion and psychopathology. *Clin Psychol Rev*. 2012;32:545–552.

41. Neff KD, Long P, Knox MC, et al. The forest and the trees: examining the association of self-compassion and its positive and negative components with psychological functioning. *Self Identity*. 2018;17:627–645.

42. Neff KD, Rude SS, Kirkpatrick KL. An examination of self-compassion in relation to positive psychological functioning and personality traits. *J Res Personality*. 2007;41:908–916.

43. Svendsen JL, Osnes B, Binder PE, et al. Trait self-compassion reflects emotional flexibility through an association with high vagally mediated heart rate variability. *Mindfulness*. 2016;7:1103–1113.

44. Brewer J. *A Simple Way to Break a Bad Habit*. Available at: https://drjud.com/a-simple-way-to-break-a-bad-habit/. Accessed February 15, 2019.

45. Kabat-Zinn J. Mindfulness-based interventions in context: past, present, and future. *Clin Psychol Sci Pract*. 2003;10:144–156.

46. Rosenberg MB. *Non-violent Communication: A Language of Life*. Encinitas: Puddle Dancer; 2005.

47. Hall ET. A system for the notation of proxemic behavior. *Am Anthropol*. 1963;65:1003–1026.

48. O'Lynn C, Krautscheid L. Original research: "how should I touch you?": a qualitative study of attitudes on intimate touch in nursing care. *Am J Nurs*. 2011;111:24–31.

49. Raja S, Hoersch M, Rajagopalan CF, et al. Treating patients with traumatic life experiences: providing trauma-informed care. *J Am Dent Assoc*. 2014;145:238–245.

50. O'Lynn C, Cooper A, Blackwell L. Perceptions, experiences and preferences of patients receiving a clinician's touch during intimate care and procedures: a qualitative systematic review. *JBI Database System Rev Implement Rep*. 2017;15:2707–2722.

51. Kelly MA, Nixon L, McClurg C, et al. Experience of touch in health care: a meta-ethnography across the health care professions. *Qual Health Res*. 2018;28:200–212.

52. Connor A, Howett M. A conceptual model of intentional comfort touch. *J Holist Nurs*. 2009;27:127–135.

53. Leder D, Krucoff MW. The touch that heals: the uses and meanings of touch in the clinical encounter. *J Altern Complement Med*. 2008;14:321–327.

54. Hertenstein MJ, Holmes R, McCullough M, et al. The communication of emotion via touch. *Emotion*. 2009;9:566–573.

55. Stevens PE. Lesbians' health-related experiences of care and noncare. *West J Nurs Res*. 1994;16:639–659.

56. Keltner D. *Born to be Good: The Science of a Meaningful Life*. New York: W.W. Norton and Co.; 2009.

57. Raja S, Shah R, Hamad J, et al. Patients' perceptions of dehumanization of patients in dental school settings: implications for clinic management and curriculum planning. *J Dent Educ*. 2015;79:1201–1207.

58. Awdish R. *In Shock: My Journey from Death to Recovery and the Redemptive Power of Hope*. New York: St. Martin's; 2017.

59. Institute of Medicine (US) Committee on Quality of Health Care in America. *Crossing the Quality Chasm: A New Health System for the 21st Century*. Washington, DC: National Academies; 2001.

60. *Jamie Moeller Dentist Reviews*. Available at: https://www.google.com/search?rlz=1C1SQJL_enUS816US816&biw=1536&bih=722&tbm=lcl&sxsrf=ALeKk00ho0sjwB-ru7w4UHO9R7WyDx720w%3A1599571056359&ei=cIRXX6PEFZy0ytMP0I6N6Ao&q=jamie+moeller+dentist+reviews&oq=jamie+moeller&gs_l=psy-ab.1.0.35i39k1j0j46i199i175k1.13772.15816.0.18158.13.13.0.0.0.0.159.1472.2j10.12.0....0...1c.1.64.psy-ab..1.12.1468...46j46i199i175i273k1j46i433k1j46i433i199i291k1j46i199i291k1j46i273k1j46i433i20i263k1j46i20i263k1j46i433i131k1j0i67k1j46i433i67k1j0i20i263k1j0i10k1j46i199i175i20i263k1j0i22i30k1.0.1JaQ7tN3uW0#lrd=0x89c7635340041f21:0x6ab3c60f278a377a,1,,,&rlfi=hd:;si:7688706757241747322;mv:[[39.150105177319034,-75.52657751990242],[39.14974522268097,-75.52704168009758]]. Accessed September 7, 2020.

61. Baile WF, Buckman R, Lenzi R, et al. SPIKES-A six-step protocol for delivering bad news: application to the patient with cancer. *Oncologist*. 2000;5:302–311.

62. Curtin S, McConnell M. Teaching dental students how to deliver bad news: S-P-I-K-E-S model. *J Dent Educ*. 2012;76:360–365.

63. Milgrom P, Weinstein P, Heaton LJ. *Treating Fearful Dental Patients: A Patient Management Handbook*. 3rd ed. Seattle: Dental Behavioral Resources; 2009.

64. Yevlahova D, Satur J. Models for individual oral health promotion and their effectiveness: a systematic review. *Aust Dent J*. 2009;54:190–197.

65. Rollnick S, Miller WR, Butler C. *Motivational Interviewing in Health Care: Helping Patients Change Behavior*. New York: Guilford Press; 2008.

66. Weinstein P. Behavioral problems in the utilization of new technology to control caries: patients and provider readiness and motivation. *BMC Oral Health*. 2006;6(suppl. 1):S5.

67. Frost H, Campbell P, Maxwell M, et al. Effectiveness of motivational interviewing on adult behaviour change in health and social care settings: a systematic review of reviews. *PLoS One*. 2018;13:e0204890.

68. Gao X, Lo EC, Kot SC, et al. Motivational interviewing in improving oral health: a systematic review of randomized controlled trials. *J Periodontol*. 2014;85:426–437.

69. Kopp SL, Ramseier CA, Ratka-Krüger P, et al. Motivational interviewing as an adjunct to periodontal therapy—a systematic review. *Front Psychol*. 2017;8:279.

70. Gillam DG, Yusuf H. Brief motivational interviewing in dental practice. *Dent J (Basel)*. 2019;7:51.

5

What We Do: Interventions for Procedural Pain and Anxiety

Preparatory Questions for Chapter 5
1. What are the procedures in your specialty that arouse physical or emotional discomfort or distress? How do you help patients minimize and manage these experiences?
2. Recall experiences in which patients were distressed due to pain or anxiety. How did that impact you? Now recall experiences of challenging procedures in which patients were comfortable and appreciative. What were these experiences like for you in comparison?

3. Are there situations in your specialty when it is necessary or appropriate to ignore a patient's pain or anxiety? If so, what situations would justify this?

As a dentist, I have always tried my best to help my patients feel comfortable while I treat them. Yet there have always been patients who—no matter what I do (or avoid doing)—complain of pain during procedures. I could bathe these patients in lidocaine, and it would not be enough! Managing pain during and after medical and dental procedures requires more than just administrating adequate local anesthesia or avoiding injury (although, these are important). It requires a multi-pronged (not literally, please!) approach. Unfortunately, many health care professionals (HCPs) still operate with a model of pain that is entirely mechanical and ignore the many factors that influence pain perception. In the words of the beloved physician and bioethicist Eric Cassell:

> *An anachronistic division of the human condition into what is medical (having to do with the body) and what is nonmedical (the remainder) has given medicine too narrow a notion of its calling. Because of this division, physicians may, in concentrating on the cure of the bodily disease, do things that cause the patient as a person to suffer.*[1]

Leaders in health care call for a change: "A cultural shift must occur at both an organizational level and at a personal level, one in which all HCPs view every procedure as a potentially painful experience for the patient, not merely a task to be performed by the HCP," and, furthermore, HCPs are called to provide "procedural comfort management" for every procedure.[2]

Medical and dental procedures, particularly those without general anesthesia or sedation, present patients with a minefield of opportunities for pain and anxiety. They range from minimally invasive procedures, such as vaccinations and radiographs, to more invasive ones, such as a biopsy, tooth extraction, or joint replacement. Procedures can be for the purpose of diagnosis, treatment, palliation, or rehabilitation and can take place in a variety of settings, including hospitals, ambulatory care centers, doctor's offices, and even at home.

PROCEDURAL PAIN

A web search of "interventions for procedural pain" yielded surprising results. Almost all articles, videos, and books I found pertained to the pediatric patient. This focus on children at the exclusion of adults is likely because children are less cooperative when they experience pain, resulting in more time, effort, and ultimately the need for sedation or restraint. The lack of attention to adults' procedural pain is evident not only in the research literature but also in practice, as reported in a position statement in the *Journal of Pain*

Management Nursing: "Few patients undergoing procedures such as venipuncture, intravenous catheter placement, fingerstick lab draws, nasogastric tube placement, or urethral catheterization received any comfort measures."[2] Why aren't adults given more consideration? Is there a belief that adults don't need or want comfort measures? Or perhaps a successful procedure is defined as one in which the patient tolerates enough to "get the job done?"

The Hidden (and Not-So-Hidden) Costs of Procedural Pain

I have heard countless stories of patients who have endured painful dental procedures. Many patients sob as they report being coerced to continue—without empathy, without options, without comfort measures—despite crying out for help. They report experiencing anxiety, fear, and trauma as a result. Unfortunately, many times the HCP doesn't receive feedback on these negative experiences because these patients (like Sally from Chapter 1 and Joyce from Chapter 3) rarely return for more treatment.

Research on the consequences of unmanaged procedural pain offers valuable insights for all HCPs. First, we know that patient satisfaction hinges on their level of comfort both during procedures and postoperatively,[3] as expressed so well by the CEO of a community health center where I worked. After I referred him to a periodontist for treatment of his gum disease, he came back raving about the doctor reporting, "The visit was painless, therefore I know she did a good job."

Next, the evidence clearly shows that procedural pain creates procedural fear and anxiety, with all of its consequent effects (Fig. 5.1). Experts in dental anxiety assert, "The most common way patients develop fear and avoidance of dentistry" is "through direct negative experiences in the dental office."[4] In particular, the negative experience of pain during procedures "has been shown to be a critical component of dental fear."[5] Renowned dental anxiety researcher Dr. Corah reports the opposite is also true: "The most important behavior

Pain ➡ Anxiety

Fig. 5.1 The Effect of Procedural Pain on Anxiety.

[to avoid dental anxiety] is the dentist's dedication to prevent pain."[6]

The fear and anxiety resulting from unmanaged procedural pain take a toll on patients and their providers as well. Fearful patients are more likely to cancel or no-show for their appointments and more likely to discontinue treatment.[7] By avoiding seeking care, fearful patients develop more serious problems, resulting in negative health care experiences, thus fueling more procedural anxiety and a vicious cycle of avoidance.[8,9]

In addition to psychological and behavioral consequences, unmanaged procedural pain causes bad things to happen in the body. For example, pain induces the stress response and its many potentially untoward effects on blood pressure, heart rate, coagulation, blood glucose, immune function, wound healing, and tumor growth.[10] In newborns and young children, whose nervous system is not completely formed, "Recurrent, poorly treated painful episodes can lead to both short and longer term hyper-sensitivity to painful stimuli, which persists into later life."[11] For patients of all ages, procedural pain can affect future procedures. "If pain is not anticipated and prevented or treated appropriately…pain levels may be higher with subsequent procedures."[2] Postoperative pain in orthopedic patients "decreases early rehabilitation and long-term joint function."[12] A review study reports that procedural pain and anxiety affect "morbidity, duration of hospital stay, and even mortality," adding, "Alleviating these factors may also lead to earlier discharge from the hospital, and thus may reduce health care costs."[13] The many consequences of unmanaged procedural pain underscore the importance of minimizing and managing pain during medical and dental procedures.

Preventing Pain: Avoiding Injury and Local Anesthetics

One general way the HCP can minimize pain during procedures is by avoiding generating pain signals from tissue injury, and this can be accomplished in several ways. First, be gentle. *Mindful procedural touch,* as described in Chapter 4, is especially warranted for procedures dealing with areas of the body that are inflamed (abscessed tooth), injured (broken arm), or intimate (pelvic exam). As an example of the importance of mindful touch, the simple act of turning a patient in the hospital bed—a task many HCPs may not even consider a procedure—was rated the most painful procedure in a study of over 6000 patients in acute and critical care.[14] Second, use *atraumatic technique.*

For example, surgeons can avoid the tearing of soft tissues, and dental hygienists can minimize gingival trauma during the scaling of the teeth. Third, use *equipment* tailored to the size and shape of each patient. Examples include the use of small-gauged needles (including butterfly needles for pediatric blood draws) and appropriately sized digital x-ray sensors (intraoral) and dental impression trays to minimize discomfort.

Unavoidable pain signals can be blocked pharmacologically with local anesthetics. Use *topical anesthetics* whenever possible, such as a eutectic mixture of local anesthetic (EMLA) or topical amethocaine for the skin and topical benzocaine for oral mucosa. Topicals are available in many formulations, including gels, sprays, creams, and patches. Topical anesthesia can be helpful for many medical and dental procedures, including injections, IV cannulation and venipuncture, nasogastric tube insertion, and urinary catheterization.[11] For ear, nose, and throat (ENT) procedures, "For the nasal cavity, cotton pledgets soaked in anesthetic spray and decongestant, or anesthetic gel, are effective. For the pharynx, an anesthetic spray is the most frequently used and effective method. For the larynx, applying local anesthesia through a catheter through the working channel of the endoscope or anesthetic injection through the cricothyroid membrane is effective"[15]; employing such techniques can obviate the need for general anesthesia and make it possible to perform procedures in an outpatient setting.

The main disadvantage of topical anesthetics is the need to wait for the onset of action. To minimize the wait, some alternatives to topical anesthetics include:

- "Injectable bacteriostatic saline or lidocaine using a small-gauge needle (e.g., >27) …for intravenous catheter insertion, suturing, biopsies, and other needlestick procedures"
- "Needleless 'injection' of 1% buffered lidocaine using the J-Tip" for IV catheter insertion.[2]

Injectable Local Anesthetics

Local anesthetics have allowed many procedures to be performed humanely and comfortably. Unfortunately, even when preceded by topical anesthetics, injection of local anesthesia can be painful, especially in sensitive parts of the body like the hands, feet, face, and mouth. Much of the pain of injection has been attributed to the acidity of local anesthetics, particularly those with epinephrine, which are about 1000 times more acidic than subcutaneous tissues.[16] (Local anesthetics are sold in an acidified formula to increase shelf-life.)[17] One simple approach to address injection pain due to local anesthetic acidity is to use a local anesthetic agent without epinephrine, which can be followed by an epinephrine-containing agent if more depth or duration of anesthesia is needed. Another very effective strategy to avoid the discomfort of local anesthesia caused by acidity involves *buffering* (increasing the pH) of the local anesthetic agent.[18]

Buffering has been reported effective in reducing injection pain in many specialties, including plastic surgery,[16] emergency medicine,[19] ophthalmology,[17,20] and dentistry.[21] Buffering of lidocaine with sodium bicarbonate is currently "commonplace for anesthetizing sensitive portions of the body such as the breasts, with evidence supporting reduced pain and anxiety during breast procedures."[22] In addition to reducing injection pain and anxiety, buffering offers two additional benefits: *quicker onset time* and the ability to *anesthetize infected tissues*, where non-buffered anesthetics are mostly ineffective.[21,23]

A standard recipe for buffered lidocaine consists of 1 mL of 8.4% sodium bicarbonate (a standard medical formulation) to 10 mL of 1% lidocaine,[16,24] resulting in about a 10% buffering agent concentration. Ratios as low as 1:40 sodium bicarbonate to lidocaine (2.5% buffering agent) have been found effective for pain reduction.[24] A 1:10 lidocaine to bicarbonate ratio "will change the mildly acidic pH of lidocaine toward a more physiological range without apparent precipitation or denaturation of the compound."[24] For clinicians using 1.8 mL local anesthetic cartridges (as in dentistry), a simple way to buffer is to add 0.1 mL 8.4% sodium bicarbonate directly to a local anesthetic cartridge.[21] This can be done easily by aspirating 0.1 mL (or 10 units) sodium bicarbonate into an insulin syringe and injecting this into the local anesthetic cartridge (which has some empty space to accommodate the added fluid volume), resulting in about a 6% concentration of the buffering agent. A small amount of lidocaine can also be expelled first to make room for more sodium bicarbonate and thus a higher concentration of buffering agent. Images of the 8.4% sodium bicarbonate and an insulin syringe, are shown in Fig. 5.2.

While the smallest available vial of 8.4% sodium bicarbonate is currently 50 mL, 4.2% is available in 5 mL vials (but requires twice as much volume to achieve the necessary pH range).[22] You can watch a demonstration of how to buffer local anesthesia by clicking the following link: https://youtu.be/5BxYfkTDZkM. There is also a mixing system developed by Onpharma that uses a specialized mixing pen.

Buffering local anesthesia has not been found to introduce unwanted side effects or increase postoperative complications, such as bleeding, swelling, or pain.[17] In addition to buffering, *warming* a buffered local anesthetic agent was found to significantly decrease pain for intradermal injections when compared to plain lidocaine, buffered lidocaine, and warmed, unbuffered lidocaine.[25]

> Note: When local anesthesia is buffered, its shelf life decreases significantly, so it must be used immediately after buffering.

Finally, injection comfort can be enhanced by *slow administration* of local. This can be accomplished with a traditional syringe or with special devices. A microprocessor-controlled delivery system[26] (the Wand) provides

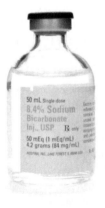
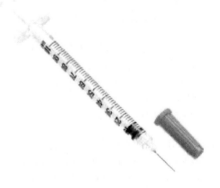

Fig. 5.2 Sodium Bicarbonate and Insulin Syringe.

a slow constant rate of local anesthetic injection with a pen-like handpiece. The Wand has been proven to be less painful than traditional injection techniques in dentistry[27] as well as eyelid surgery.[28]

More Than Just Stimulus and Response: Gate Control Theory of Pain

Although local anesthesia, as well as mindful touch, atraumatic technique, and properly-sized equipment, are all are very important and work well for many patients, they don't manage procedural pain all the time. Through the years, I have encountered many dental patients for whom no amount of numbing medication or numbing techniques work—whether I use a little or a lot, cold or warm, fast or slow, buffered or unbuffered, these patients will still complain of pain or discomfort, sometimes even before I touch their tooth! Unfortunately, many HCPs, in their attempts to control procedural pain, stop here. It seems the prevailing approach to procedural pain control is based on a model of pain as simply a direct response to a physical stimulus. This model logically leads to an approach to procedural pain management limited to pharmacologic means (anesthetics and analgesics) and avoiding tissue injury (mindful touch, atraumatic technique, proper equipment). Unfortunately, this pain model is incomplete, inaccurate, and aligns with a centuries-old theory of pain—one that has long been disproven.

The Specificity Theory of Pain, proposed by Descartes in 1664, depicted the mind and body as completely separate and described pain as an entirely physical phenomenon whereby a pain stimulus generates a signal which is detected by a pain receptor in the brain.[29] Yet, evidence shows pain is much more complex. For example, a doctor in World War II noted that anxious patients required more opioids than severely injured calm patients.[30] In addition, "The degree of pain reported does not depend exclusively on the extent of the tissue injury."[31] Descartes' model also fails to explain how pain can be reduced by a placebo medication, and it fails to explain the phenomenon of phantom pain, whereby pain is perceived from a part of the body that no longer exists, as from an amputated limb.

More than 50 years ago, a new theory helped to explain the complex nature of pain perception, and today it is still "accepted as common knowledge."[32] The Gate Control Theory of Pain, proposed by Melzack and Wall

in 1965, has profound practical implications for all HCPs. In their words,

Evidence fails to support the assumption of a one-to-one relationship between pain perception and intensity of the stimulus. Instead, the evidence suggests that the amount and quality of perceived pain are determined by many psychological variables in addition to the sensory input.[33]

According to this theory, "There is a transmission station in the spinal cord that influences the flow of nerve impulses to the brain,"[29] and this transmission station is called a "gate." Fig. 5.3 depicts a pain signal originating from the mouth and traveling to the brain.

There are two general ways to *close the gate* for transmission of pain signals from the site of the stimulus to the brain: "bottom-up" and "top-down." Bottom-up approaches consist of non-pain sensations in the same area as the pain sensations. Thus, during a painful medical procedure, such as an injection, pain perception can be lessened by providing other stimuli such as pressure, cold, or vibration in the same area (more in the upcoming section on non-pain stimuli). The second means of closing the gate is top-down: "The brain can send electrical messages down nerve pathways to close the gate and shut out or reduce the flow of nerve impulses to the brain…for example, positive mood, distraction, and deep relaxed breathing can act to close or partially close the gate"; conversely, "Strong emotions like fear, anxiety, and expecting the worst can open the gate."[29] The top-down means of closing the gate are rated as the most influential: "Of these contributors to a patients' perception of pain, the psychological factors—especially anxiety—show the

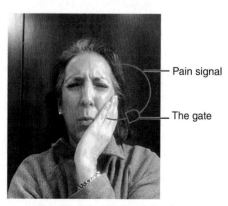

Fig. 5.3 Pain Signal and the Gate.

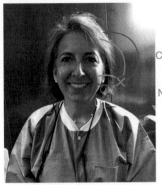

Cognitive/psychological factors
("top down")

Non-pain sensations
("bottom up")

Fig. 5.4 Two General Ways to Close the Gate.

strongest association."[34] Fig. 5.4 illustrates the two general ways of closing the gate.

Gate control theory fundamentally changed our understanding of pain perception. The main shift is the realization that "Pain is not injury…it's our brain's assessment of danger. That's why there is no exact relationship between how strong a stimulus is, the amount of injury it causes if any, and the amount of pain we feel."[29] Further, "Anxiety, depression, worry, and other psychological factors which had been considered 'reactions to pain' came to be viewed as integral to processing of pain-related information."[32]

So, when an HCP ignores the many psychological factors that contribute to pain perception (e.g., anxiety, depression, worry) and considers only mechanical contributors to pain (intensity of stimulus/tissue injury) and pharmacologic means to block pain signals (local anesthesia), they are operating with a pain model from 1664—analogous to using leeches to treat an infection! *The validation of gate control theory should inspire and impel all HCPs to consider the many non-pharmacologic means to avoid opening the gate and the many means to close the gate to pain transmission.* Now, let's explore the psychological factor that affects pain the most, *anxiety*.

Note: Gate control theory has been more recently expanded into the Neuromatrix Theory of Pain. Neuromatrix theory does not negate or invalidate gate theory, but rather it refines and expands the model to explain other pain phenomena such as chronic pain and phantom pain.[35] For the purposes of this chapter, we will focus on Melzack's pain model in its earlier, simpler iteration, gate control.

UNDERSTANDING AND ASSESSING PROCEDURAL ANXIETY

Anxiety and pain perception are closely linked. Numerous studies have found significant correlations between anxiety and self-reported pain both *during* procedures[36,37] and *postoperatively.*[38–43] A systematic review reports that in fact, "Anxiety was *the most common predictor* of postoperative pain and was shown to have a positive correlation with pain intensity" (emphasis added).[44]

Does the increased pain associated with higher anxiety translate into more pain medication use? Indeed, researchers report, "The higher the preoperative anxiety the greater requirement of postoperative analgesia."[38] A review article on anxiety in interventional radiology procedures reports, "Procedural anxiety has been found to increase the use of medications and lengthen procedure time."[45]

Gate control theory explains how anxiety increases pain perception (Fig. 5.5)—by opening the gate to pain transmission. Further, reducing anxiety closes the gate to pain (Fig. 5.6) and reduces both the need for anesthesia and analgesia[38] and mortality risk after surgery.[46]

To better understand how to reduce procedural anxiety, let's first look at what makes patients anxious about procedures, who is most likely to be anxious, and how to identify these individuals and their fears.

What Evokes Procedural Anxiety?

According to research, there is a particular time that is most stressful for patients—the time immediately *before procedures.*[47] There is also a particular procedure in medicine and dentistry that is almost universally feared—*injections.* In fact, needles are rated as one of the top ten fears of all fears (including non-medical ones like snakes and fear of heights).[48] An estimated 4% of the US population has a specific phobia called *blood-injection-injury*; these patients "experience marked and persistent fear or apprehension when confronted with stimuli such as blood, injuries, wounds, mutilations,

Pain ⟵ Anxiety

Fig. 5.5 Effect of Anxiety on Pain (a).

↓ Pain ⟵ ↓ Anxiety

Fig. 5.6 Effect of Anxiety on Pain (b).

needles, or injections."[49] Researchers report the most commonly feared procedure in dentistry is the injection of local anesthesia.[50,51]

Dental research has much to offer on the topic of procedural anxiety, given that "dental care has historically been characterized as generating more fear and anxiety than other forms of health care."[52] During dental procedures, "Helplessness and distress may be triggered lying in a defensive position, the dentist bending over from behind with instruments and hands in the patient's mouth, inhibiting verbal exchange."[53] (An excellent resource for people with dental phobia and dental fear can be found at www.dentalfearcentral.org.) A literature review cites the following sources of procedural anxiety and phobia in dentistry:

Previous negative or traumatic experience, especially in childhood (conditioning experiences), vicarious learning from anxious family members or peers, individual personality characteristics such as neuroticism and self-consciousness, lack of understanding, exposure to frightening portrayals of dentists in the media, the coping style of the person, perception of body image, and the vulnerable position of lying back in a dental chair.[54]

The anxiety of parents/caregivers of children (and special needs patients) can fuel anxiety in the patient, as noted above. Many times, I have witnessed parents of my dental patients making potentially triggering comments in front of their children like, "I hate the dentist, it always hurts." Research has found parental anxiety correlates with their children's pain *during* procedures (e.g., intravenous cannulation)[55] and with *pre- and postoperative pain.*[56] Therefore, "Targeting parents' preprocedural anxiety might be beneficial to the parents as well as the children undergoing a distressing medical procedure."[57]

Deborah Jastrebski, founder of Practice without Pressure (PWP), a method of companioning special needs people through medical and dental procedures, reports anxiety is common in caregivers, parents, and guardians (CPG) of people who have struggled with previous procedures, and she affirms the challenges posed by this. Here are some of her recommendations to HCPs and their team:

- *Reassure* the CPG starting before coming in and every step of the way ("We will work through this")
- *Take leadership* of the procedure ("Let us take the lead")
- Set limits (e.g., separating CPG from the patient at times, using hand signals to indicate no talking)
- Engage the CPG in *modeling* procedures for the patient[58] (more on modeling in the section on gradual exposure).

Of all the sources of procedural anxiety and fear, "*Direct negative experiences* in the dental office" are "the most common way patients develop fear and avoidance of dentistry" (emphasis added).[4,7] Medical reports echo the findings that procedural anxiety originates from *previous negative health care experiences.*[59] Such information underscores the importance of providing comfort measures to minimize pain and anxiety during medical and dental procedures.

The Effects of Trauma and Abuse on Procedural Anxiety

In addition to a history of negative health care experiences, trauma unrelated to health care is also a predictor of procedural anxiety. Examples of traumatic events include "child abuse or neglect, domestic violence, sexual assault, elder abuse, and exposure to combat."[60] Trauma can occur in different ways, including "directly experiencing or witnessing a traumatic event, or learning that the event occurred to a family member or close friend."[61] (Based on this definition, anyone who consumes a regular diet of news media may have some degree of trauma!) Patients from ethnic groups who have a history of medical maltreatment may experience anxiety about receiving substandard care or of being harmed during a procedure. Note that people who experience trauma related to poverty, racism, or war may not have the chance to have closure on a traumatic event if they continue to live in the oppressive conditions associated with the event.[61] People with special needs and children whose parents are stressed due to poverty or depression are at higher risk for abuse.[60] For trauma survivors, health care experiences that are negative or insensitive to their needs can result in feeling revictimized, resulting in what is called "secondary victimization."[60]

As a public health dentist dealing mostly with patients of lower socioeconomic levels and minority populations, I was never surprised by the high rates of trauma and abuse among my patients, knowing the potentially traumatizing effects of poverty and racism. What did surprise me was the prevalence of trauma in the general population of the United States. In the United States, "10 to 20 percent of men… reported combat exposure" and "one in every five U.S. women… reported having been sexually assaulted as an adult."[60]

Trauma often leaves long-term physiologic and psychologic effects. For example, "Traumatic events, particularly recurrent trauma over the lifespan can cause the sympathetic nervous system and the hypothalamic-pituitary-adrenal axis to become chronically activated."[62] In addition to physiologic consequences, patients with a history of trauma may also experience anxiety and fear extending far beyond the common fears such as needles and injections. Many medical and dental procedures—due to the invasion of personal space, the need to touch, and the vulnerable position of patients—trigger fears and the memories of trauma in survivors. Research from dentistry has reported significantly higher dental fear scores in patients exposed to sexual abuse compared to the general population.[63]

The woman in the next recording (Video 5.1) is a survivor of childhood abuse. Listen to her description of what triggers her anxiety during health care encounters. The two main triggers for this survivor include touch, namely "being handled roughly," and the HCP's voice when it is "mean, harsh, or uncaring."

Trauma-informed care requires universal precautions—assuming every patient has experienced some type of trauma until proven otherwise. Patient-centered communication (including the ISLEEP skills) and other interventions for procedural pain and anxiety (IPPAs) help create a sense of safety, agency, and trust with trauma survivors and all patients.

Questions for Reflection:
1. As an HCP, how do you know if a patient is anxious before, during, and after a procedure?
2. Researchers have noted, "When providers are themselves survivors of traumatic events, they may feel uncomfortable talking about these issues for fear of retriggering their own feelings."[60] Do you have a history of trauma, yourself? If so, how does this impact your ability to address your patients' trauma?

Screening for Anxiety, Trauma, and Abuse

Patients benefit from "early identification and assessment" of anxiety and phobia.[53] Several written scales and questionnaires have been developed in medicine and dentistry that can be very helpful in uncovering patients' procedural anxiety. The gold standard for many years has been the State-Trait Anxiety Inventory (STAI).[64] Because of its length, however (20 questions), this scale may not be practical to many clinicians. In contrast, a one-item self-report instrument called the Visual Analog Scale for Anxiety (VAS-A) shown in Fig. 5.7 allows for easy identification of patients with high procedural anxiety.[47] The VAS-A consists of a 0 to 100 scale on which the patient simply marks a point on a 100 mm line.

Values above 46 are considered clinically meaningful.[65] This scale has been proven valid and correlates significantly with a dental questionnaire called the Corah Dental Anxiety Scale.[65]

Could an anxiety questionnaire increase anxiety? Several studies have investigated the effects of administering the Modified Dental Anxiety Scale (MDAS), the gold standard for dental anxiety screening.[66] Research shows that the MDAS not only did increase state anxiety[67–69] but was actually associated with *decreased* state anxiety when comparing pre- to postoperative anxiety scores.[70] Further, studies have tested the impact of a patient handing their completed MDAS to the different members of the care team. A randomized controlled trial (RCT) found significantly lower postoperative anxiety in patients who handed their MDAS *directly to the dentist* compared with patients who handed it to the receptionist.[71] Further, a study found significantly lower dental anxiety 3 months later in patients "who were provided 'space' to *discuss their anxiety*" (emphasis added); it seems the key element is to "respond to the patient…rather than passively noting the dental anxiety rating."[70]

In addition to an anxiety scale before any procedure, the HCP should obtain two other key pieces of information: first, patients' *specific worries and fears* related to

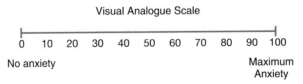

Fig. 5.7 Visual Analogue Scale for Anxiety. (Source: Kindler CH, Harms C, Amsler F, et al. The visual analog scale. *Anesth Analg.* 2000;90:706–712.)

the procedure, and second, *what would make them more comfortable*, including patients' own remedies. These questions can be asked either verbally or in writing. The following form (Fig. 5.8) provides a simple, efficient way to gather this essential information before procedures (also found in Appendix K).

The form above can be customized to your health care specialty. For example, for Question #2, you might list some of the common fears of patients you treat, such as fear of needles or disrobing during procedures. Among trauma survivors, common fears include "having their bodies exposed, fear of powerlessness or being alone with an unknown provider, fear of having something inserted into their body, fear of not being able to breathe/swallow, fear of being touched."[62] Dental patients with a history of sexual abuse commonly fear "having to lie down for treatment, having objects put into their mouths, the dentists' hand over the mouth or nose, not being able to breathe or swallow and worry that the dentist may get angry."[60] Under Question #3 ("What can we do to make you more comfortable"), you might also list specific comfort measures your team can offer, such as

music, a warm blanket, and sunglasses; but, only include things you can provide consistently.

While routine screening of trauma is appropriate and commonly performed by primary care and mental health professionals, it is not recommended for all HCPs. One study, for example, found that childhood sexual abuse survivors "felt it would be inappropriate for a dentist to ask a direct question about abuse," but "most advocated for the inclusion of more limited forms of inquiry that included *questions about patients' discomfort or sensitivity with components of the exam or treatment* such as disrobing and touch of specific body parts" (emphasis added).[72] Question #2 of the preprocedural screening form above would satisfy this wish.

Experts suggest that any HCP who works with high-risk populations should perform routine screening for trauma and abuse. A recommended tool to screen for childhood trauma is the Adverse Childhood Experiences (ACEs) Questionnare, which can be found at https://www.chcs.org/media/TA-Tool-Screening-for-ACEs-and-Trauma_020619.pdf and in Appendix L.

Preprocedural Screening

Because anxiety, trauma, and abuse are common and affect one's health and health care experiences, we ask all patients the following questions:

1) Please mark on the line your level of anxiety about your upcoming procedure.

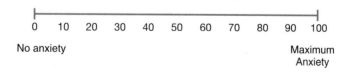

No anxiety   Maximum Anxiety

2) What worries you about your upcoming procedure? _____

3) What can we do or offer you to make you more comfortable? _____

4) Is there anything else you would like us to know? _____

NOTE: The information you share is confidential and will enable us to care for you in a way that is more sensitive to your needs.

Fig. 5.8 Preprocedural Screening for Anxiety.

The ACEs Questionnaire consists of 10 questions, such as, "Did a parent or other adult in the household often or very often…Swear at you, insult you, put you down, or humiliate you? or Act in a way that made you afraid that you might be physically hurt?" and "Did you live with anyone who was a problem drinker or alcoholic or who used street drugs?" The questions are answered with a yes or no, but to allow for more privacy, patients may be given the option to simply tally their total number of yesses out of the possible 10. For the patient who discloses a history of trauma or abuse in the past or the present, be prepared to follow up with additional questions and local referral resources. For current referral resources in the United States, visit the National Center for Domestic Violence, Trauma, and Mental Health website at http://www.nationalcenterdvtraumamh.org/survivors/.

In summary, minimizing procedural pain brings many benefits, including reduced anxiety, reduced need for medication, reduced untoward physiologic reactions, reduced stress to the HCP, and, best of all increased satisfaction to patients and providers alike. There are three main ways to reduce pain, including:

1. *Minimize painful stimuli* with mindful touch, atraumatic technique, proper equipment, and local anesthesia (bottom-up).
2. *Apply non-pain stimuli* (bottom-up).
3. *Manage psychological factors,* namely, reducing anxiety and increasing relaxation (top-down).

Pain and anxiety are so closely intertwined that they are inextricable. Earlier, we saw that minimizing procedural pain also minimizes patients' procedural anxiety. Gate control explains how the reverse is also true—reducing anxiety diminishes pain perception by closing the gate on pain signals. This bidirectional relationship between pain and anxiety (Fig. 5.9) makes it difficult, if not impossible, to classify specific interventions as either pain management or anxiety management. Therefore, the general techniques described next and the more specific techniques described later in this chapter will all be classified as "interventions for procedural pain and anxiety management." Let's now take a look at

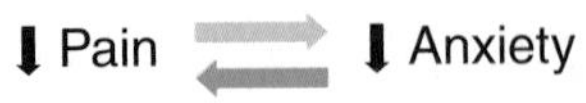

Fig. 5.9 Bidirectional Relationship Between Procedural Anxiety and Pain.

a variety of bottom-up and top-down means of reducing pain and anxiety.

INTERVENTIONS FOR PROCEDURAL PAIN AND ANXIETY

Many approaches have been explored to manage procedural anxiety and pain, not all of which are ideal for all medical and dental procedures. *Pharmacologic approaches* to pain and anxiety management, while they can be helpful at times, introduce risks of medication side effects and drug interactions as well as medication costs. Oversedation "can increase procedural risks by depressing the cardiovascular and respiratory systems"[45] and can "delay the patient's recovery."[73] Finally, the opioid overdose epidemic, which has wreaked havoc on our society, highlights the importance of seeking non-pharmacologic approaches to pain and anxiety management.

Many *psychological techniques* are available, such as systematic desensitization and cognitive rehearsal, but they may not be practical because they require significant time outside of the procedure.[74] Hypnosis has also been shown very helpful in managing procedural pain and anxiety, especially in burn care,[75,76] and while it may not require a lot of time outside of the procedure, it does require special training for the practitioner.

The interventions for procedural pain and anxiety (IPPAs) included in this chapter are non-pharmacological, time-efficient, cost-effective, and simple to employ during tests and procedures. The Joint Commission "supports a multimodal approach using both pharmacologic and non-pharmacologic strategies to effectively manage pain."[77] My wish is for you to acquire a varied and rich repertoire of tools that you and your whole team can draw on to facilitate comfortable, pleasant experiences for your patients and yourselves as well.

General Strategies: Provider Demeanor and Office Environment

Before discussing specific interventions, let's discuss general approaches that have been shown to reduce anxiety and pain: first, the general *demeanor* of the HCP and the whole team. It is "extremely important that the clinician assume a calm, confident demeanor and not appear hurried."[78] A study of 250 dental patients measured the correlation between dentist behaviors and two dependent variables: reduction in anxiety and patient satisfaction; calm manner correlated with both.[6] Calm demeanor is especially important when sharing relaxation techniques with patients as reported by dentist and meditation teacher, Dr. John Lovas. "Dentist-directed relaxation techniques are considered to be most effective when the dentist teaches the technique primarily by embodying its result."[79] Not only the HCP but *every member of the health care team* contributes to the patient's experience of care by embodying calm.

In addition to the general demeanor of the team members, many aspects of the *office atmosphere* can contribute to a calm and comfortable experience. Consider the many sights, sounds (including the words you use), and smells of your office. A review article on anxiety reduction during interventional radiology procedures offers many strategies including "avoid holding patients in high-traffic, noisy areas."[45] When fear-inducing instruments or equipments are needed, like needles and scalpels, keep them out of sight, and avoid talking about them openly in ways patients can understand. For example, a skilled dental assistant would avoid asking the dentist within earshot of the patient, "Do you want a long or a short needle?" or "What kind of scalpel?" (unfortunately this has happened before!). Other general office environment strategies include soft music, avoiding bright lights, muting the sounds of treatment with doors, office décor, and scents such as lavender.[54]

Offer *comfort measures* when possible. For example, when bright lights are unavoidable, provide sunglasses. When patients must disrobe, provide soft textiles, warm ambient temperature, and/or warm blankets. Finally, whenever possible, allow the patient to be in an upright position, as this "promotes a sense of control and security."[80]

Experiment

Invite everyone on your team to take a tour of your office as if you were the patient. From the entrance of the building or office to the reception room, the treatment areas, and everything in between.

- *Notice what you see, smell, hear, and touch. Notice the temperature (too cold, too hot?)*
- Try changing into the clothing (gown, drape, etc.) you offer to your patients.
- If your patients are required to lie down at any point, notice the view from that place and position.
- Make a list of items that could potentially arouse anxiety or cause discomfort.

Brainstorm with your team possible ideas for enhancing the patient experience. Have fun, be creative!

Now, let's focus on the following interventions for procedural pain and anxiety (IPPAs):

- ISLEEP Communication Skills
- Progressive Muscle Relaxation
- Diaphragmatic Breathing
- Mindfulness of the Breath and Body
- Gradual Exposure
- Non-pain Stimuli
- Distraction
- Mental Imagery
- Nonverbal Communication
- Touch: Expressive, Mindful Procedural, and Reiki
- Postoperative Communication

Returning to the tree metaphor once more, let's tie together what we have learned in previous chapters and see where the IPPAs fall into the tree model. Fig. 5.10 shows the relationship between what we are (EASE [equanimity, attentiveness, self-awareness, and empathy]), what we say (ISLEEP), and what we do (IPPAs). Through regular mindfulness practice, we cultivate the qualities of mindfulness or EASE. When we are mindful, we are better able to discern and be motivated to meet the needs of each patient, moment by moment. The fruits and flowers of mindfulness are our words (ISLEEP) and our actions (IPPAs). Table 5.1 includes a mnemonic to help remember these eleven categories of IPPAs.

Aside from non-pain stimuli and touch, which are bottom-up approaches to pain management, all the other interventions are top-down. Whether the HCP acknowledges it or not, there are many potential forces both on the patient's end and on the HCP's end that can inadvertently open the gate to pain transmission. These top-down forces account for the wide range of pain perception that patients experience with the same procedure. The interventions we will discuss can help counteract and reverse such gate-opening forces. For example, a patient's future-oriented, catastrophizing thoughts, like, "I won't be able to handle the pain," will have the effect of opening the gate; *mindfulness* will help close the gate by centering in the present. As another example, coercing a patient to do something uncomfortable will open the gate, but offering the patient the option to stop—ISLEEP skill *power*—and *gradual exposure* can counteract this effect. Lastly, the gate-opening effects of feeling alone or minimized can be avoided with *empathy* (ISLEEP skill), *touch*, and *postoperative communication*.

Each of the above techniques will be accompanied by videos to illustrate specific applications. The dental

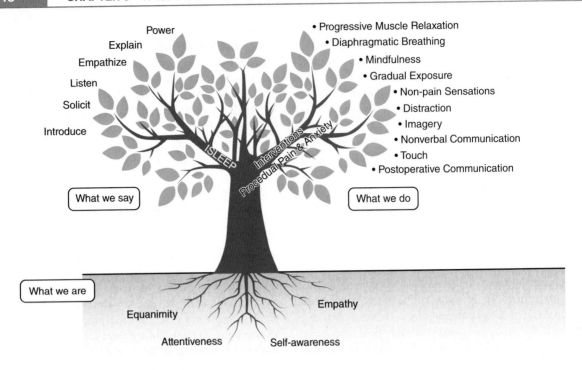

Fig. 5.10 Tree Metaphor Including What We Are, What We Say, and What We Do.

TABLE 5.1 Mnemonic for Interventions for Procedural Pain and Anxiety (IPPAs)	
IPPA	**Mnemonic**
ISLEEP skills	Inflicting
Progressive muscle relaxation	Pain
Diaphragmatic breathing	Doesn't
Mindfulness	Make
Gradual exposure	Guests
Non-pain stimuli	Nice
Distraction	Doing
Imagery	Interventions
Nonverbal communication	Needed
Touch	To
Postoperative communication	Please

profession provides many opportunities for pain and anxiety and, thus, an abundance of opportunities to employ IPPAs. Through the generosity of my dental patients, I can offer videos demonstrating these techniques in live patient encounters in the dental setting.

Even if you are not a dental professional, you are likely familiar with the dental setting as a patient and may be able to relate to the scenarios depicted. My hope is that you will be inspired to explore your own unique applications of these interventions in your own health care setting.

First, let's listen to what my patient Nicholas has to say about the question, *"What helped you overcome severe anxiety and pain during dental procedures"* (Video 5.2 from 0 to 3:30). Nicholas describes several techniques that helped him, including a non-pain stimulus (shaking the cheek) and diaphragmatic breathing—"when you told me to take the deep breaths, the pain was less." Both techniques will be discussed in more depth soon. Of all the factors that put him at ease, Nicholas' favorite is clearly the ISLEEP skill *explain*, so let's start with ISLEEP skills as an intervention for procedural pain and anxiety.

ISLEEP Communication Skills

According to research, the ISLEEP skills from Chapter 3 have the effect of decreasing pain and anxiety and therefore can function as *anxiolytics* and *analgesics* during procedures—without having to take a pill! Here's what a review of 51 studies and more than 5000 patients found: that providing patients information (ISLEEP skill *explain*), as well as being empathetic and positive are all important "to *reduce pain* intensity" (emphasis added).[81]

Explain

Let's start with Nicholas' favorite ISLEEP skill. In Video 5.2 above, he describes the importance of *explaining*, and he defines very clearly the things he likes to have explained to him: "*What's going to happen before you do it…prewarning me of pain, and what I can do to alleviate it.*" A position statement by the American Society for Pain Management Nursing asserts: "The lack of acknowledgment by HCPs that pain may occur during or after a procedure" comprises *one of the most important determinants of pain* because it precludes "the necessary anticipation, prevention, and management of potential or actual procedural pain" (emphasis added).[2] On the other hand, "Explaining and preparing the patient provides an opportunity to inform the patient about what will occur and what to expect…this serves to reduce the patient's anxiety and provides cues about how to cope with the situation."[74] This reduction in anxiety that results from explaining is the likely mechanism for reducing pain, according to gate control theory.

Note that more is *not* always better when it comes to explaining. Recall the story of the oral surgery resident in Chapter 3 who scared a patient by explaining how he was going to "flap the gum and file down the bone." This is an example of too much information. So, try to tailor the level of detail and amount of information to the patient's needs and tolerance level.

For the patient with a traumatic history, explaining is essential and should include which body parts will be touched during an examination or procedure.[62] Explaining to such patients, "You can trust me, you are safe" can actually trigger fear and anxiety because in many cases the perpetrators of the abuse said similar words "when just the opposite was true."[82] Trust is not asserted but rather something earned by acting trustworthy over a period of time.

Introduce/Interconnect

The ISLEEP skill *introduce/interconnect* can greatly impact procedural pain and anxiety. Martha B, CNM, describes the experience of her patient in the OR right before a complicated surgery:

> *The entire team who would be working in the OR came and stood around her and introduced themselves briefly and had a moment of pause and intention and a kind of prayer (not specific to any religion) together with the patient. She describes her anxiety reducing as she felt they saw her, cared about her outcome, and were going to do their absolute best for her.*

Solicit

People with a history of anxiety, trauma, or abuse don't present with a sign on them saying, "I have a trauma history," nor do they usually volunteer these issues, as we discussed in Chapter 3. Such patients may appear calm, cool, and collected. Many times, my dental residents are surprised when I tell them the patient whom they just treated has severe anxiety or has a trauma history: "I would have never known… the patient seemed so at ease," reported one resident. People often hide their fears, and, without skillful soliciting, the HCP will not uncover important issues that color a patient's experience.

The following patient with a history of childhood abuse has a request for all HCPs pertaining to the ISLEEP skill *solicit* (Video 5.1a from 14:05 to end). Although this individual fears she would "shut down" if she were asked directly about her childhood abuse, she definitely wants her HCP to know about her anxiety, and she would like to share about it both verbally and in writing.

Before a procedure, the HCP can ask about "what 'rules' you need me to follow and what coping strategies might be useful for you."[53] As discussed in Chapter 3, *soliciting* with open-ended questions such as, "How anxious are you about today's visit?" or "What bothers you most," may be more effective than a yes-or-no question. Some patients, however, may be reticent no matter how the question is asked. For such patients, it may be more effective to solicit fears in writing before a procedure, such as a questionnaire. The woman in the previous audio recording reports, "If I write it then it's easier to talk about."

During a medical or dental procedure, the HCP can *solicit* the patient's comfort level such as, "Are you okay? How are you doing?" Patients appreciate it when HCPs check in frequently, especially during uncomfortable procedures. When the HCP knows what is anxiety-producing or painful to the patient in the moment, there is the opportunity to adjust, offer comfort measures, and express empathy.

Empathize/Validate

What do you do with the information you have solicited about anxiety, trauma, or abuse? *Empathizing and validating* the patient's fears provides a means to not only comfort but even to reduce pain, as evidenced by a study of patients in oncology wards: "Development of the nurse-patient empathic communication is very important for patients because it relieves mental stress, *reduces anxiety*, gives *pain control*, and increases emotional compatibility and hope (emphasis added)."[83]

Video 5.4 shows my colleague, Dr. Garces, a highly rated dentist, in a reenactment of a real consultation with a patient (played by myself). The patient was an active, middle-aged man who presented with the request to remove all his teeth and make complete dentures. Through her skillful soliciting, listening, empathizing, and validating, Dr. Garces was able to learn important things about the patient. Although he seemed so calm and cool, he was actually extremely anxious due to the trauma he had experienced at multiple points in his life. Dr. Garces and I both viewed this patient's radiographs with wet eyes as we identified metal plates in his facial bones—the result of injuries sustained during repeated assaults in childhood by a family member.

At the time this was recorded, Dr. Garces was not yet familiar with the ISLEEP model, yet this interaction demonstrates all the ISLEEP skills. Her strongest skill in my view is *empathize/validate*. Video 5.3 provides a brief background to the scenario in Video 5.4.

> **Exercise:**
> See if you can identify the ISLEEP skills captured in this Video 5.4. Identify the words and the nonverbal communication that convey empathy and validation of the patient. See Appendix M for an outline of the ISLEEP skills demonstrated in this dialogue.

A couple of notes about this scenario: first, the patient did not disclose everything immediately, and this is a common pattern. Because of this, the HCP must be gentle yet persistent while sensing and respecting when a patient does not want to disclose more. Fortunately, in this case, Dr. Garces was patient yet persistent in her inquiry. After several rounds of *soliciting, listening,* and *empathizing,* she was able to uncover the most severe trauma of this patient, enabling her to offer care for his concerns. Finally, as we saw earlier, the words, "You're safe with me" or "You can trust me," as Dr. G told this patient, can be triggering to a survivor of abuse because many times, they heard the same words from their abusers. Luckily, this patient was not deterred by these words. In fact, he returned to the clinic shortly after this initial consultation with Dr. G. Not only was he able to undergo impressions and extractions, but he even asked to do more the same visit since he was feeling so well! This is a great example of how the mindful presence of the HCP and skillful use of ISLEEP communication skills can forge a bond of trust in a short time that overcomes even great obstacles.

Power of the Patient

Arguably the most important ISLEEP skill for managing procedural pain and anxiety is affirming the *power* of the patient, especially for a patient with a history of trauma. "Trauma survivors often report that a lack of control in medical settings increases their anxiety,"[62] as well as affects "their sense of safety and treatment adherence."[84] A sense of perceived control minimizes fear *even in the face of pain* because "pain experienced by a patient in control is not likely to lead to fear," as dental fear experts report.[4]

Perceived control of pain not only reduces anxiety, but also reduces pain perception because "it changes the 'meaning' of the pain making it less threatening."[85] An interesting neuroimaging study had subjects experience a painful stimulus (electrical shock to hand) with and without the ability to stop it; the identical stimulus was rated as *less intense* when the participant had the power to control it.[85] Another study found that subjects who had a choice about coping strategies were able to *tolerate higher levels* of arm shock and reported *less pain*[86]—a vivid example of the mutability of the experience of pain.

How does the HCP affirm the power of the patient to help reduce anxiety and pain? Previous ISLEEP skills can affirm the patient's power indirectly. For example, by *soliciting* the patient's fears, preferences, and comfort level and by *explaining* what will be done, what it will feel like, and what the patient can do to alleviate discomfort, the HCP implicitly affirms the patient's power.

HPCs can more explicitly offer patients a sense of control and power by *offering options* during exams and procedures. Be creative! Possible options include "shifting an item of clothing out of the way rather than putting on a gown," "sitting in a chair instead of on an exam table," leaving the exam room door ajar, allowing a support person to accompany the patient, and the option to signal if discomfort arises.[62] You might also offer options about which arm the patient would prefer to use for an IV catheter or blood-pressure cuff, what position they'd prefer to be in the bed or chair, and more. I was offered some interesting options during a dreaded pelvic ultrasound. My wonderful ultrasound technician gave me control of the hardest part of the procedure (I inserted the ultrasound transducer myself). She also allowed me to use a sheet as a curtain between me and her, which created a boundary and a sense of safety for me. Thank you, ultrasound tech! Having my power affirmed by giving me these options made a huge difference in my psychological and physical comfort.

In conclusion, by *soliciting* skillfully and *listening* mindfully, the HCP can uncover the fears, needs, and wishes of their patients. By *empathizing, validating,* and affirming the patient's *power*, procedures can be experienced with less stress, less pain, and more ease for all.

Progressive Muscle Relaxation

NOTE: In Chapter 2, you learned several practices for your own self-care, which can also be helpful to patients for procedural pain and anxiety management. These include the *body scan, progressive muscle relaxation (PMR), Emotional Freedom Technique (EFT Tapping), diaphragmatic breathing, and awareness of the breath and body.* Your own personal practice and proficiency in these practices will allow you to share them with your patients more naturally. Consider providing patients with instructions on relaxation techniques in written, audio, or video format. (Feel free to share the videos from this book.) The waiting time before procedures is an opportune time for a patient to learn and practice these techniques on their own.

Remember that one cannot be physically relaxed and anxious at the same time. This underscores the value of simply relaxing the body to relax the mind, thereby closing

the gate on pain transmission from the "top down." Progressive muscle relaxation trains us to relax the body by learning to recognize how it feels when the body is tense and then releasing that tension. (See more on PMR in Chapter 2.) Videos 5.5 to 5.9 pertain to progressive muscle relaxation and are tailored to patients for their use during health care procedures. Video 5.5 offers a brief description of the practice.

Progressive muscle relaxation can be practiced while waiting for a procedure to begin, as demonstrated in Video 5.6, and during many procedures, as demonstrated in Video 5.7 (dental filling). Notice how the inhalation coincides with tensing muscles and the exhalation with relaxing.

Video 5.8 offers a couple of important tips for the patient, and Video 5.9 guides the patient through a 15-minute PMR practice, which can be used during many health care procedures to reduce anxiety and pain.

Reflection:

(1) What challenging procedures do you perform before and during which patients could practice PMR to help them relax?

(2) When could your patients receive instructions on PMR? (e.g., at home, in the reception room, etc.)

(3) How could the instructions be shared (e.g., live instruction by a team member or video)?

Diaphragmatic Breathing

Experts in dental anxiety assert, "The most important and fundamental way of helping patients to relax is to teach them *proper breathing techniques*" (emphasis added).[54] Why is breathing so helpful? The many reactions comprising stress reactivity, or "fight, flight, freeze," are a function of the autonomic nervous system and, by definition, not consciously controllable, with one exception: the breath. Breathing into the lower abdomen, or diaphragmatic breathing, activates the parasympathetic nervous system by activating the phrenic plexus,[79] thus rapidly inducing physiologic relaxation. As we discussed with PMR, physiologic relaxation precludes anxiety; in other words, "once a person is physically relaxed, it is impossible to be psychologically upset at the same time."[54] In this way, diaphragmatic breathing is an excellent way to "close the gate" on the transmission of pain signals to the brain from the top down.

Diaphragmatic breathing can be taught to patients of any age, even as young as 3 years.[80] Children (and the young at heart) can be instructed to *blow imaginary bubbles or birthday candles*, or they can be instructed to exhale to the *count of four and inhale to the count of four*.[80] Not only the patient but also caregivers, parents, and guardians (CPGs) can benefit at times from deep breaths before, during, or after a challenging procedure. Deborah Jastrebski, an expert in health care for people with special needs, frequently invites CPGs to "all take a deep breath now," to diffuse the charge of emotions and help everyone relax.[58]

I like to train patients in this technique as I work, without taking any extra time, as demonstrated in Video 5.10. Despite the challenges of an intraoral injection, this young patient was able to tolerate the procedure quite well.

The next example (Video 5.11) demonstrates a special type of diaphragmatic breathing, called "*ujjayi breathing*" (from the yoga tradition) and nicknamed "ocean breath" or "Darth Vader breath." It involves exhaling as if you were fogging up a mirror, but with the mouth closed. The constriction of the throat facilitates a slowing down and deepening of the breath, which may explain why ujjayi breathing is touted for its calming and blood-pressure-lowering effects.[87] Although usually done with the mouth closed, this dental patient practices it with the mouth open as she receives an intraoral injection. Notice how easily breathing instructions can be woven into the course of treatment. Notice, also, the patient's positive experience of this potentially difficult injection (inferior alveolar nerve block), reporting with relief, "I didn't really feel it!"

A couple of other interesting breathing techniques involving the diaphragm include the "*cough trick*" and the *Valsalva maneuver*. The cough trick involves having the patient cough twice and introducing the painful stimulus on the second cough. In the Valsalva maneuver, the patient takes a deep breath and then a forceful holding of the breath, during which a momentary painful procedure is performed.[88] Both of these techniques may be helpful for short procedures such as vaccinations, venous cannulation, or venipuncture.

Mindfulness of the Breath and Body Sensations

In the words of Lao Tsu, "If you are depressed you are living in the past. If you are anxious you are living in the future. If you are at peace you are living in the present."[89] The effects of living in the past and future on the perception of pain were illustrated so vividly by a patient I met only once many years ago but whom I will never forget.

> *Peggy was a middle-aged woman who had been feeling mild discomfort on swallowing for several months. When she finally had it checked by a specialist she received a dire diagnosis—stage 4 laryngeal cancer. She presented to me just days after her diagnosis and was angry and terrified. The sensation in her throat that previously had been a minor irritation now consumed her.*

It is unlikely that the pain in Peggy's throat changed the moment she learned of her diagnosis. What changed was her thoughts *about* the sensations. Thoughts of the past ("I should have quit smoking") and thoughts of the future ("I'm going to die") changed her experience of her throat dramatically, and in an instant, her whole world was turned upside-down—understandably so!

Renowned physician and bioethicist Eric Cassell helps to understand the role of our thoughts and interpretations as they relate to pain by making a distinction between pain and suffering. He points out how pain can be great yet not cause suffering, as in the case of a mother giving birth to a baby. Conversely, pain can be slight yet cause tremendous suffering, as in the story of Peggy. Further, Cassell notes how suffering is very future-oriented:

> *Suffering has a temporal element. In order for a situation to be a source of suffering, it must influence the person's perception of future events. ('If the pain continues like this, I will be overwhelmed'...) If the pain cannot be controlled, I will not be able to take it.') At the moment when the patient is saying, 'If the pain continues like this, I will be overwhelmed,' he or she is not overwhelmed. Fear itself always involves the future.*[1]

During challenging medical and dental procedures, turning toward the present-moment sensations of the breath and the body naturally diminishes the effect of future-oriented thoughts, thereby diminishing anxiety and pain. Because it is not possible to feel the breath and body sensations in the past or the future—only in the present—mindfulness of the breath and body naturally brings us into the present. Dr. John Lovas, a dentist, dental educator, and meditation teacher, echoes Cassell: "Focusing detailed attention specifically on the physical sensations of the breath anchors patients in their bodies and in the present moment, whereas anxiety takes them out of the present and into their fear of future events."[79] We can think of mindfulness of the breath and body as a way of letting go of the second arrows (thoughts *about* the pain, the event, etc.) as we discussed in Chapter 4. We can also think of mindfulness as a top-down way of closing the gate on pain. An interesting study of endoscopy patients found a large range of pain for the same procedure and reported that "catastrophizing thoughts account for between-subject differences in endoscopy pain."[36]

During fight or flight reactivity, breathing becomes shallow, rapid, and localized to the upper chest—a signature breathing pattern I witness frequently in dental patients. When these patients are invited to notice their breath and feel the sensations, they often are surprised to find how constricted their breathing pattern is. In fact, many find they are hardly breathing at all! The moment of awareness provides the opportunity to resume normal breathing function, which naturally supports both physical and psychological comfort.

The instructions for mindfulness of the breath and body are simple: *"Gather the attention and rest it on the sensations of the breath and the body."* Alternatively, *"Check in with your breathing. See if you can notice where your belly is in the breathing cycle—going up, or down or in between."* The sensations of the breath are a helpful anchor for many (and the most common anchor in the mindfulness meditation tradition) since the breath is dynamic, cyclical, and always present. Focusing on sensations of the breath—particularly sensations in the belly—also encourages diaphragmatic breathing, which, as we saw previously, induces parasympathetic function. In fact, mindfulness of the breath can be even more effective at promoting diaphragmatic breathing than direct instructions to breathe with the belly, which can trigger resistance.

Video 5.12 shows Mark, a patient with a long history of dental phobia. As a choir director, Mark understands the value of proper breathing. I first invite him to breathe diaphragmatically. Then, I invite him to simply bring awareness to his breathing. Despite his fear, he is able to follow his breath and tolerate the intraoral injection quite well. Afterward, his words capture how thoughts *about* our experience trigger more stress than the experience itself: "the dread was worse than the physical sensations." In contrast, mindfulness of the present-moment sensations of the breath help us find calm.

> **Experiment: Language for Mindfulness of the Breath**
> When instructing a patient in awareness of the breath, the choice of language is important. Direct commands tend to arouse resistance, while gentle invitations promote willingness. Compare your own reactions to the following two sets of instructions:
> 1. *Breathe. Feel your breath. Breathe in. Breathe out.* (Commanding)
> 2. *If you could just bring your attention to the breath, allowing it to be as it is. If you notice tension, if you can, let it go; if not, let it be.* (Invitational—directly from the video above)

Next, you will see another patient with a severe fear of needles. Video 5.13 demonstrates both diaphragmatic breathing and awareness of the breath during an intraoral injection. Again, notice the invitational language used to guide the patient's attention to the breath.

In addition to mindfulness of the breath, *mindfulness of the body sensations* allows the patient to stay present during stressful procedures and thereby reduces anxiety and pain. Another practice we discussed, PMR, also involves awareness of body sensations, but this practice requires subtle movements (while tensing a part of the body), and therefore is not the best practice for procedures requiring total stillness (e.g., during a magnetic resonance imaging [MRI]). In contrast, mindfulness of the body is done with the body in stillness. Simple, short invitations such as, *"If you find it helpful, tune into the sensations of your feet,"* or *"You might check in with the contact points of your body with the chair."* Try to call attention to parts of the body that are distant from the area involved in the procedure. Alternatively, the patient can be led through a full body scan (see Chapter 2) by a team member or a pre-recorded guide.

Treating patients who are anxious or in pain can be very stressful for the HCP. Sometimes I wonder whose blood pressure is higher—the patient's or my own! Each time the HCP invites a patient to bring attention to their breath or body sensations, it also provides the HCP an opportunity to bring attention to their own breath and body sensations. Often, I find I am not breathing at all, and these moments give me the precious opportunity to take some life-sustaining breaths, helping me to calm down and focus.

Gradual Exposure

For the anxious patient, and especially for the person with a history of trauma, abuse, or special needs, *gradual exposure* can make the difference between a procedure being traumatizing, revictimizing, and painful or being comfortable, confidence-building, and successful. The pioneering work of Deborah Jastrebski has demonstrated over and over the power of gradual exposure techniques for health care procedures, especially in patients with special needs. Her practice model, PWP, employs a "practice specialist" who coaches patients in "practice sessions" before procedures as well as during their medical and dental procedures.[58] Through a relationship of trust and many gradual exposure techniques, numerous PWP patients have experienced dramatic conversions—from severe anxiety and trauma (usually due to being treated with coercion and restraint) to being able to undergo difficult procedures (blood draws, pelvic exams, and dental restorations) with dignity and success. Let's look at some different ways to practice gradual exposure in health care.

For many patients, *modeling* is a good first step toward completing a challenging procedure. The model can be live or prerecorded (video). Also, the model can be a peer or a trusted person. Research with filmed modeling shows that "Children who observed a peer modeling appropriate behavior during oral care had lower anxiety levels."[7] Modeling helps reduce the fear of the unknown and helps the patient learn "what is considered appropriate behavior…and what can be expected in the upcoming treatment session."[54]

Modeling should be done at whatever distance and/or barrier is needed for the patient's comfort, as demonstrated by Jastrebski and her dental patient with special needs named Donna. This patient's anxiety and gag reflex were so severe, she could not even witness a model undergoing dental impression without gagging! The turning point for Donna was being able to watch from the distance she needed to feel safe and not induce gagging (even if it means watching from behind a glass door—as was the case for one patient!) From there, Donna was able to come closer and closer to her goal of getting dentures until she was able to regain her smile—a triumph for her and her caregivers.

In addition to modeling, another way to practice gradual exposure is by breaking procedures down into *small steps* and *short (but increasing) time increments*. By doing so, aversive stimuli such as the dental handpiece (drill) can be more easily tolerated, as illustrated in Video 5.14. Notice how gradual exposure can be easily

woven into the course of treatment without requiring much extra time. (See timeframe 2:30 to 3:30.)

In the previous example, the exposure to the dental handpiece was approached in three stages:
1. Turning on the handpiece near the tooth without touching
2. Touching the tooth with the handpiece on for 1 second
3. Touching the tooth with the handpiece on for 5 to 10 seconds

If needed, I could have backed up even one more step and simply placed the handpiece in the mouth without turning it on. The more severely affected a person is by their emotional, cognitive, or mental conditions, the smaller the steps. For example, the patient we met earlier named Joyce needed to have dentures made but was initially too terrified to even sit in the dental chair. Starting with a conversation about her fears and the events which contributed to her phobias, we eventually built a relationship of trust. She started denture fabrication by simply holding the dental impression tray in her own hand. Next, she placed the tray in her own mouth for a few seconds, then for a longer time. Through gradual exposure, Joyce was able to overcome her traumatic past and gain comfort with dental impressions.

Note that unlike a neurotypical patient like Joyce, patients with special needs should not be asked to touch equipment to avoid the confusion that can arise from being invited to touch medical equipment at certain times (during practice) and then being forbidden to touch at others (during procedures). In the case of Donna's impressions, after observing impressions on a model, Donna experienced having a practice specialist insert the impression tray in her mouth for 1 second, followed by increasing time intervals, until she could tolerate it for the full duration of a denture impression. The final preparation step towards the impression for Donna was the transfer of the trust between Donna and her practice specialist to the dentist with the *"trust bridge"*— the moment when the practice specialist touches the dentist's hand while the dentist touches Donna.[58]

A final success story illustrating the use of gradual exposure techniques is that of Emily, a 10-year-old with Down syndrome. Emily was traumatized as a result of multiple dental experiences with restraint. The first encounter allowed the practice specialist to assess her fear, get to know her as a person, and meet her where she was comfortable—in her van in the parking lot! From there, Emily was encouraged to come closer to the entrance of the building and then back to her safe place in the van. With trust as a foundation, gradual exposure techniques made it possible for Emily to learn to sit in the dental chair, recline the chair, and do many other necessary tasks. After several practice sessions, she is now able to experience routine dental care with ease and confidence.

NOTE: Some dental insurance companies in the United States, both private and government-subsidized, offer reimbursement for practice sessions under the code "behavioral management."

The key to building trust with gradual exposure is to "do only what you say, nothing more" and when necessary, go back to earlier steps, even if it means going back to performing the task for 1 second.[58] Also, rewards in the form of praise or gifts can be very motivating, especially for children. Jastrebski reports that many patients with special needs benefit from being able to see their reward as they are doing the task.[58]

Gradual exposure employs two ISLEEP skills. First, *explain*—what you will do, what sensations the patient will feel, and the duration. Second, *power* of the patient—for example, allowing the patient to stop at any time with a signal (such as raising their hand or using a stop card as in PWP). Patient *power* is also affirmed by asking permission to progress to the next step. (As discussed in Chapter 3, asking permission can be problematic with young children and patients with special needs, who benefit from a gentle but firm and more directed approach.) Because it reframes procedures in a safer, more empowering way, gradual exposure decreases anxiety and, by doing so, can also close the gate on pain transmission.

While gradual exposure may require more time short term, in the long run, it can save not only time but also energy, money, and medico-legal risks associated with sedation and restraint. Most importantly, patients avoid being traumatized and gain competence and confidence as their trust grows. In closing, "Gradual exposure to anxiety-producing situations" is a key skill for doctor-patient relationships.[52]

> **Reflection:**
> What are some of the challenging procedures that you do and how could you implement the principle of gradual exposure, such as modeling and small steps to make it easier for patients?

Non-Pain Stimuli

I once heard of a veterinarian who routinely punched his horses while performing an injection. I mention this not to promote punching patients (please, no!) but to offer an excellent example of gate control of procedural pain with *non-pain stimuli*. This is not a new technique: "That touch inhibits pain has been a central tenet of pain research for half a century."[90] A common example you may have done to yourself—rubbing an injury to diminish pain, something many of us do instinctively. While psychological techniques close the gate in a "top-down" approach, *non-pain stimuli* represent a "bottom-up" approach.

General examples of non-pain stimuli include *shaking, pressure, vibration, heat, and cold.* How does a non-pain stimulus diminish pain? Based on the gate control theory, non-nociceptive (non-painful) input closes the gate to painful input, preventing pain signals from traveling up to the central nervous system.[29] More specifically, "Activity in large diameter, low-threshold mechanoreceptors (touch-related) nerve fibers could inhibit the transmission of action potentials from small-diameter higher threshold nociceptive (pain-related) fibers."[91]

The location of the non-pain stimulus matters. Pain researchers have found that "tactile inputs inhibited pain perception segmentally, but not when tactile and nociceptive inputs were delivered to different dermatomes."[90] The same researchers found that as the distance between the non-nociceptive stimulus and the painful stimulus increases, the perceived pain level increases as well. This underscores the importance of keeping the non-pain stimulus in the same dermatome and in close proximity to the pain stimulus. Also, it is recommended to apply the non-pain stimulus proximal to the pain or "between the pain and the brain."[92]

"I hate needles!" "I am terrified of the needle." "How many shots do I have to get?" As a dentist, I hear these words almost daily, like the refrain of a song. Just the sight or the thought of a needle can send some patients into a panic. (Tip: Keep needles and other potentially fear-inducing instruments out of sight. When a patient—usually a child—requests to see the syringe, you can show the "squirter" with the cap on.) My dental patients are big fans of bottom-up gate control for intraoral injections. Two examples of non-pain stimuli for intraoral injections include:

1. Shaking the cheek or lip
2. Applying pressure with the blunt end of an instrument (particularly for palatal injections)

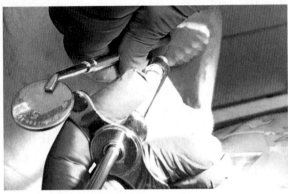

Fig. 5.11 Non-Pain Sensation for Injection Pain: Pressure.

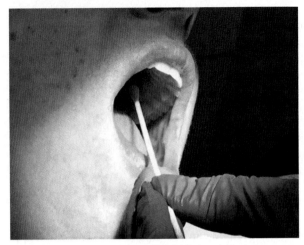

Fig. 5.13 Application of Cold Before Injection.

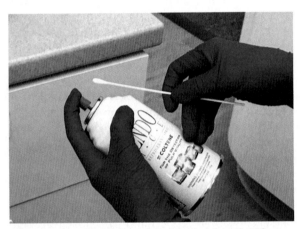

Fig. 5.12 Non-Pain Sensation for Injection Pain: Cold Spray.

Here is the video of Mark again (Video 5.12a), this time to illustrate shaking of the cheek during injection (see minute 1:50).

Fig. 5.11 illustrates the application of pressure to the hard palate to close the gate during a palatal injection. While this may not block the pain completely, it can greatly diminish it. Another non-pain sensation that can help close the gate for palatal injections is a cold spray, as shown in the Figs. 5.12 and 5.13.

Many different non-pain sensations have been employed in medicine to effectively manage procedural pain. Here are just a few examples:

- *Pinching* the skin at the site of an injection[93]
- *Cold spray:* "Proven efficacy in reducing the needle insertion pain for intravenous cannulation and venepuncture (sic)"[11]

- *Cold packs* for chest tube removal (rated one of the most painful experiences in critical care units) 20 minutes prior[94,95]
- *Heat:* Use of a radiant warmer for neonates 2 minutes prior to injection[96]
- *Mechanical vibration* during heel sticks for neonates[97,98]
- *Pulsed electrical currents* (high-frequency transcutaneous electrical nerve stimulation) for chest tube removal[99]
- *Cold and vibration combination* for needle procedures in children ("Buzzy," a device that looks like a bumblebee with cold-pack removable wings and a vibrating body)[100]

In conclusion, non-pain stimuli represent an easy, time-efficient, non-pharmacologic means of managing procedural pain. They are most effective when applied in the same dermatome, between the pain and the brain, and as close to the pain stimulus as possible.

> **Reflection:**
> Consider the painful sensations induced by procedures you do for your patients. What non-pain sensations could you or a team member provide to help close the gate on the transmission of the pain signals?

Distraction for Managing Anxiety, Pain, and the Gag Reflex

My colleague, Megha, describes an incident when she was about 8 years old in which she accidentally fell and landed on her face. Her spectacles lacerated her eyebrow and created a bloody mess. Despite the challenges of receiving sutures at this young age, Megha doesn't remember any pain during the procedure. "The only thing I recall from this experience was the caring and friendly nature of the doctor. He was kind and respectful and seemed genuinely interested as we talked about school and friends." She reports the doctor's conversation was so engaging that she experienced no pain. This story is an example of top-down gate control of pain with *distraction.*

Studies confirm the effectiveness of distraction for both pediatric and adult patients. Distraction has been rated "the most effective non-pharmacological intervention for mitigating pain and anxiety experienced by pediatric patients undergoing needle-related procedures."[101] (A heart-warming demonstration of distraction and non-pain stimuli can be seen in a video of a doctor injecting a baby at https://youtu.be/jSeO62o6V2o.) The efficacy of distraction for pain is based not only on self-reported pain but also on physiologic measures such as pulse rates.[102] In addition to diminishing pain and anxiety, distraction provides the unique benefit of decreasing the gag reflex, as we shall soon see.

Passive Distraction: Music

Several means of passive distraction have been proven effective with children, including "listening to music, watching cartoons… mother-directed distractions, such as soothing."[101] *Music* has been found helpful in reducing procedural pain and anxiety in adults as well, and my personal experience offers an example.

In my early twenties, I was faced with the decision to extract my impacted wisdom teeth with conscious sedation or without. As I weighed the options, I struggled with competing, negative mental images—on one hand, a picture of me fully awake to the sounds and sensations of drilling and hammering and on the other hand, images of being sedated, limp as a ragdoll, vulnerable, and defenseless. I chose to skip sedation and instead try some headphones piping in my favorite classical piano music. Each time I heard drilling or other unpleasant sounds or sensations I consciously shifted my attention to the music. By focusing on the music, I was able to tolerate the whole procedure surprisingly well.

Research confirms the benefits of music for procedural pain and anxiety management in adults. While one review study did not find benefits of music for adults undergoing venipuncture,[88] many studies report

benefits to adults undergoing invasive procedures. For example, a systematic review found music helpful for adults with dental anxiety and recommended providing headphones to adults during procedures.[103] Another review study of 73 RCTs involving adult surgical patients found the following benefits: *decreased postoperative pain, anxiety, analgesic medication use,* and *increased patient satisfaction.*[104] A review of over 80 RCTs of adult surgical patients (including patients undergoing general anesthesia, regional anesthesia only, and both general and regional) found evidence that music interventions significantly *decrease anxiety and pain* (mean decrease in anxiety of 21 mm and a mean decrease of 10-mm pain on 100-mm visual analogue scales) compared to controls.[13] Additional benefits of music include *decreased delirium, decreased hospital stay,* and *increased foot movement after hip and knee surgery.*[13] Here is interesting evidence that the effect of music is more than just placebo: five studies reported that patients who were exposed to music only while under general anesthesia experienced a statistically significant *decrease in pain.*[13]

Music is more than just a distraction—otherwise, there would be no difference between the effects of music and the effects of noise from traffic! How does music affect anxiety and pain? A review study reports, "The primary way by which music listening affects us biologically is via modulation of stress response."[105] Common parameters measured by researchers include plasma cortisol (day surgery patients[106] and amniocentesis patients[107]), salivary cortisol (colonoscopy patients[108]), heart rate and arterial pressure (endoscopy patients).[109]

Are there certain features of music listening—type, duration, timing—that are particularly helpful? Apparently, a wide variety of music interventions have been found effective as reported by two review studies. One found "no significant association between the effect of music interventions and age, sex, choice and timing of music, and type of anesthesia"[13] and another reports, "Choice of music and timing of delivery made little difference to outcomes." Yet another review of research on music for procedures reported two important findings: *anxiety* decreases most when music listening occurs *preoperatively,* and *pain* decreases most when music listening is *postoperative*[104]; further, music seems to be most beneficial when *patients choose music from a list* than when they choose "freely"[13] or when the music is assigned to them.[106]

Children's distraction needs seem to differ from adults' needs. One review study showed music was helpful in decreasing children's vaccination pain.[110] However, a systematic review of the effectiveness of music interventions on dental anxiety found inconclusive evidence for children (although helpful for adults).[103] Perhaps children require engaging more senses than just listening to be fully distracted from an anxiety-provoking or prolonged procedure. This theory is supported by a systematic review and meta-analysis which found "lower dental anxiety in the audiovisual method groups" in children aged 4 to 10 years.[111] Another review study reinforced these findings, reporting significantly *lower anxiety and pulse rate* associated with audiovisual distraction as well as "improving children's cooperation."[112] Apparently, the more engaging the distraction, the more helpful it is for procedures with children. This leads us to active distraction and an interesting technology proven helpful for all ages.

Active Distraction: Virtual Reality and Pet Therapy

Virtual reality (VR) is an audiovisual technology that immerses patients in an interactive, three-dimensional experience by projecting vivid images directly into specialized goggles shown in Fig. 5.14. The most dramatic example of VR's usefulness I have witnessed involved a 10-year-old boy undergoing IV catheter insertion while playing a VR video game. The child's complete comfort during the procedure was revealed in his question to the nurse after she was done: "When are you going to do it?"

Systematic reviews of VR report several positive findings: "VR-based interventions reduced pain for patients undergoing medical procedures,"[113] and it is effective in pediatric patients.[114] Applications of VR for pain management include "chemotherapy, physical therapy, burn wound changes, and surgery,"[115] otolaryngology office-based procedures,[116] and interventional radiology procedures.[45] Finally, a dental study of VR reported patients experienced less pain and anxiety based on both subjective and objective measures such as heart rate.[30] Virtual reality is an exciting new form of "non-pharmacological analgesic and anxiolytic intervention."[116]

Another interesting form of active distraction has proven helpful for procedural pain and anxiety—pet therapy (PT). Decreased blood cortisol levels and

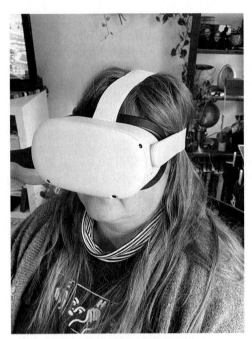

Fig. 5.14 VR Goggles.

decreased distress were noted in a study of children in venipuncture.[117] A meta-analysis of 28 studies with all age groups reports, "Significant differences occurred in heart rate, self-reported anxiety, and self-reported stress after PT exposure compared to before PT."[118] Dog lovers might argue that the rich experience of enjoying a pet is more than just a distraction!

Active Distraction for the Gag Reflex

The gag reflex can pose an obstacle to many procedures, especially in emergency medicine, otolaryngology (ENT), and dentistry. The gag reflex can be either somatic in origin (physical triggers) or psychogenic (mental or psychological triggers).[119] Distraction represents one of three general categories of strategies to reduce gagging for patients with a gag reflex of psychogenic origin (other strategies include relaxation and desensitization techniques).[120]

My favorite way to distract a patient with a strong gag reflex is with *active distraction* using simple movements of the body. Unlike VR and other forms of distraction, this approach doesn't require any technology. Even the most severe gaggers are able to successfully complete procedures using active distraction with body movements, such as those demonstrated in Video 5.15. The bilateral nature of the movements shown in this video may account for their effectiveness.

The patient you will see in Videos 5.16 and 5.17 had me worried at first. Fabrication of his dentures required keeping the impression tray in his mouth for about 5 minutes, but he wasn't able to keep the trays in his mouth for more than 5 seconds before gagging! I wondered how we would get through it, until I remembered the active distraction technique shown in the next video. The movements distracted him so well that it's hard to believe gagging was ever a problem for him by his ease during the impression. This simple distraction technique has helped him and many others overcome the gag reflex during their procedure.

As always, offer the patient gentle, invitational instructions instead of commands. For example, before starting a procedure, the HCP or team member can say a simple preparatory statement like, *"I may offer some movement instructions to make the procedure more comfortable. You can choose to follow them if you feel it would be helpful."* This provides the patient the option to participate or not (affirming the power of the patient) and allows for a smooth transition into what might seem to the patient like an exercise routine! Suggested instructions include: *"Try holding one foot up. Stay there for a count of 5 or until you feel tired, then switch to the other leg. Or if you prefer, wiggle the toes of one foot then switch to the other."* Some other active distraction remedies that have been proven effective for gagging during procedures include:

- Patient taps their temples while repeating an affirmation[121]
- Patient breathes audibly through the nose while tapping the foot on the floor rhythmically[122]

The more challenging the task, the more it will occupy the patient's attention and reduce the gag reflex.

Several interesting studies have explored other forms of active distraction to address gagging in children. One dental study involved children *counting geometrical shapes and colors* and found a statistically significant reduction in median gag reflex score.[123] Another dental study used a *puzzle ball game* in which children matched colorful geometric shapes with similarly shaped openings in a ball.[124] In this RCT, all study subjects exhibited significantly less gagging,

and, more importantly, all study subjects, including those who experienced gagging, were able to complete the procedure successfully.

> **Reflection:**
> Consider what possible forms of distraction, both active and passive, you and your team could offer your patients to help manage their procedural anxiety and pain.

Mental Imagery

Whether the HCP acknowledges the power of mental imagery or not, patients engage in mental imagery spontaneously and usually not in a way that is helpful! It's human nature—as soon as we know we are going to undergo a procedure, we start to imagine what it will be like based on what we know from our past experience and that of others. Mental imagery can also be triggered by language a patient hears from their HCP or a team member. For example, if a dentist is extracting a patient's tooth and tells their assistant (in front of the patient—true story), "I need a scalpel and a long needle," you can be sure the patient will have some imagery about that! Does a patient's mental imagery affect their procedural pain and anxiety? Before answering that question, let's try an experiment.

> **Experiment:**
> Take a moment to imagine holding a lemon in your hand. Notice the color, shape, and size. Imagine feeling the temperature and the texture of the lemon's surface against your skin. Imagine cutting a slice of the lemon. Hold the slice in your hand and notice how the slice glistens with lemon juice. Imagine bringing the lemon slice up to your nose and inhaling the fresh citrus smell. Now take a bite out of the slice, imagining the juice in your mouth and the tart, lemon flavor.

You may have noticed some changes in your body as you imagined this scenario—maybe increased salivation or the impulse to swallow. How can a mere mental image—a "thought with sensory qualities"[125]—induce physiologic changes? As it turns out, the human brain processes *imagined* experiences in much the same way as *actual* experiences.[126–128] More importantly, as the brain processes these imagined experiences, the human body reacts similarly to how it would if the experiences were real, as the lemon experiment demonstrates. This has very important implications for pain and anxiety management in health care.

Researchers report, "It is well established that mental imagery can both exacerbate and alleviate acute and chronic pain."[129] For example, one study had patients receive a painful stimulus on their arm while imagining either a protective glove or a painful lesion on their arm; when subjects imagined the protective glove, they experienced *less pain*.[129] In another study, subjects immersed their hand in ice water and compared the effects of imagining their hand wearing a warm, protective glove versus no imagery or control imagery (imagining hand only). Again, subjects focusing on positive imagery experienced less pain.[126]

There are several explanations for the mechanism by which mental imagery works to lessen pain. Positive mental imagery induces "physiological relaxation by lowering sympathetic nervous system and increasing parasympathetic nervous system response through neurochemical and peptide changes."[12] Mental imagery can also work by inducing a placebo-like effect to "reduce

experimentally evoked pain as well as acute and chronic clinical pain."[126] Whether it relaxes the body or suggests a positive outcome, positive mental imagery is a potentially powerful means of closing the gate on pain transmission.

Now let's look at some ways to harness the benefits of positive mental imagery and ways to limit the effects of patients' negative imagery.

Guided Imagery

One approach which has long been touted for its calming effect is *guided imagery*. The patient is instructed either by a live professional or with a recording to imagine a pleasant scene, such as a beach, meadow, or forest, and to imagine it vividly using all the senses—imagine what it looks like, smells like, sounds like. Guided imagery practice is usually preceded by relaxation practices like deep breathing or progressive muscle relaxation.

Experts recommend using "patients' spontaneous coping imagery if they have developed any."[127] Allowing the patient to choose their own positive imagery as opposed to a scripted or audio-recorded scenario avoids

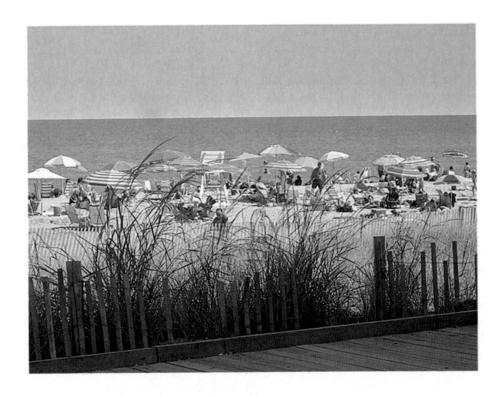

the risk of evoking a negative reaction to an assigned image (e.g., if the patient is invited to imagine a beach scene and they don't like the beach or they had a bad experience associated with a beach).

Research has found many benefits of guided imagery. For example, an RCT of patients undergoing gallbladder removal found guided imagery was associated with *decreased stress* and improved *wound healing*.[130] Additional research has found "*pain relief, decreased anxiety, and decreased length of stay*" in joint replacement patients[131] and as much as 50% *reduction in narcotic medication* use in surgical patients.[12] Finally, the value of guided imagery "as a complementary approach to drug analgesia in *postoperative pain control*" has been affirmed in a review.[132] Many times, guided imagery can be practiced at the same time as a diagnostic or therapeutic procedure. Other protocols that have been tested include playing a recording daily for several days before and after surgery.[130]

While I enjoy guided meditation as a way to relax, there are times when it feels aversive. For example, being asked to imagine a beautiful beach when I am faced with the impending doom of my annual pelvic exam feels aversive and even dismissive. Perhaps my own negative imagery is dominating my experience of the moment. When a patient's own negative imagery is too strong, it may be helpful to address it more directly, as we will discuss in the next section.

Spontaneous Negative Mental Imagery

A common, universal form of mental imagery is worrying.[125] Worry is based entirely on thoughts and mental imagery and includes images of related past experiences and future negative events. For example, worry about a dental appointment may be associated with images of a foot-long needle. Such images have the potential to open the gate to pain transmission and thereby increase pain perception.

The HCP can help minimize the effect of spontaneous negative imagery in several ways. First, avoid language that could evoke negative mental images when describing procedures to patients (e.g., "I'm going to shape your gums," instead of "I'm going to flap your gums and file down the jawbone."). Second, pay attention to the language used while communicating with team members during procedures. For example, instead of saying, "Please pass the scalpel," you might say, "Can I have a number 12, please."

As we noted earlier, medical and dental procedures can evoke mental imagery spontaneously, and when this happens, it may be helpful to bring these images into awareness and to work with them. Experts report that simply describing the mental image can help "disentangle cognitions from reality," and patients have described relief upon noticing their negative mental images.[127] However, focusing on negative mental images also has the potential to increase patients' pain and anxiety.[133,134] In these cases, it is beneficial to invite patients to notice and then reshape or *rescript* their own negative mental images into positive ones, as described next.

Imagery rescripting. Imagery rescripting or interactive guided imagery has been applied successfully to treat many psychological disorders, including posttraumatic stress disorder (PTSD), phobias, eating disorders, and nightmares.[135] A variation of imagery rescripting called anodyne imagery has been used effectively for interventional radiology procedures and was found to significantly reduce medications needed.[73]

Here's an approach to imagery rescripting. Before a challenging medical or dental procedure (the same day or another day beforehand), allow the patient to sit quietly and settle before inviting them to notice any negative images associated with the procedure. Through gentle questions, invite the patient to imagine a new, positive version of the same story. Experts report the importance of "not deviating too much from the original imagination."[135] Example questions include: "*How would you rather see the image? How would you prefer it to have been? Describe in full what this image would entail.*"[134] Encourage patients to summon up images of people and beings that they find supportive, including saints, angels, God, deities, pets—whatever they believe would be helpful.

Research supports the practice of imagery rescripting for pain management. A study of pain patients found that negative pain-related images "occur repeatedly and spontaneously" and that the practice of rescripting was "fast and appeared pleasurable to the participants."[134] Working with a patient's *own images* provides "relief of intrusive recurring images"[136] and provides "remarkable reductions in emotion, cognitions, and *pain levels*" (emphasis added).[134] Mental imagery is a great way to harness the power of the mind to decrease anxiety and close the gate on pain signal transmission.

Experiment:

Find a private place, and take a moment to quiet the mind and body. Call to mind an upcoming stressful event, such as a medical/dental procedure or a stressful school or work-related event. (Choose an event that is not the highest level of stress but something manageable.) Rate your level of stress on a scale of 1 to 10. Notice any spontaneous negative images that arise, perhaps involving pain or failure. If it helps, close your eyes and explore all the senses. What do you see, hear, smell, feel?

Now imagine the same scene, but this time, you and/or another person/being that you find supportive (either real or imagined), change the course of events to a positive outcome. Imagine the scenario in detail with all your senses. Feel the experience in the body. Now rate your stress level again. Take a moment to journal the experience:

(1) How did your stress level change in this exercise?

(2) What procedures do you perform at work that could produce negative mental imagery for your patients?

(3) How could you help your patients become aware of their negative mental images and rescript them to positive ones (e.g., in writing/verbally, with a team member/with the provider, before or during the procedure)?

Nonverbal Communication: Posture, Tone of Voice, Eye Contact

Nonverbal communication plays a significant role in all human relations. In fact, "Most human communication and interaction is nonverbal…not only are nonverbal cues processed faster but they also have a greater impact on the perceiver than corresponding verbal statements."[137] In medicine, researchers report nonverbal communication "has significant implications for patient satisfaction, health outcomes, and malpractice claims."[137] Nonverbal communication has the power to soothe or scare, thereby closing or opening the gate to pain signal transmission. An instrument developed in dentistry to evaluate "therapeutic communication skills" identified several key nonverbal communications, including "making regular eye contact," "having a pleasant tone of voice," and "having a professional appearance."[138] (This instrument also identified the importance of "being gentle"—mindful procedural touch—during procedures, as discussed previously

in Chapter 4.) A review study on communication skills reported, "Smiling, forward-leaning, and eye contact has been demonstrated to correlate with patient satisfaction."[139] Let's consider some of these nonverbal communications and how they might affect procedural anxiety and pain.

Many times, I have noticed HCPs and trainees standing over their patients as they talk, which, from a distance, looks like they are lecturing the patient. Standing over a patient can exaggerate a sense of hierarchy and intimidate a fearful patient. *Body posture*, especially "sitting down with patients at eye level," can be helpful to "convey both interest in and time for patients," reports Helen Riess.[137] Sitting doesn't take more time, yet research has found that it creates the perception of a longer visit. A randomized, controlled study of adult postoperative inpatients found, "Patients perceived the provider as present at their bedside longer when he sat, even though the actual time the physician spent at the bedside did not change significantly whether he sat or stood. Patients with whom the physician sat reported a more positive interaction and a better understanding of their condition."[140]

When asked what makes them comfortable, patients often mention the *tone of voice of their HCP*. Listen to Joyce in Video 5.18 as she describes this key nonverbal communication element. The patient reports, "Your voice meant a great deal. It wasn't demanding. It meant a great deal to have a soft voice tell you, "Will you do this for me?" Dentist, educator, and meditation teacher John Lovas states, "Borrowing from hypnosis, clinicians should try to make sure that their *tone of voice and body language* are intentionally and consistently soothing, monotonous, and congruent with achieving their goal of *relaxing* and *reassuring* the patient" (emphasis added).[79] An interesting study of malpractice trends among surgeons has found indirect evidence of the importance of tone of voice: "Dominant tones correlated with patients filing lawsuits, whereas tones conveying warmth and anxiety about a patient's condition were correlated with no litigation history."[137] Although causality cannot be concluded, the strong correlation between tone of voice and patient dissatisfaction is compelling.

Eye contact is a particularly powerful nonverbal communication, which can serve to connect—or distance—providers and patients. Note that some forms of eye contact in medicine actually are distancing. "Medical gaze" is described by philosopher Michel Foucault as dehumanizing because the patient is viewed as a body and object for study, instead of a person.[141] In contrast, research has found the affirming effects of eye contact when it demonstrates awareness of the patient's presence.[142] During the Covid-19 pandemic, faces were covered by masks, making eye contact even more critical to being able to connect.

Eye contact is a simple way for the professional to comfort a patient who is anxious or in pain. A host of physiologic and psychologic benefits of eye contact have been identified:

> *Eye gaze and retinal lock between an anxious person and a trusted 'other' has a direct effect on the synchronization of the right brain hemispheres and the quieting of the sympathetic nervous system and the amygdala, changing the 'fearful effect' and increasing the ability to deal with trauma. Thus it enables the caregiver or trusted 'other' to 'soothe.'*[143]

Note that some cultures may forbid eye contact between certain groups, such as men with women or patients with the doctor. When in doubt, take cues from the patient and sense what is comfortable for them.

Unfortunately, modern health care poses many obstacles to eye contact between HCPs and patients. During consultations, the use of *computers* for documentation and for reviewing test results and images takes the HCP's eyes off the patient. At other times, eye contact may not be possible (e.g., a dentist needing to focus on patient's tooth) or may not be appropriate (e.g., while examining an intimate area like the genitals). Also, the use of surgical, dental, and hygiene *loupes* can block the clinician's eyes and, even worse, create an intimidating sight for the patient. Compare the four pictures in Fig. 5.15 showing a dentist with and without personal protective equipment (PPE). (Note: Photos pre-date the Covid-19 pandemic.)

Exercise:

Imagine yourself sitting in the dental chair before a procedure. You are anxious due to a history of traumatic dental experiences. Now look at each of the pictures of your dentist in Fig. 5.14, one at a time. How does each picture impact you?

Diminished eye contact in general has been noted in younger generations, a trend attributed to the

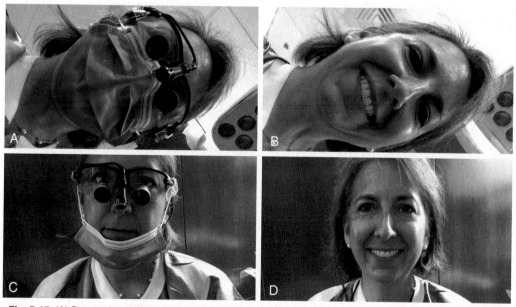

Fig. 5.15 (A) Dentist from above with PPE. (B) Dentist from above without PPE. (C) Dentist from side with PPE. (D) Dentist from side without PPE. *PPE, Personal protective equipment.*

habitual use of digital communications instead of face-to-face. Nonverbal communications expert Janine Driver suggests this interesting tip to help remember to make eye contact: "When you walk into the room… go in with the intention of remembering the person's eye color."[144]

When eye contact is not possible during a procedure, the HCP should try to find opportunities to engage with eye contact immediately before and after procedures to connect and build trust. During these procedures that preclude eye contact, touch can be a powerful means to connect and to comfort as discussed in the next section.

Reflection:

(1) Consider the procedures you do that are challenging for patients and some nonverbal ways you can convey care, such as eye contact and seated posture.

(2) What are possible times, during the encounter, that you could sit with a patient at eye level and make eye contact without any physical obstacles (such as, equipment, computers, furniture)?

Touch: Expressive, Mindful Procedural, and Reiki

Touch…is the primary language of compassion, love, and gratitude.[145]

Touch can enrich the patient's and the provider's experience of health care, as the following scenario illustrates.

Before I begin working on a dental crown for my patient, Sarah, she shares with me her anxiety about the procedure. I explain to her what she will feel and invite her to stop me any time she needs a break. While working on her tooth, I notice her belly isn't moving at all: a cue that she is holding her breath, perhaps due to anxiety. I want to connect with her somehow, but eye contact from such a close distance would be awkward, and talking isn't possible with her mouth full right now. So, while waiting for her crown impression to set, I hold the impression tray with one hand and rest my other hand on her shoulder gently, connecting with my wish for her to be at ease. Soon, I see her belly start to rise and fall again, and I feel a calm, soothing sensation in the region of my heart.

Throughout history, healers have used the power of touch to comfort and heal the sick. Unfortunately, today there are many obstacles to touch in health care. In our age of high-tech medicine and dentistry, the hands of the HCP are often tied to a computer keyboard or other mechanical device. In addition, fears of being misunderstood keep HCPs from touching patients—many are concerned about "sexual harassment, the legal repercussions of touching, and uncertain boundary issues."[146] As a result, touch "is currently underutilized by many doctors."[147]

Yet, the power of touch to comfort is undeniable. We know this instinctively, which is why we hug a baby when they are crying and why we reach out to touch our friends on the shoulder when they are upset. Researchers report, "Patients…say they expect to be touched and appreciate the way it humanizes their care."[147] Interestingly, the power of touch has been measured even in unconscious patients: in a study of patients who had been resuscitated, those who had received caring touch were found to be more aware of their providers' "interest, concern and caring for them," even though few had any recollection of being touched.[148] Touch transcends words and consciousness, and because of this, it is particularly helpful for "distressed patients with whom verbal communication is limited, inadequate, or unnecessary."[149]

Science is uncovering many measurable benefits of the ancient practice of laying on of hands to reduce both *pain and anxiety*. For example, studies of babies undergoing heel sticks and other painful procedures have shown that babies who are held during the procedure experience *less pain* as measured by reduced crying and heart rate.[150,151] The benefits of touch for *anxiety* have also been measured: a study investigated the brain activity of women who were anticipating a painful electric stimulus. Subjects were observed while holding their spouse's hand, a stranger's hand, and no hand. Functional MRI (real-time imaging) showed reduced activity in the part of the brain related to reactions to threat in the women who were holding hands with a stranger and a statistically significant reduction when holding hands with their spouse.[152] Several studies report, "Touching may induce a direct *reduction* of arousal in the recipient's physiology," such as reduced heart rate (emphasis added).[153] Other benefits of touch include "reduction of stress, pain and depression; and enhancement of immunity."[143]

Caring touch is calming, soothing, and increases trust because it involves the mammalian caregiving network and the "love hormone" oxytocin. Interestingly, this is the same mechanism of *compassion* that we saw in Chapter 2. "The stroking of touch-sensitive neurons in the skin sends signals to one region of the brain—the orbitofrontal cortex, which *activates the release of oxytocin and endorphins*. At the same time, pleasurable touch *reduces activation of the HPA axis*, the provenance of stress and anxiety" (emphasis added).[145] A review study reports other mechanisms of the effect of touch on pain: "Increased serotonin and decreased substance P may explain [touch's] pain-alleviating effects."[154] The benefits of expressive touch for pain can also be explained with gate control theory. Any touch—whether expressive (caring) touch or procedural touch—that conveys care has the potential to close the gate to pain transmission from the top down. Also, because touch is a non-pain stimulus, it has the potential to close the gate from the bottom up.

What kind of touch qualifies as caring touch? Unfortunately, an intention of care during touch from an HCP is not a guarantee of the perception of care by the patient, which is why the experience of touch is so complicated. In the same way that the experience of physical pain is more than just a painful stimulus and response, the experience of touch is experienced differently by different people and even by the same person at different times. We know this instinctively, which is why we don't offer the same hug that we would give a crying child to our professor or department chair when they are upset!

The experience of both painful stimuli and caring touch stimuli are a combination of bottom-up factors (the quality of the touch stimulus) moderated by top-down influences such as mood, beliefs, social norms, expectations, et cetera.[155] Dr. Paula Barry points out, "It is important to note that the physical touch or hug effects are positive only in those that there is a caring relationship not from unwanted touching. In fact, undesired physical contact can have the opposite effect by increasing cortisol levels and stress."[156]

The bottom line is that the HCP needs to try to understand each patient's preferences and boundaries and to act—or not act—accordingly. In the absence of explicit instruction from patients, HCPs can look for cues from patients, and in the absence of clear cues, the HCP can *solicit* patients' preferences on touch. For example, if a dental assistant notices a patient clutching the armrests, they could ask, "Would it be helpful if I put my hand on your shoulder or hand your hand?"

Research on touch in health care has identified several general patient preferences. One study reported, "patients accept unnecessary touch only when the relationship has developed."[157] Other studies report patients do not like being "handled carelessly"[142] and prefer a touch that is "firm but not rough, unhurried but not so slow that it lingers."[158] Touch from overhead (the predominant posture in dentistry and other specialties) "is associated with the exertion of power,"[149] which underlines the importance of affirming the *power of the patient* (the P in ISLEEP), especially when touching. Video 5.19 captures an example of caring touch as well as affirming the *power of the patient* by asking permission: "Are you okay with me bringing the chair back?"

The HCP is not the only person who can provide caring touch to alleviate procedural pain and anxiety—it can also come from any trusted person. For example, a parent could provide caring touch to their child, a caregiver to a special needs patient, and a significant other or friend to an adult patient. Touch from a trusted person could be offered before, during, or after a challenging procedure. Also, as we learned in Chapter 4 (self-compassion), an individual can offer *themself* care with their own touch. During a stressful procedure, a patient could be invited to "gently place your hand on your belly or heart if it feels comforting to you. Feel the contact, feel the warmth, imagine positive energy flowing into your body with every breath."

A final note: Expressive touch has benefits to the giver of the touch as well, as captured in the opening story with Sarah—the calm feeling in my heart as I touched her with an intention of care. Compassion even without touch is associated with oxytocin and dopamine, as we saw in Chapter 2. Adding the inherently intimate and immediate experience of touch only magnifies the effects of compassion.

In conclusion, caring touch can offer patients relief from anxiety and pain during medical and dental procedures. It has the potential to close the gate on pain transmission both bottom-up (non-pain sensation of touch) as well as top-down (psychological effects of caring). The subjectivity of the experience of touch requires understanding each patient's personal touch preferences. Taking cues from the patient and soliciting their wishes allows the patient to lead the delicate dance of touch.

Experiments: Expressive (Caring) Touch

1. Mindful self-compassion teacher Mila de Koning, co-author of *Heart for the Doctor*, explains to her class participants that when you touch yourself with self-compassion you get an immediate "oxytocin shot." Touch can be a powerful means of soothing oneself, especially during stressful situations. Try this experiment with touch:

   Sit quietly in a private space and allow the attention to settle on the breath, the body, or sounds. Notice how you are feeling right now. Like a mother comforts her child with touch, try gently placing a hand on your heart or another area that would feel comforting. Feel the sensations of the touch, including perhaps warmth, the texture of clothing, pulse of the heart, the chest rising and falling with the breath. Connect with an intention of care and acceptance for yourself (including the part of you that protests self-compassion!) Notice what arises. You might take a moment to journal whatever you notice.

2. Consider procedures that you perform that are anxiety-provoking or painful for patients. (a) Is there a time when you could invite the patient to place a hand on themself to provide themself with an "oxytocin shot?" (b) Is there a time before, during, or after the procedure when it would be possible for someone (HCP, team member, family, or friend) to offer the patient a caring touch?

Reiki

Scenario: *A patient presents for a dental extraction, and it needs to be extracted as soon as possible since the patient is in pain and has an abscess. Unfortunately the patient's blood pressure is too high to proceed. If their blood pressure does not decrease, the appointment will have to be rescheduled.*

This is a common scenario in my dental practice, and when it arises, I offer patients reiki, a relaxation technique involving touch. Reiki is a simple, non-invasive, non-pharmacologic way to help patients manage pain and anxiety. After less than 5 minutes of a reiki treatment, most patients' blood pressure decreases (at times dramatically!) thus allowing for treatment to proceed as planned. Also, patients frequently report decreased anxiety and a greater sense of calm and ease. For me, it is refreshing to be able to transcend the confines of procedural

touch to offer another form of touch, one that helps soothe and calm both the patient and myself.

Reiki originated in Japan, and it involves the practitioner's hands either contacting or hovering over different areas of the patient's body in a sequence. The belief is that the practitioner channels energy "to promote or facilitate self-healing in the patient."[159] A systematic review of RCTs found reiki decreased pain and anxiety as well as depression, stress, and hopelessness.[159] According to reiki teachers Barnett and Chambers, the main mechanism of action of reiki is through induction of the relaxation response, which in turn releases endorphins and improves immune function.[160]

Reiki requires at least one of three levels of training. Level one can be completed in 10 to 12 hours of training (which can be done in as little as 2 days), according to my teacher Myra Reichel, a seasoned reiki master. Training includes "attunements" of students by the teacher, without which "a person cannot be said to be practicing reiki, even if they learn the technical aspects of where to put their hands."[161] While attunement and technique are important, the most important aspect of reiki is the *intention of care* for the client. This emphasis on an intention of care makes reiki a form of compassion practice, and, as we saw in Chapter 2, compassion brings benefits, such as a positive mood and decreased stress, not only to the recipient but also to the practitioner.

My experience with Reiki has been very positive, not only for supporting my patients but also for my own well-being. After my first class with Myra, I felt peaceful and relaxed; I went straight from the reiki class to my doctor for a routine physical exam, where my blood pressure, which was normally around 100/60, was measured at 75/45! When I administer reiki to myself (a standard practice), it helps me be calm and focused. Similarly, when I practice reiki on my dental patients, it also calms and focuses me and fosters compassion for the person in the dental chair. I encourage all HCPs to explore this fascinating healing modality for their own benefit and that of their patients. Figs. 5.16 and 5.17 illustrate reiki treatment for a dental patient.

Postoperative Communication

Few patient care practices generate as much goodwill and gratitude from patients as a postoperative phone call. Research has found evidence that postoperative communication can close the gate on pain transmission remotely after the patient has left the office! A cluster of

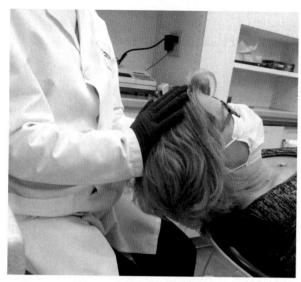

Fig. 5.16 Reiki for Dental Patient 1.

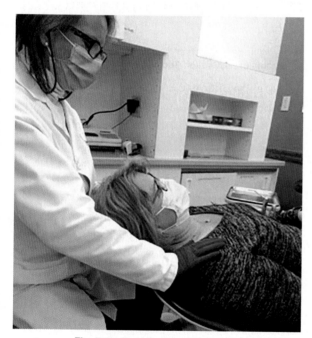

Fig. 5.17 Reiki for Dental Patient 2.

were significantly decreased in the postoperative call group ($P < 0.001$) compared to the no-call group."[162] Another study, an RCT, compared the effects on orthodontic patients of no postoperative communication with daily calls or text for 7 days. "Participants in both the telephone call group and text message group reported a lower level of pain than participants in the control with a larger and more consistent effect for the telephone call group."[163] Similarly, other orthodontic studies have compared the effects of text messages versus no communication and found significantly *lower pain* in the group receiving postoperative texts.[43,164]

No rigorous medical studies were identified investigating the analgesic effects of simple postoperative texts or phone calls; however, some research has explored automated text messages to parents of children before and after tonsillectomy surgery. "Parents reported that [short message service] reminders increased feelings of security and calm, prevented panic, and reduced stress when caring for their child."[165] (As we discussed earlier, reducing parental anxiety can also reduce the child's anxiety.) A more complex form of communication—ACT therapy, a mindfulness-based psychological intervention—was investigated in an RCT involving patients receiving surgery for orthopedic trauma and found *lower pain* associated with 2 weeks of twice daily text messages of ACT. Further, the group receiving the texts used 36.5% *fewer pain pills* than the no-call group.[166] Future research in medicine could explore text messages, phone calls, and in-person postoperative communication (e.g., after hospital-based procedures) as a means of reducing procedural pain and anxiety.

When communicating with a patient after a procedure, the ISLEEP model can provide the HCP and members of their team with a helpful road map:

- *Introduce:* give your name and role
- *Solicit and Listen:* comfort level, adherence to homecare recommendations, questions
- *Empathize:* especially with discomfort or other challenges
- *Explain:* review homecare recommendations; possible postoperative signs, symptoms, and challenges; and how to manage
- *Power:* offer recommendations/suggestions (not commands), offer options

Listen to the following simulated phone call between me and a dental patient several hours after a root canal (Video 5.20).

dental studies have found evidence for the effects of postoperative communications on pain. An age-matched and sex-matched study of 118 periodontal surgery patients compared patients who received a call within 24 hours postoperatively with patients who did not receive a call. It found, "Pain and analgesics used

In summary, research strongly supports the practice of postoperative communications, not only to reduce pain but for a host of other benefits as well. "Structured telephone calls after painful procedures have been shown to be helpful in oral and general health-care delivery to reassure and encourage patients, disseminating information about expected discomfort, reinforcing home-care regimens, and *reducing pain*" (emphasis added).[34] Postoperative communication represents patient-centered care at its best.

Experiment:
(1) What procedures do you do that create anxiety or pain for patients and that could be followed up with postoperative communication?
(2) What form of communication could you use (e.g., text, phone call)?
(3) Which team members could do this and when?

INTEGRATING INTERVENTIONS FOR PROCEDURAL PAIN AND ANXIETY WITH PATIENT STORIES

Just like a surgeon needs an armamentarium of surgical instruments, every HCP needs an armamentarium of techniques for managing procedural pain and anxiety. A calm, comfortable patient is more satisfied, requires less medication, and has a physiology that is more stable and more amenable to healing. Admittedly, there are times, such as emergency situations, in which procedural pain is unavoidable. Yet, with care, creativity, and a combination of interventions, you can aim for a positive—or at least tolerable—experience for your patients every time. As the saying goes, "Shoot for the moon. Even if you miss, you'll land among the stars."[167]

Documenting IPPAs

We have discussed a variety of ways to close the gate as well as ways to avoid opening the gate, both bottom-up and top-down. Table 5.2 summarizes all the interventions by category (top down or bottom up). As you try different interventions for your patients, be sure to document in the patient chart what techniques you employed and how well they worked. This will allow you and other providers to use this information to tailor the approach to the patient's needs. Fig. 5.18 shows an example of how to document IPPAs.

TABLE 5.2 Summary of IPPAs by Category (Top Down or Bottom Up)

IPPA	Bottom Up	Top Down
ISLEEP skills		X
Progressive muscle relaxation		X
Diaphragmatic breathing		X
Mindfulness of breath and body		X
Gradual exposure		X
Non-pain stimuli	X	
Distraction		X
Mental imagery		X
Nonverbal communication		X
Touch (expressive and mindful procedural)	X	X
Postoperative communication		X

IPPAs, Interventions for procedural pain and anxiety.

Example: Restoration, Tooth #19

Name: Charles Gordon

DOB: 8/26/60

S: Pt presents with unlocalized sensitivity lower left teeth for the past month

O: Radiograph (PA #19) reveals periapical region WNL. No swelling or sinus tract LL. Caries #19-0, percussion negative.

A: Restoration needed. Pt opts for composite.

P: Topical benzocaine applied. 1.7 ml lidocaine 2% with epi 1:100,000 via IAN block. Caries removed, etch, prime and bond. Flowable and packable composite. Finish and polish. Postop instructions given.

IPPA: *Diaphragmatic breathing (preop), non-pain stimuli (shaking cheek), mindfulness of breath and body*

Fig. 5.18 Documenting Interventions for Procedural Pain and Anxiety.

To review and reinforce all the ISLEEP skills and IPPAs, let's look at three patient-centered health care experiences. First, Video 5.21 is a conversation with a patient with a history of dental phobia who just had a dental restoration (filling). My questions to her was,

"What was helpful to you during the procedure?" The second is an interview of a woman with a history of childhood abuse (see Video 5.22, audio only). She tells the story of "My very best experience with a doctor before surgery." The last example is a revision of the opening story of Sally (beginning of Chapter 1). For each example, try to identify the ISLEEP communication skills and IPPAs. See Appendix N for summaries, transcripts, and answers.

NOTE: You may notice that the boundaries between different ISLEEP skills and IPPAs are sometimes blurry. For example, an HCP might *interconnect* by *soliciting* personal information like "Have you lived in this area for a long time?" Another example includes affirming a patient's *power* by *explaining* what a patient can do if they experience discomfort during a procedure or by practicing *gradual exposure*. A final example—as an HCP *touches* a patient in pain to comfort them, the HCP might be expressing *empathy*. Because of the overlap of many of the different skills and techniques, there may be several possible labels for the many of the skills and techniques illustrated in the three stories. Don't belabor. Simply notice as many communication skills and IPPAs as you can.

Sally's Visit to the Dental Clinic (New, Improved Version of Chapter 1 Story)

Stabbing, throbbing toothache in the middle of the night, again. Sally had been having pain for months in her lower left back tooth. She couldn't afford treatment and dreaded having dental work done ever since her traumatic dental experience as a child. So, she medicated herself for months and went to the ER once, too. Finally, she couldn't take it anymore.

The dental clinic nearby was swamped on the day of her appointment. After being greeted warmly by the receptionist, she hears her name and sees a woman smiling at her _____ (Intervention for PPA) from the door to the clinic.

Assistant: Hi, my name is Ashley and I am a dental assistant. _____ (ISLEEP skill). Is this your first time at our clinic?_____ (ISLEEP skill).

Sally: *Nods, butterflies in her stomach.*

A: Welcome! I see you have come from a distance. How was your drive? _____ (ISLEEP skill).

S: I got stuck in a bad traffic jam.

A: It's getting harder to drive in this area with so much traffic! _____ (ISLEEP skill).

Are you ready to follow me to our room? _____ (ISLEEP skill).

S: *Nods and follows the assistant down a long hall to the treatment room.*

A: What brings you here today?_____ (ISLEEP skill).

S: Bad pain in this broken tooth. It's been going on for months. *Points to the upper left tooth.*

A: That sounds really uncomfortable! I'm sorry you've been having this problem_____ (ISLEEP skill). How has this affected you in the day-to-day? _____ (ISLEEP skill).

S: I can't sleep at night, which makes it hard to deal with my kids and my job.

A: That sounds really hard. _____ (ISLEEP skill). It would be helpful to get a picture of the tooth so we can see the parts that are under the gum. _____ (ISLEEP skill) Is that okay? _____ (ISLEEP skill).

S: *Nods in approval.*

A: I'm going to recline the chair a bit and put a heavy shield on you now_____ (ISLEEP), okay? _____ (ISLEEP skill)

S: Actually, I have a bad neck. Do you have a pillow? It would help a lot.

A: Sure! *She tucks a pillow behind Sally, who adjusts it a bit until comfortable.* Ready? _____ (ISLEEP skill) *Ashley rests her hand gently on Sally's shoulder as she lowers the chair into position.* _____ (Intervention for PPA).

I'm going to place this x-ray device next to the tooth, and then I'll need you to hold still until you hear the beep. _____ (ISLEEP skill). Ready?_____ (ISLEEP skill)

S: *Gagging a bit.*

A: I have a suggestion—something that helps a lot of people in this situation. Would you like to try holding your foot up for about 10 seconds?_____ (IPPA and ISLEEP skill). Perfect, thank you!

Ashley leaves to get Dr. M.

Dr. M: Hello, Sally! Welcome to our clinic. I'm Dr. M. _____ (ISLEEP skill). I understand you have a painful tooth. Sorry to hear about that!_____ (ISLEEP skill). *He sits down making eye contact.* _____ (IPPA). Can you tell me what the symptoms have been? _____ (ISLEEP skill).

S: A lot of pain for months. I've been taking a lot of pain meds, but it doesn't always help. I wish I could get the tooth out.

Dr. M: Sounds really uncomfortable! _____ (ISLEEP skill). If it's okay _____ (ISLEEP skill; hint: asking permission) I would like to look in your mouth now to see what our options are _____ (ISLEEP skill).

S: Okay.

Dr. M performs an intraoral exam.

Dr. M: Unfortunately, it looks like the tooth is not salvageable. Our options are to do nothing, which I would not recommend since the infection will continue to grow, or to take the tooth out, which we could do today. _____ (2 ISLEEP skills).

S: I think I would like to take it out now.

Dr. M: Okay. What concerns or worries do you have about getting the tooth out? _____ (ISLEEP skill).

S: I am terrified of needles! I had a bad experience as a child and have been terrified ever since.

Dr. M: I can imagine how hard it would be for you after a bad childhood experience. It makes sense! _____ (ISLEEP skill). I will do everything possible to make it easy for you _____ (ISLEEP skill). And you can stop me at any time—if you can't talk just raise your hand. _____ (ISLEEP skill). Here's what I can do for you: we can numb the tooth with a gel, then the numbing medicine. After a few minutes, we will test the tooth to make sure it is numb. You will feel some pressure even if you are totally numb._____ (ISLEEP skill) My assistant, Ashley, and I work with a lot of people who have dental anxiety, and we are here to support you. I encourage you to take a few deep breaths, filling up the belly like a balloon_____ (IPPA). Would you like to try it right now with me? _____ (ISLEEP skill) We know that this kind of breathing helps the body to relax. Many people tend to hold their breath when they are nervous, so I will remind you every now and then to notice and feel your breath_____ (IPPA).

A: Sally, I would like to go over the risks of the tooth extraction and then we will get your blood pressure _____ (ISLEEP skill). Is that okay?_____ (ISLEEP skill). *After obtaining consent and preoperative vital signs…*Would

you be interested in some headphones with music or nature sounds? _____(IPPA).

S: That would be great! *She scans the options.* I love the beach. I'll try this one with ocean sounds and music.

A: Enjoy! Many people find it helpful to imagine the beach with all the senses…what it smells like, feels like, and sounds like. _____ (IPPA).

Dr. M returns.

Dr. M: I'm going to put the chair back now_____ (ISLEEP skill), okay? _____ (ISLEEP skill). Here is the numbing gel. _____ (ISLEEP skill).

He gently retracts Sally's cheek as he tunes into the sensations of warmth and reconnects with an intention of care. _____ (IPPA).

Dr. M: Now I'm going to give you the numbing medicine and you may feel a slight pinch_____ (ISLEEP skill). If it's okay, _____ (ISLEEP skill) I'm going to wiggle your cheek to make it more comfortable. _____ (ISLEEP skill). *He begins to inject local anesthesia while wiggling the cheek. _____ (IPPA). While injecting slowly….*Check-in with your breathing. See if you can notice where your belly is in the breathing cycle—going up, or down or in between. _____ (IPPA) How was that? _____ (ISLEEP skill).

S: Not bad at all! Thank you!

Dr. M: Let's wait a few minutes now for the tooth to numb and then check to make sure it is comfortable for you. _____ (ISLEEP skills).

After a few minutes:

Dr. M: Are you ready? _____ (ISLEEP skill).

S: Ready as I'll ever be.

Dr. M: I'm going to apply a little pressure first. _____ (ISLEEP skill) How's does this feel? _____ (ISLEEP skill).

S: Fine.

Dr. M: Okay. I'm going to apply a little more pressure now. And now I'm going to apply pressure for a few seconds. _____ (IPPA—hint: going a step further than last time). Are you still doing okay? _____ (ISLEEP skill).

Assistant: Check in with your breathing. See if you can soften your belly and let the air flow down there. _____ (IPPA)

After a short time, the tooth is out.

Dr. M: Are you doing okay? _____ (ISLEEP skill).

Thank you for your trust in us. You did it! Ashley will give you some instructions on how to care for yourself at home. _____ (ISLEEP skill). What questions do you have before I go? _____ (ISLEEP skill).

S: Can I make an appointment to have all my teeth fixed here? I am so grateful for your help today. You and Ashley were great!

A few hours later Dr. M calls Sally _____ (Intervention for PPA).

Dr. M: Hello this is Dr. M from the dental clinic calling for Sally _____ (ISLEEP skill).

S: Thank you so much for calling!

Dr. M: How is the area we worked on…feeling comfortable? _____ (ISLEEP skill)

S: Yes, I am doing great. Thank you so much.

Dr. M: You are welcome. Glad to hear you are feeling well. You must be relieved _____ (ISLEEP skill).

S: I am!

Dr. M: Take good care and don't hesitate to call if any questions or issues arise! _____ (2 ISLEEP skills)

See Appendix N for answers.

Reflection Questions:

1. How do you think this approach would impact Sally's future dental and medical experiences?
2. What obstacles do you see in your work situation to adopting a more patient-centered approach as illustrated above? How can you overcome them?
3. Create a story in your own health care specialty that demonstrates the ISLEEP communication skills and several IPPAs.

REFERENCES

1. Cassel EJ. The nature of suffering and the goals of medicine. *N Engl J Med.* 1982;306:639–645.
2. Czarnecki ML, Turner HN, Collins PM, et al. Procedural pain management: a position statement with clinical practice recommendations. *Pain Manag Nurs.* 2011;12:95–111.
3. Riley JL III, Gordan VV, Rindal DB, et al. Dental Practice-Based Research Network Collaborative Group. Components of patient satisfaction with a dental restorative visit: results from the Dental Practice-Based Research Network. *J Am Dent Assoc.* 2012;143:1002–1010.
4. Milgrom P, Weinstein P, Heaton LJ. *Treating Fearful Dental Patients: A Patient Management Handbook.* 3rd ed. Seattle: Dental Behavioral Resources; 2009.
5. Randall CL, Shaffer JR, McNeil DW, et al. Toward a genetic understanding of dental fear: evidence of heritability. *Community Dent Oral Epidemiol.* 2017;45:66–73.
6. Corah NL, O'Shea RM, Bissell GD, et al. The dentist-patient relationship: perceived dentist behaviors that reduce patient anxiety and increase satisfaction. *J Am Dent Assoc.* 1988;116:73–76.
7. King D. Anxiety control. In: Daniel S, Harfast S, eds. *Dental Hygiene: Concepts, Cases, Competencies.* 1st ed. St. Louis: Mosby; 2002:576–854.
8. Ronis DL. Updating a measure of dental anxiety: reliability, validity, and norms. *J Dent Hyg.* 1994;68:228–233.
9. Armfield JM, Stewart JF, Spencer AJ. The vicious cycle of dental fear: exploring the interplay between oral health, service utilization and dental fear. *BMC Oral Health.* 2007;7:1.
10. Hamunen K, Kontinen V, Hakala E, et al. Effect of pain on autonomic nervous system indices derived from photoplethysmography in healthy volunteers. *Br J Anaesth.* 2012;108:838–844.
11. Wilson-Smith EM. Procedural pain management in neonates, infants and children. *Rev Pain.* 2011;5:4–12.
12. Forward JB, Greuter NE, Crisall SJ, et al. Effect of structured touch and guided imagery for pain and anxiety in elective joint replacement patients—a randomized controlled trial: M-TIJRP. *Perm J.* 2015;19:18–28.
13. Kühlmann AYR, de Rooij A, Kroese LF, et al. Meta-analysis evaluating music interventions for anxiety and pain in surgery. *Br J Surg.* 2018;105:773–783.
14. Puntillo KA, White C, Morris AB, et al. Patients' perceptions and responses to procedural pain: results from Thunder Project II. *Am J Crit Care.* 2001;10:238–251.
15. Wellenstein DJ, van der Wal RAB, Schutte HW, et al. Topical anesthesia for endoscopic office-based procedures of the upper aerodigestive tract. *J Voice.* 2019;33:732–746.
16. Frank SG, Lalonde DH. How acidic is the lidocaine we are injecting, and how much bicarbonate should we add? *Can J Plast Surg.* 2012;20:71–73.
17. Ing EB, Philteos J, Sholohov G, et al. Local anesthesia and anxiolytic techniques for oculoplastic surgery. *Clin Ophthalmol.* 2019;13:153–160.
18. Cepeda MS, Tzortzopoulou A, Thackrey M, et al. Adjusting the pH of lidocaine for reducing pain on injection. *Cochrane Database Syst Rev.* 2010;(12):CD006581.
19. Davies RJ. Buffering the pain of local anaesthetics: a systematic review. *Emerg Med (Fremantle).* 2003;15:81–88.
20. Gostimir M, Hussain A. A systematic review and meta-analysis of methods for reducing local anesthetic injection pain among patients undergoing periocular surgery. *Ophthalmic Plast Reconstr Surg.* 2019;35:113–125.

21. Goodchild JH, Donaldson M. Novel direct injection chairside buffering technique for local anesthetic use in dentistry. *Compend Contin Educ Dent.* 2019;40:e1–e10.

22. Simmons CL, Harper LK, Holst KJ, et al. Bargain hunting for buffered lidocaine: a collaborative discovery of cost-saving strategies that can improve patient care. *J Breast Imaging.* 2021;3:93–97.

23. Arora G, Degala S, Dasukil S. Efficacy of buffered local anaesthetics in head and neck infections. *Br J Oral Maxillofac Surg.* 2019;57:857–860.

24. Richtsmeier AJ, Hatcher JW. Buffered lidocaine for skin infiltration prior to hemodialysis. *J Pain Symptom Manag.* 1995;10:198–203.

25. Colaric KB, Overton DT, Moore K. Pain reduction in lidocaine administration through buffering and warming. *Am J Emerg Med.* 1998;16:353–356.

26. Clark TM, Yagiela JA. Advanced techniques and armamentarium for dental local anesthesia. *Dent Clin North Am.* 2010;54:757–768.

27. Garret-Bernardin A, Cantile T, D'Antò V, et al. Pain experience and behavior management in pediatric dentistry: a comparison between traditional local anesthesia and the Wand Computerized Delivery System. *Pain Res Manag.* 2017;2017:7941238.

28. Lee EW, Tucker NA. Pain associated with local anesthetic injection in eyelid procedures: comparison of microprocessor-controlled versus traditional syringe techniques. *Opthal Plast Reconstr Surg.* 2007;23:37–38.

29. LeFort SM, Webster L, Lorig K, et al. *Living A Healthy Life with Chronic Pain.* Boulder: Bull Publishing; 2015.

30. Beecher HK. Anxiety and pain. *JAMA.* 1969;209:1080.

31. Beecher HK. Relationship of significance of wound to pain experienced. *J Am Med Assoc.* 1956;161:1609–1613.

32. Katz J, Rosenbloom BN. The golden anniversary of Melzack and Wall's gate control theory of pain: celebrating 50 years of pain research and management. *Pain Res Manag.* 2015;20:285–286.

33. Melzack R, Wall PD. Pain mechanisms: a new theory. *Science.* 1965;150:971–979.

34. Bartlett BW, Firestone AR, Vig KW, et al. The influence of a structured telephone call on orthodontic pain and anxiety. *Am J Orthod Dentofacial Orthop.* 2005;128:435–441.

35. Melzack R. Pain and the neuromatrix in the brain. *J Dent Educ.* 2001;65:1378–1382.

36. Lauriola M, Tomai M, Palma R, et al. Procedural anxiety, pain catastrophizing, and procedure-related pain during EGD and colonoscopy. *South Med J.* 2020;113:8–15.

37. Lee KC, Bassiur JP. Salivary alpha amylase, dental anxiety, and extraction pain: a pilot study. *Anesth Prog.* 2017;64:22–28.

38. Stamenkovic DM, Rancic NK, Latas MB, et al. Preoperative anxiety and implications on postoperative recovery: what can we do to change our history. *Minerva Anestesiol.* 2018;84:1307–1317.

39. Ahmadi M, Kiakojori A, Moudi S. Association of anxiety with pain perception following periodontal flap surgery. *J Int Soc Prev Community Dent.* 2018;8:28–33.

40. Wang TF, Wu YT, Tseng CF, et al. Associations between dental anxiety and postoperative pain following extraction of horizontally impacted wisdom teeth: a prospective observational study. *Medicine (Baltimore).* 2017;96:e8665.

41. Feinmann C, Ong M, Harvey W, et al. Psychological factors influencing post-operative pain and analgesic consumption. *Br J Oral Maxillofac Surg.* 1987;25:285–292.

42. Sobol-Kwapinska M, Bąbel P, Plotek W, et al. Psychological correlates of acute postsurgical pain: a systematic review and meta-analysis. *Eur J Pain.* 2016;20:1573–1586.

43. Mendonça DL, Almeida-Pedrin RR, Pereira NC, et al. The influence of text messages and anxiety on pain perception and its impact on orthodontic patients routine. *Dental Press J Orthod.* 2020;25:30–37.

44. Ip HY, Abrishami A, Peng PW, et al. Predictors of postoperative pain and analgesic consumption: a qualitative systematic review. *Anesthesiology.* 2009;111:657–677.

45. Makary MS, da Silva A, Kingsbury J, et al. Noninvasive approaches for anxiety reduction during interventional radiology procedures. *Top Magn Reson Imaging.* 2020;29:197–201.

46. Zemła AJ, Nowicka-Sauer K, Jarmoszewicz K, et al. Measures of preoperative anxiety. *Anaesthesiol Intensive Ther.* 2019;51:64–69.

47. Kindler CH, Harms C, Amsler F, et al. The visual analog scale allows effective measurement of preoperative anxiety and detection of patients' anesthetic concerns. *Anesth Analg.* 2000;90:706–712.

48. Horn A. *Phobias: The Ten Most Common Fears People Hold.* ABC News. https://www.abc.net.au/news/2015-05-01/ten-of-the-most-common-phobias/6439210. Accessed March 3, 2021.

49. Ritz T, Meuret AE, Ayala ES. The psychophysiology of blood-injection-injury phobia: looking beyond the diphasic response paradigm. *Int J Psychophysiol.* 2010;78:50–67.

50. Rajwar AS, Goswami M. Prevalence of dental fear and its causes using three measurement scales among children in New Delhi. *J Indian Soc Pedod Prev Dent.* 2017;35:128–133.

51. Armfield JM, Milgrom P. A clinician guide to patients afraid of dental injections and numbness. *SAAD Dig.* 2011;27:33–39.

52. Orsini CA, Jerez OM. Establishing a good dentist-patient relationship: skills defined from the dental faculty perspective. *J Dent Educ.* 2014;78:1405–1415.

53. Torper J, Ansteinsson V, Lundeby T. Moving the four habits model into dentistry. Development of a dental consultation model: do dentists need an additional habit? *Eur J Dent Educ.* 2019;23:220–229.

54. Appukuttan DP. Strategies to manage patients with dental anxiety and dental phobia: literature review. *Clin Cosmet Investig Dent.* 2016;8:35–350.

55. Oommen S, Shetty A. Does parental anxiety affect children's perception of pain during intravenous cannulation? *Nurs Child Young People.* 2020;32:21–24.

56. Yayan EH, Zengin M, Düken ME, et al. Reducing children's pain and parents' anxiety in the postoperative period: a therapeutic model in Turkish sample. *J Pediatr Nurs.* 2020;51:e33–e38.

57. Bearden DJ, Feinstein A, Cohen LL. The influence of parent preprocedural anxiety on child procedural pain: mediation by child procedural anxiety. *J Pediatr Psychol.* 2012;37:680–686.

58. Jastrebski D. *Practice Without Pressure | Disabilities | Education.* Available at: https://www.practicewithoutpressure.com/. Accessed January 12, 2022.

59. CF Foundation. *Procedural Anxiety.* Available at: https://www.cff.org/Life-With-CF/Daily-Life/Emotional-Wellness/Procedural-Anxiety/. Accessed February 25, 2021.

60. Raja S, Hoersch M, Rajagopalan CF, et al. Treating patients with traumatic life experiences: providing trauma-informed care. *J Am Dent Assoc.* 2014;145:238–245.

61. Treleaven DA. *Trauma-Sensitive Mindfulness: Practices for Safe and Transformative Healing.* New York: WW Norton and Company; 2018.

62. Raja S, Hasnain M, Hoersch M, et al. Trauma informed care in medicine: current knowledge and future research directions. *Fam Community Health.* 2015;38:216–226.

63. Willumsen T. Dental fear in sexually abused women. *Eur J Oral Sci.* 2001;109:291–296.

64. Spielberger CD, Gorsuch RL, Lushene RE, et al. *Manual for the State-Trait Anxiety Inventory (Form Y1-Y2).* Palo Alto: Consulting Psychologists Press; 1983.

65. Facco E, Stellini E, Bacci C, et al. Validation of visual analogue scale for anxiety (VAS-A) in preanesthesia evaluation. *Minerva Anestesiol.* 2013;79:1389–1395.

66. Humphris GM, Morrison T, Lindsay SJ. The Modified Dental Anxiety Scale: validation and United Kingdom norms. *Community Dent Health.* 1995;12:143–150.

67. Humphris GM, Clarke HM, Freeman R. Does completing a dental anxiety questionnaire increase anxiety? a randomised controlled trial with adults in general dental practice. *Br Dent J.* 2006;201:33–35.

68. Humphris GM, Dyer TA, Robinson PG. The modified dental anxiety scale: UK general public population norms in 2008 with further psychometrics and effects of age. *BMC Oral Health.* 2009;9:20.

69. Humphris GM, Hull P. Do dental anxiety questionnaires raise anxiety in dentally anxious adult patients? A two-wave panel study. *Prim Dent Care.* 2007;14:7–11.

70. Hally J, Freeman R, Yuan S, et al. The importance of acknowledgement of emotions in routine patient psychological assessment: the example of the dental setting. *Patient Educ Couns.* 2017;100:2102–2105.

71. Dailey YM, Humphris GM, Lennon MA. Reducing patients' state anxiety in general dental practice: a randomized controlled trial. *J Dental Res.* 2002;81:319–322.

72. Stalker CA, Russell BD, Teram E, et al. Providing dental care to survivors of childhood sexual abuse: treatment considerations for the practitioner. *J Am Dent Assoc.* 2005;136:1277–1281.

73. Lang EV, Hamilton D. Anodyne imagery: an alternative to i.v. sedation in interventional radiology. *AJR Am J Roentgenol.* 1994;162:1221–1216.

74. Ayer WA. *Psychology and Dentistry: Mental Health Aspects of Patient Care.* New York: Haworth Press; 2005.

75. Wright BR, Drummond PD. Rapid induction analgesia for the alleviation of procedural pain during burn care. *Burns.* 2000;26:275–282.

76. de Jong AE, Middelkoop E, Faber AW, et al. Non-pharmacological nursing interventions for procedural pain relief in adults with burns: a systematic literature review. *Burns.* 2007;33:811–827.

77. Lewis MJM, Kohtz C, Emmerling S, et al. Pain control and nonpharmacologic interventions. *Nursing.* 2018;48:65–68.

78. Krupat E, Frankel R, Stein T, et al. The Four Habits Coding Scheme: validation of an instrument to assess clinicians' communication behavior. *Patient Educ Couns.* 2006;62:38–45.

79. Lovas JG, Lovas DA. Rapid relaxation–practical management of preoperative anxiety. *J Can Dent Assoc.* 2007;73:437–440.

80. Royal Children's Hospital Melbourne. *Clinical Guidelines (Nursing): Procedural Pain Management.* Available at: https://www.rch.org.au/rchcpg/hospital_clinical_guideline_index/procedural_pain_management/. Accessed December 7, 2020.

81. Mistiaen P, van Osch M, van Vliet L, et al. The effect of patient-practitioner communication on pain: a systematic review. *Eur J Pain.* 2016;20:675–688.

82. Schachter CL, Stalker CA, Teram E, et al. *Handbook on Sensitive Practice for Health Care Practitioners: Lessons from Adult Survivors of Childhood Sexual Abuse.* Ottawa: Public Health Agency of Canada; 2008.

83. Kesbakhi MS, Rohani C. Exploring oncology nurses' perception of the consequences of clinical empathy in patients and nurses: a qualitative study. *Support Care Cancer.* 2020;28:2985–2993.

84. Schachter CL, Radomsky NA, Stalker CA, et al. Women survivors of child sexual abuse. How can health professionals promote healing? *Can Fam Physician.* 2004; 50:405–412.

85. Wiech K, Kalisch R, Weiskopf N, et al. Anterolateral prefrontal cortex mediates the analgesic effect of expected and perceived control over pain. *J Neurosci.* 2006; 26:11501–11509.

86. Rokke PD, Fleming-Ficek S, Siemens NM, et al. Self-efficacy and choice of coping strategies for tolerating acute pain. *J Behav Med.* 2004;27:343–360.

87. Iyengar BKS. *Light on Yoga: Yoga Dipika.* New York: Schocken Books; 1979.

88. Boerner KE, Birnie KA, Chambers CT, et al. Simple psychological interventions for reducing pain from common needle procedures in adults: systematic review of randomized and quasi-randomized controlled trials. *Clin J Pain.* 2015;31:S90–S98.

89. *Lao Tzu Quotes.* Available at: https://www.goodreads.com/author/quotes/2622245.Lao_Tzu. Accessed September 21, 2020.

90. Mancini F, Nash T, Iannetti GD, et al. Pain relief by touch: a quantitative approach. *Pain.* 2014;155: 635–642.

91. Tashani O, Johnson M. Transcutaneous electrical nerve stimulation (TENS): a possible aid for pain relief in developing countries? *Libyan J Med.* 2009;4:62–65.

92. Texas Children's Hospital. *'Buzzy' Device Reduces Pain and Anxiety for Kids Getting Shots at Hospital.* Available at: https://www.texaschildrens.org/blog/2013/02/buzzy-device-reduces-pain-and-anxiety-kids-getting-shots-hospital. Accessed December 13, 2020.

93. Haussler KK. The role of manual therapies in equine pain management. *Vet Clin North Am Equine Pract.* 2010;26:579–601.

94. Mazloum SR, Gandomkar F, Tashnizi MA. The impact of using ice on quality of pain associated with chest drain removal in postcardiac surgery patients: an evidence-based care. *Open Nurs J.* 2019;12:264–271.

95. Demir Y, Khorshid L. The effect of cold application in combination with standard analgesic administration on pain and anxiety during chest tube removal: a single-blinded, randomized, double-controlled study. *Pain Manag Nurs.* 2010;11:186–196.

96. Zahed Pasha Y, Ahmadpour-Kacho M, Hajiahmadi M, et al. Effect of heat application during intramuscular injection of vitamin K in pain prevention in neonates. *Iranian J Neonatol.* 2017;8:31–35.

97. Baba LR, McGrath JM, Liu J. The efficacy of mechanical vibration analgesia for relief of heel stick pain in neonates: a novel approach. *J Perinat Neonatal Nurs.* 2010; 24:274–283.

98. McGinnis K, Murray E, Cherven B, et al. Effect of vibration on pain response to heel lance: a pilot randomized control trial. *Adv Neonatal Care.* 2016;16:439–448.

99. Malik V, Kiran U, Chauhan S, et al. Transcutaneous nerve stimulation for pain relief during chest tube removal following cardiac surgery. *J Anaesthesiol Clin Pharmacol.* 2018;34:216–220.

100. Jones C. The Buzzy: revolutionary acute pain management or simple distraction. *Sci Based Med.* 2014. Available at: https://sciencebasedmedicine.org/the-buzzy-revolutionary-acute-pain-management-or-simple-distraction/. Accessed December 11, 2020.

101. Wong CL, Lui MMW, Choi KC. Effects of immersive virtual reality intervention on pain and anxiety among pediatric patients undergoing venipuncture: a study protocol for a randomized controlled trial. *Trials.* 2019;20:369.

102. Bukola IM, Paula D. The effectiveness of distraction as procedural pain management technique in pediatric oncology patients: a meta-analysis and systematic review. *J Pain Symptom Manag.* 2017;54:589–600.e1.

103. Moola S, Pearson A, Hagger C. Effectiveness of music interventions on dental anxiety in paediatric and adult patients: a systematic review. *JBI Libr Syst Rev.* 2011; 9:588–630.

104. Hole J, Hirsch M, Ball E, Meads C. Music as an aid for postoperative recovery in adults: a systematic review and meta-analysis. *Lancet.* 2015;386:1659–1671.

105. Finn S, Fancourt D. The biological impact of listening to music in clinical and nonclinical settings: a systematic review. *Prog Brain Res.* 2018;237:173–200.

106. Leardi S, Pietroletti R, Angeloni G, et al. Randomized clinical trial examining the effect of music therapy in stress response to day surgery. *Br J Surg.* 2007;94:943–947.

107. Ventura T, Gomes MC, Carreira T. Cortisol and anxiety response to a relaxing intervention on pregnant women awaiting amniocentesis. *Psychoneuroendocrinology.* 2012;37:148–156.

108. Uedo N, Ishikawa H, Morimoto K, et al. Reduction in salivary cortisol level by music therapy during colonoscopic examination. *Hepatogastroenterology.* 2004;51:451–453.

109. Wang MC, Zhang LY, Zhang YL, et al. Effect of music in endoscopy procedures: systematic review and meta-analysis of randomized controlled trials. *Pain Med.* 2014;15:1786–1794.

110. Birnie KA, Noel M, Chambers CT, et al. Psychological interventions for needle-related procedural pain and distress in children and adolescents. *Cochrane Database Syst Rev.* 2018;10:CD005179.

111. Barreiros D, de Oliveira DSB, de Queiroz AM, et al. Audiovisual distraction methods for anxiety in children during dental treatment: a systematic review and meta-analysis. *J Indian Soc Pedod Prev Dent.* 2018;36:2–8.

112. Zhang C, Qin D, Shen L, et al. Does audiovisual distraction reduce dental anxiety in children under local anesthesia? A systematic review and meta-analysis. *Oral Dis.* 2019;25:416–424.

113. Georgescu R, Fodor LA, Dobrean A, et al. Psychological interventions using virtual reality for pain associated with medical procedures: a systematic review and meta-analysis. *Psychol Med.* 2020;50:1795–1807.

114. Eijlers R, Utens EMWJ, Staals LM, et al. Systematic review and meta-analysis of virtual reality in pediatrics: effects on pain and anxiety. *Anesth Analg.* 2019;129:1344–1353.

115. Wiederhold MD, Gao K, Wiederhold BK. Clinical use of virtual reality distraction system to reduce anxiety and pain in dental procedures. *Cyberpsychol Behav Soc Netw.* 2014;17:359–365.

116. Gray ML, Goldrich DY, McKee S, et al. Virtual reality as distraction analgesia for office-based procedures: a randomized crossover-controlled trial. *Otolaryngol Head Neck Surg.* 2021;164:580–588.

117. Vagnoli L, Caprilli S, Vernucci C, et al. Can presence of a dog reduce pain and distress in children during venipuncture? *Pain Manag Nurs.* 2015;16:89–95.

118. Ein N, Li L, Vickers K. The effect of pet therapy on the physiological and subjective stress response: a meta-analysis. *Stress Health.* 2018;34:477–489.

119. Forbes-Haley C, Blewitt I, Puryer J. Dental management of the "gagging" patient—an update. *Int J Dental Health Sci.* 2016;3:423–431.

120. Dickinson CM, Fiske J. A review of gagging problems in dentistry: 2. Clinical assessment and management. *SADJ.* 2006;61:258–262, 266.

121. Boitel RH. Gagging problem in prosthodontic treatment. *J Prosthet Dent.* 1984;51(6):854–855.

122. Kovats JJ. Clinical evaluation of the gagging denture patient. *J Prosthet Dent.* 1971;25:613–619.

123. Debs NN, Aboujaoude S. Effectiveness of intellectual distraction on gagging and anxiety management in children: a prospective clinical study. *J Int Soc Prev Community Dent.* 2017;7:315–320.

124. Dixit UB, Moorthy L. The use of interactive distraction technique to manage gagging during impression taking in children: a single-blind, randomised controlled trial. *Eur Arch Paediatr Dent.* 2021;22:219–225.

125. Bresler D. *Physiological Consequences of Guided Imagery.* Practical Pain Management. Available at: https://www.practicalpainmanagement.com/treatments/complementary/biobehavioral/physiological-consequences-guided-imagery. Accessed April 15, 2021.

126. Peerdeman KJ, van Laarhoven AIM, Bartels DJP, et al. Placebo-like analgesia via response imagery. *Eur J Pain.* 2017;21:1366–1377.

127. Berna C, Tracey I, Holmes EA. How a better understanding of spontaneous mental imagery linked to pain could enhance imagery-based therapy in chronic pain. *J Exp Psychopathol.* 2012;3:258–273.

128. McNorgan C. A meta-analytic review of multisensory imagery identifies the neural correlates of modality-specific and modality-general imagery. *Front Hum Neurosci.* 2012;6:285.

129. Fardo F, Allen M, Jegindø EM, et al. Neurocognitive evidence for mental imagery-driven hypoalgesic and hyperalgesic pain regulation. *Neuroimage.* 2015;120:350–361.

130. Broadbent E, Kahokehr A, Booth RJ, et al. A brief relaxation intervention reduces stress and improves surgical wound healing response: a randomised trial. *Brain Behav Immun.* 2012;26:212–217.

131. Antall GF, Kresevic D. The use of guided imagery to manage pain in an elderly orthopaedic population. *Orthop Nurs.* 2004;23:335–340.

132. Felix MMDS, Ferreira MBG, da Cruz LF, et al. Relaxation therapy with guided imagery for postoperative pain management: an integrative review. *Pain Manag Nurs.* 2019;20:3–9.

133. Philips HC. Imagery and pain: the prevalence, characteristics, and potency of imagery associated with pain. *Behav Cogn Psychother.* 2011;39:523–540.

134. Philips C, Samson D. The rescripting of pain images. *Behav Cogn Psychother.* 2012;40:558–576.

135. Maier A, Schaitz C, Kröner J, et al. Imagery rescripting: exploratory evaluation of a short intervention to reduce test anxiety in university students. *Front Psychiatry.* 2020;11:84.

136. Smucker MR. *Common Language for Psychotherapy (CLP) Procedures. Imagery Rescripting Therapy.* Available at: https://www.commonlanguagepsychotherapy.org/assets/accepted_procedures/imagery_rescripting.pdf. Accessed April 19, 2021.

137. Reiss H. *The power of empathy.* TedXMiddlebury. Available at: https://www.youtube.com/watch?v=baHrcC8B4WM. Accessed August 4, 2021.

138. Wener ME, Schönwetter DJ, Mazurat N. Developing new dental communication skills assessment tools by including patients and other stakeholders. *J Dent Educ.* 2011;75:1527–1541.

139. McKenzie CT. Instructor and dental student perceptions of clinical communication skills via structured assessments. *J Dent Educ.* 2016;80:563–568.

140. Swayden KJ, Anderson KK, Connelly LM, et al. Effect of sitting vs. standing on perception of provider time at bedside: a pilot study. *Patient Educ Couns.* 2012;86:166–171.

141. Foucault M. *The Birth of the Clinic: An Archaeology of Medical Perception.* London: Tavistock; 1973.

142. Stevens PE. Lesbians' health-related experiences of care and noncare. *West J Nurs Res.* 1994;16:639–659.

143. Kerr F, Wiechula R, Feo R, et al. The neurophysiology of human touch and eye gaze and its effects on therapeutic relationships and healing: a scoping review protocol. *JBI Database System Rev Implement Rep.* 2016;14:60–66.

144. Pierre-Bravo D. *Here are the Biggest Body Language Mistakes Millennials Make.* NBC News. Available at: https://www.nbcnews.com/know-your-value/feature/here-are-biggest-body-language-mistakes-millennials-make-ncna816581. Accessed February 21, 2021.

145. Keltner D. *Born to be Good: The Science of a Meaningful Life.* New York: W.W. Norton and Co.; 2009.

146. Connelly JE. The power of touch in clinical medicine. *Pharos Alpha Omega Alpha Honor Med Soc.* 2004;67:11–13.

147. Cocksedge S, George B, Renwick S, et al. Touch in primary care consultations: qualitative investigation of doctors' and patients' perceptions. *Br J Gen Pract.* 2013;63:e283–e290.

148. Tippett J. Providing comfort in the resuscitation room. *Accid Emerg Nurs.* 1994;2(3):155–159.

149. Kelly MA, Nixon L, McClurg C, et al. Experience of touch in health care: a meta-ethnography across the health care professions. *Qual Health Res.* 2018;28:200–212.

150. Gray L, Watt L, Blass EM. Skin-to-skin contact is analgesic in healthy newborns. *Pediatrics.* 2000;105:e14.

151. Johnston C, Campbell-Yeo M, Disher T, et al. Skin-to-skin care for procedural pain in neonates. *Cochrane Database Syst Rev.* 2017;2:CD008435.

152. Coan JA, Schaefer HS, Davidson RJ. Lending a hand: social regulation of the neural response to threat. *Psychol Sci.* 2006;17:1032–1039.

153. Greenbaum PE, Lumley MA, Turner C, et al. Dentist's reassuring touch: effects on children's behavior. *Pediatr Dent.* 1993;15:20–24.

154. Field T. Touch for socioemotional and physical well-being: a review. *Develop Rev.* 2010;30:367–383.

155. Ellingsen DM, Leknes S, Løseth G, et al. The neurobiology shaping affective touch: expectation, motivation, and meaning in the multisensory context. *Front Psychol.* 2016;6:1986.

156. Penn Medicine. *Can You Kiss and Hug Your Way to Better Health?* Available at: https://www.pennmedicine.org/updates/blogs/health-and-wellness/2018/february/affection. Accessed January 6, 2022.

157. Loveridge N. The therapy of touch. *Emerg Nurse.* 2000;7:9–13.

158. O'Lynn C, Krautscheid L. Original research: 'how should I touch you?': a qualitative study of attitudes on intimate touch in nursing care. *Am J Nurs.* 2011;111:24–31, quiz 32–33.

159. Lee MS, Pittler MH, Ernst E. Effects of reiki in clinical practice: a systematic review of randomised clinical trials. *Int J Clin Pract.* 2008;62:947–954.

160. Barnett L, Chambers M. *Reiki: Energy Medicine.* Rochester: Healing Arts; 1996.

161. vanderVaart S, Gijsen VM, de Wildt SN, et al. A systematic review of the therapeutic effects of Reiki. *J Altern Complement Med.* 2009;15:1157–1169.

162. Touyz LZ, Marchand S. The influence of postoperative telephone calls on pain perception: a study of 118 periodontal surgical procedures. *J Orofac Pain.* 1998;12:219–225.

163. Cozzani M, Ragazzini G, Delucchi A, et al. Self-reported pain after orthodontic treatments: a randomized controlled study on the effects of two follow-up procedures. *Eur J Orthod.* 2016;38:266–271.

164. Keith DJ, Rinchuse DJ, Kennedy M, et al. Effect of text message follow-up on patient's self-reported level of pain and anxiety. *Angle Orthodontist.* 2013;83:605–610.

165. Farias N, Rose-Davis B, Hong P, et al. An automated text messaging system (Tonsil-Text-To-Me) to improve tonsillectomy perioperative experience: exploratory qualitative usability and feasibility study. *JMIR Perioper Med.* 2020;3:e14601.

166. Anthony CA, Rojas EO, Keffala V, et al. Acceptance and commitment therapy delivered via a mobile phone messaging robot to decrease postoperative opioid use in patients with orthopedic trauma: randomized controlled trial. *J Med Internet Res.* 2020;22:e17750.

167. Kukolic S. *Shoot for the Moon.* Huffington Post. Available at: https://www.huffpost.com/entry/shoot-for-the-moon_b_59721cd0e4b06b511b02c2c9. Accessed March 4, 2021.

EVALUATING PATIENT-CENTEREDNESS

Ironically, the tools for evaluating patient-centeredness in health care have not been themselves patient-centered. Until recently, there has been a "tendency to evaluate aspects of clinical encounters using criteria developed by managers or professionals in contrast to those based on active input from patients in the development of evaluation criteria."[1] Yet, research has shown that health care professionals (HCPs) are not always the best judges of quality of care. The large-scale study by Riley et al. found that of the 726 patients who were dissatisfied, dentists were unaware in 684 cases, amounting to 94% of cases![2] One explanation offered by investigators: "Health care providers generally are poor judges of their patients' actual preferences, in part because patients often are unable or unwilling to express their expectations and needs."[3] Experts assert, "Patients' experiences may be a more appropriate measure of the patient–clinical relationship than observations from another professional."[1] For measuring provider empathy, a systematic review found, "patient assessment, in contrast to self-report, is the most salient dimension."[4]

Researchers over the past few years have developed several assessment instruments for gathering patient feedback about health care. First, the Consultation And Relational Empathy (CARE) measure is a 10-item patient questionnaire for measuring patients' perceptions of relational empathy in the consultation. It has been found to be a valid and reliable measure in medicine.[5] Subsequently, the CARE measure was tested with dental students and was found to be both valid and reliable for the dental setting as well.[6]

The questions on the CARE measure correspond very closely to each of the six ISLEEP skill categories. For example, CARE measure question #2 asks how the doctor was at "letting you tell your story," which corresponds closely to the ISLEEP skill, *listening*; the ISLEEP skill, *explain*, is captured in CARE question #8, which asks how well the doctor "explained things clearly." See Appendix O for the CARE measure and corresponding ISLEEP skill to each question. The strong correlation between this patient satisfaction measure and the ISLEEP model suggests that the HCP's proficiency in the ISLEEP skills, while not a direct measure of the patient experience, is a good predictor of patient satisfaction.

Unfortunately, current communication evaluation tools in health care, including the CARE measure, focus entirely on the *consultation* and do not capture the many aspects of communication particular to medical and dental *procedures*. Future research could test a revised version of the CARE measure that includes questions pertaining to procedures. Two such possible questions, derived from a 20-point survey of factors correlating with dental patient satisfaction, include (a) *How my health care provider limited my fear and anxiety,* and (b) *How my provider limited pain during the procedure.*[2] Questions such as these would capture the challenges particular to medical and dental procedures.

Another communication evaluation instrument which incorporates patient preferences, the Patient Communication Assessment Instrument (PCAI), was developed expressly for dentistry. The PCAI identifies six factors "significantly associated with communication skills" and identifies questions for the dental patient associated with each factor.[7] Like the CARE measure, the questions of the PCAI also correspond very closely to the six skills of ISLEEP, suggesting that proficiency in ISLEEP skills would predict a positive patient experience.

Appendix C provides an evaluation tool for ISLEEP skills.

HUMANITY OF THE PATIENT AND THE HCP

One of the essential qualities of the clinician is interest in humanity, for the secret of the care of the patient is in caring for the patient.[8]

Francis Peabody

For while our aspiring doctors will be appreciated by patients for their astute diagnosis or successful treatment, they will be loved for their listening ear and gentle touch.[9]

Tod Worner

Health care providers internalize the model of health care imparted by their education and training; thereby, the culture of education sets the tone for the professional culture beyond. As long as educational systems continue to promote a reductionist model of illness and focus entirely on scientific knowledge and technical skills, medicine and dentistry will be confined to a limited, mechanistic approach, and attempts to provide patient-centered care will continue to be an uphill, countercurrent endeavor. A mechanistic approach to health care, at the exclusion of the humanistic aspects, denies patients and providers the full potential of the therapeutic relationship and creates what has been called, "an unfortunate conundrum":

> Health care providers "express their caring by conscientiously doing what they have been taught to do—pursue diagnostic assessment and treatment—yet patients perceive this as uncaring because their needs to be heard and understood are not met. Patients feel unacknowledged; physicians feel unappreciated. Both are hurt by a model of practice that is too narrowly focused on the biology of disease rather than the experience of illness."[10]

Conversely, an educational culture that elevates the care of the whole person would promote a patient-centered professional culture, as described by physician and educator Dr. Tod Worner:

> "Education done properly…involves not solely passing along facts and details" but also "reminding the student to 'remember the goal.'…not to simply give them fish, nor simply to teach them how to fish, but even more, to remind them steadily why they are fishing in the first place."[9]

In addition, the education and training of a humanistic HCP must include developing the qualities and communication skills of a healer delineated in this book. Such an education would allow patients and providers to enjoy the full potential of whole person care.

The call to embrace humanity in health care is not limited to the patient, alone. Humanism in health care requires moving beyond a view of the HCP as a receptacle of knowledge or a skilled technician to embracing the whole professional—strengths and weaknesses. Many are drawn to the healing professions as a result of their own wounds, and these challenges are compounded by the mounting stresses of the health care industry in our times. The vulnerability of the HCP is evidenced by the current rates of burnout, mental health disorders, and suicide.

A focus on self-care and self-compassion for the HCP is a natural and requisite expression of a whole person orientation to patient care. There are so many means to self-care and self-compassion, and I encourage you to find your own unique path. The paths to healing are many and include meditation, support groups, psychotherapy, prayer, journaling, exploring nature, art, and music.

Mindfulness and self-compassion practice are especially beneficial to the HCP. They support personal well-being on all levels—physical, mental, and emotional—while also cultivating compassion for others. In the words of the great meditation teacher Gunaratana, "When you have learned compassion for yourself, compassion for others is automatic. An accomplished meditator has achieved a profound understanding of life, and he inevitably relates to the world with a deep and uncritical love."[11]

So, practice the meditations, study your ISLEEP charts, and master interventions for procedural pain and anxiety. Then, set aside the maps and models, tables and charts of what you should say and do. Be present with a kind intention to others and yourself, and let the curiosity and kindness of Presence show you the way.

REFERENCES

1. Wener ME, Schönwetter DJ, Mazurat N. Developing new dental communication skills assessment tools by including patients and other stakeholders. *J Dent Educ.* 2011; 75:1527–1541.

2. Riley JL III, Gordan VV, Rindal DB, et al.; Dental Practice-Based Research Network Collaborative Group. Components of patient satisfaction with a dental restorative visit: results from the Dental Practice-Based Research Network. *J Am Dent Assoc.* 2012;143:1002–1010.

3. Riley JL III, Gordan VV, Hudak-Boss SE, et al.; National Dental Practice-Based Research Network Collaborative Group. Concordance between patient satisfaction and the dentist's view: findings from The National Dental Practice-Based Research Network. *J Am Dent Assoc.* 2014;145:355–362.

4. Hemmerdinger JM, Samuel DR, Stoddart SDR, Lilford RJ. A systematic review of tests of empathy in medicine. *BMC Med Educ.* 2007;7(24).

5. Mercer SW, Maxwell M, Heaney D, et al. The Consultation And Relational Empathy (CARE) measure: development and preliminary validation and reliability of an empathy-based consultation process measure. *Fam Pract.* 2004;21:699–705.

6. Babar MG, Hasan SS, Yong WM, et al. Patients' perceptions of dental students' empathic, person-centered care in a dental school clinic in Malaysia. *J Dent Educ.* 2017; 81:404–412.

7. Schönwetter DJ, Wener ME, Mazurat N. Determining the validity and reliability of clinical communication assessment tools for dental patients and students. *J Dent Educ.* 2012;76:1276–1290.

8. Peabody F. *The Care of the Patient. JAMA.* 1927;88(12): 877-882.

9. Worner T. *What's gone wrong in the training of doctors and how to make it right.* Available at: https://aleteia.org/blogs/catholic-thinking/whats-gone-wrong-in-the-training-of-doctors-and-how-to-make-it-right/. Accessed April 19, 2022.

10. Suchman AL, Markakis K, Beckman HB, Frankel R. A model of empathetic communication in the medical interview. *JAMA.* 1997;277:678-682.

11. Gunaratana H. *Mindfulness in Plain English.* Boston: Wisdom; 2002.

Mindfulness Resources

COURSES

- Mindfulness-based Stress Reduction (MBSR) Available Worldwide
- Mindful Self-compassion Courses See www.mindfulmsc.org

GUIDED MEDITATIONS

1. www.headspace.com includes a smartphone app
2. http://health.ucsd.edu/specialties/mindfulness/programs/mbsr/Pages/audio.aspx: MBSR course meditations, including body scan, sitting practice, yoga.
3. www.centerformsc.org

SUGGESTED BOOKS

- *Mindfulness: A Practical Guide to Finding Peace in a Frantic World*; Williams and Penman
- *Mindfulness in Plain English*; Gunaratana: can download free from internet (also available in paperback)
- *Real Happiness*; Sharon Salzberg
- *Full Catastrophe Living*; Jon Kabat-Zinn

(Text for the 8 week MBSR course)

- *How to Meditate*; Pema Chödrön

ISLEEP Summary Chart

ISLEEP Skill	Components
I. *Introduce/Interconnect*	• *Introduce* self by name and title and address patient by name and title (Mr./Mrs.) or ask "how would you like to be called?" • *Interconnect* with the patient as a person (e.g., not just a tooth problem) • *Introduce* the planned procedure/purpose for visit
S. *Solicit*	• *Before/after procedures*: solicit questions/concerns/fears using open-ended questions (why, what, where, when, how) • *During procedures:* solicit comfort level using closed-ended questions (yes/no)
L. *Listen*	• Focusing with Mindfulness: **S.T.O.P.** = Stop, Take a breath, Observe/open the heart, Proceed • Demonstrating active listening sitting still, at eye level, making eye contact, leaning forward, nodding, mirroring (words and body language) • Attire: without gloves and goggles, clean, professional Note: when possible, give the patient a chance to tell their story uninterrupted
E. *Empathize/Validate*	• *NONVERBAL:* Body language mirrors the patient's emotions • *VERBAL:* "It must be hard to feel so _____." "It makes sense that you would feel_____."
E. *Explain/Reassure*	• *Before tx:* explain how you can address the need/want/fear, tx options, risks and benefits • *During exam:* what you are looking for • *During tx:* what sensations will be felt (**especially** discomfort) • *After tx:* what to expect Note: use language the patient can understand
P. *Power of the patient*	• *Before and after tx*: offer recommendations and suggestions (not commands) • *During tx:* - make requests NOT commands: "Could/would you, _____," "When you're ready, please _____." - ask permission: "I'm going to_____, is that alright/ok?" - give options: "Can you keep going or do you need a break?" especially for pain during procedures: e.g., "Would you like to try again, wait a moment, or more numbing medicine?"

ISLEEP Evaluation Worksheet

ISLEEP Skill	Positive		Suggestions for Improvement	
	Hands off	Hands on	Hands off	Hands on
I. *Introduce/Interconnect*				
S. *Solicit*				
L. *Listen*				
E. *Empathize/Validate*				
E. *Explain*				
P. *Power of the Patient*				

© Carmelina D'Arro, DMD 2015, 2018, 2019.

ISLEEP Skills for the Consultation (With Examples)

ISLEEP Skill	Consult/tx Plan	Examples
I. *Introduce/Interconnect*	*(See Appendix B)*	
S. *Solicit*	• Chief complaint • Symptoms	NOTE: The consultation features soliciting with open-ended questions usually beginning with "what" or "how"
	• Concern/fears————— →	*What if anything makes you anxious? How can I make it easier for you?*
	• Needs, wants, values——— →	*What, from your point of view, matters most for your teeth? What do you wish for your mouth?*
	• Beliefs about condition/tx options/ prevention strategies →	*What have you heard about root canals? What is your understanding about the cause of cavities? What do you know about dentures?*
	• How they experience the condition/tx options/prevention strategies →	*How does this condition impact you?*
	• Questions about condition/treatments/ prevention strategies————— → • Potential barriers to care (social determinants) ————— →	*What questions do you have about_____ i.e., gum disease?* *What could get in the way of completing your treatment: time, money, transportation?*
L. *Listen*	*(See Appendix B)*	
E. *Empathize/Validate*	*(See Appendix B)*	
E. *Explain/Reassure*	• Treatment options • Risks/benefits of each option • Use visuals (pictures, decision boards, option grids) • Check understanding———— →	*Could you tell me how you understand the treatment choices I've presented to you?*
P. *Power of the Patient*	Ask permission to give information → Patient chooses tx when ready———— →	*Can I tell you about some options for restoring this tooth?* *Are you ready to decide? Do you need more time/information? What would be your preference?*

ISLEEP Skills for Pre- and Postoperative Phases (With Examples)

ISLEEP Skill	Treatment Visit: Preop and Postop	Example
I. *Introduce/Interconnect*	*(See Appendix B)*	
S. *Solicit*	**Preop:**	
	• Questions————→	*What questions do you have about the procedures for today?*
	• Fears/concerns————→	*What, if anything, are you concerned/worried/anxious about?*
	• Requests for comfort measures ————→	*What can I do or avoid doing to make you more comfortable?*
	Postop:	
	• Questions————→	*What questions do you have now that we are done for today?*
	• Feedback on experience————→	*How was today's visit for you? What could I do next time to make it easier for you?*
L. *Listen*	*(See Appendix B)*	
E. *Empathize/Validate*	*(See Appendix B)*	
E. *Explain/Reassure*	**Preop:**	
	• Procedure and rationale	
	• Review risks and benefits	
	• How you will address fears ————→	*(e.g., for fear of needle) To make it as comfortable as possible, I will rub a numbing gel, and, as I give the Novocain, I will use a shaking technique.*
	• What the patient can do to alleviate pain and anxiety————→	*Many patients tend to hold the breath, so I will remind you from time to time to check in with your breathing and try to allow it to flow, as much as possible (Mindfulness of breath).*
	Postop:	
	• Postop—What to expect————→	*Numbness should wear off in a couple hours. Please call if you have any questions or concerns.*
	• After hours care————→	*Please call this number if you have an urgent need after hours.*
P. *Power of the Patient*	Agree on a STOP signal (esp. for pain or anxiety)	*Please raise your hand if you need to stop at any time because you are uncomfortable or you just need a break.*

ISLEEP Skills for Hands on Mode (With Examples)

ISLEEP Skill	Treatment Visit: During Procedure or Clinical Exam	Examples
I. Introduce/ Interconnect	Continue interconnect during procedure breaks (e.g., waiting for local anesthesia)	*How is your family doing? What are you looking forward to in the coming weeks?*
S. Solicit	Comfort level (physical/ emotional) Details about discomfort	*Are you doing OK? Still comfortable?* (ask frequently, especially when patient cannot talk) *I'm sorry something is bothering you. Can you tell me what it is?*
L. Listen	Tune in to non-verbal cues of discomfort, pain, or anxiety	For example, noticing patient not breathing diaphragmatically, or clutching armrests, tensing body
E. Empathize/ Validate	When patient expresses discomfort	*I see that something is bothering you. I can understand why this would be hard for you/why you would be uncomfortable?*
E. Explain/ Reassure	EXAM: what looking for (i.e., decay, defective restorations) EXAM and PROCEDURES: • What sensations will be felt *(especially uncomfortable)* • What the patient can do to help with pain and anxiety - Diaphragmatic breathing - Mindfulness of breath - Distraction	*Checking the soft parts of the mouth, now the teeth for new decay, now old fillings to make sure they are still sealed and intact. You will feel _____ (air, pressure, water spray, pinch) now.* *If it's possible, allow the belly to be soft and to flow up and down with each breath. Check in with your breathing. Notice what it feels like. Notice if you are holding your breath.* For example, for x-rays or dental impressions: *You can try to hold a leg up. When you get tired, switch legs.*
P. Power of the Patient	• Ask permission • Make requests • Give options (especially when uncomfortable) • Gradual exposure	(Before starting) *If it's OK, I'm going to recline the chair now.* (During tooth preparation) *Can I continue a little longer? If it's possible, please open a little wider/turn your head.* (Anytime: remind about stop signal) *Please stop me if you need a break or if something bothers you.* (Pain during tooth preparation) *I'm sorry it's bothering you. Would you like me to numb the tooth more or maybe try again?* (During tooth preparation) *I'm going to turn on the handpiece near the tooth without touching. Is that OK? Now I will touch for 1 s, OK? Now for 5 s at a time, and you can stop me any time.*

Explain Using Lay Terminology

Medical Term	Lay Language
Edema	Swelling
Antibiotics	Medication to kill or stop growth of bacteria
Benign	Not dangerous
Fast	Go without food and water
Glucose	Sugar
Negative lab result	Nothing is detected (e.g., no infection is present)
Positive lab result	Something is detected (e.g., infection is present)
CVA (Cerebral Vascular Accident)	Stroke
Incontinence	Not able to control urine or bowel movements

Dental Term	Lay Language
Composite restoration	White filling, tooth-colored filling
Extraction	Tooth removal
Alveoloplasty	Shaping the gums
Local anesthesia	Numbing medicine
Topical anesthesia	Numbing gel
Administer anesthesia	To numb
Gingival recession	Gums falling/moving down
Soft tissues	Soft parts of the mouth—gums/cheeks/tongue
Scaling and root planing	Treatment of gum disease*
Irreversible pulpitis/pulp necrosis/chronic PA (periapical) periodontitis/acute PA periodontitis	Infection
Gingival graft	Gum patch
Acid etch	Gel cleanser
Post and core	Special filling with an anchor to support filling/crown
Recall visit	Recare/maintenance

Note: *"Deep cleaning"* does not capture the value or importance: sounds optional (like most cleanings in life!)

Summary of ISLEEP Skills in All Phases of Care

ISLEEP Skill	"HANDS OFF" Consultation	"HANDS OFF" Treatment Visit: Preop and Postop	"HANDS ON" Clinical Exam and Treatment Visit (During Procedure)
I. *Introduce/Interconnect*	Address by name, interconnect, clarify agenda for visit	Address by name, interconnect, clarify agenda for visit	Continue interconnect during procedure breaks (e.g., waiting for local anesthesia)
S. *Solicit*	• Chief complaint • Symptoms • Concerns/fears • Needs, wants, values • Beliefs about condition/tx options • Experience of the condition/tx • Questions	Preop (written or verbal): • Questions • Fears/concerns • Requests for comfort measures Postop: • Questions • Feedback on experience	Comfort level (physical and emotional) Details about discomfort
L. *Listen*	Tune in Demonstrate attention and care	Tune in Demonstrate attention and care	Especially if patient can't talk, tune in to nonverbal cues about discomfort, pain, anxiety
E. *Empathize/Validate*	Demonstrate understanding and acceptance	Demonstrate understanding and acceptance	Demonstrate understanding and acceptance (especially when patient expresses discomfort)

E. *Explain/Reassure*	• Treatment options
	• Risks/benefit
	• Use visuals
	• Check understanding of info
	NOTE: *Avoid details about procedures*
		Preop:
		• Review procedure and rationale
		• Review risks and benefits
		• How will you address pain and anxiety
		• What patients can do to alleviate pain and anxiety
		Postop:
		• What to expect and how to cope
		• After hours support
			CLINICAL EXAM: Describe what looking for (e.g., decay, defective restorations, oral cancer)
			EXAM and PROCEDURES:
			• What sensations will be felt (especially if uncomfortable)
			• What the patient can do to help with
			  - Breathing techniques
			  - Mindfulness
			  - Distraction

P. *Power of the Patient*	Patient chooses tx based on their preferences, needs, and values NOTE: *Recommendations and suggestions (not commands)*	Agree on a stop signal (for pain or anxiety)	• Ask permission • Make requests • Give options • Gradual exposure

ISLEEP Applied to Motivational Interviewing

ISLEEP Skill	Motivational Interviewing Skill	Examples
I. *Introduce/ Interconnect*		
S. *Solicit*	• **"DARN"** **D**esires	**D**: What do you want, like, wish, hope for, etc.? How much do you wish to change the health of your teeth?
	Ability	**A**: What is possible? What can or could you do?
	Reasons	**R**: Why would you make this change? What are the benefits?
	Need	**N**: How important is this change? How much do you need to do it?
	• Importance of change to patient	• How important is it for you to avoid losing more teeth?
	• Confidence in ability to change	• How confident are you that you could quit smoking if you decided to?
	• Pros and cons of the behavior	• What do you like about smoking? (Pros) What's the downside? (Cons)
	• Rulers (asking the questions on a scale of 1–10 and then ask why not a lower number)	• You estimate your desire to quit smoking a 5 out of 10. Why not a lower number? (Solicits change talk)
L. *Listen*	• Reflect resistance to change	• It takes more time and effort to brush and floss than you have. It hasn't seemed a good time to quit smoking until now.
	• Reflect change talk (DARN, commitment, and steps to take) • Summarize	• You want to quit smoking because it's important to set a good example to your kids (desire and reason).
E. *Empathize/ Validate*	NOTE: Avoid scare tactics and shame	• It's hard to change habits and routines, especially with all the stressors you are dealing with at this time.

Continued

ISLEEP Skill	Motivational Interviewing Skill	Examples
E. *Explain/Reassure*	• Ask what the patient already knows • Ask permission to provide info • Provide info that patient asks for • Ask for their response to the info • Talk about what others do (instead of suggesting what the patient should do) • Check for understanding	• What do you know about the effects of smoking? • Could I tell you about some ways to avoid cavities? • What would you most like to know about? • What do you make of that? What does this mean for you? What more would you like to know? • Some patients in your situation reduce sugar intake, brush more often, or use more fluoride products. • Does this make sense? Is there any part that you didn't understand or would like to ask more about?
P. *Power of the Patient*	• Offer choices: offer multiple choices at once (instead of one at a time) • Patient chooses next step *NOTE: Avoid suggesting what the Patient should do (unlike treatment planning)*	• (Caries prevention) Would you like to try reducing sugar intake, brush more often, or use more fluoride products? • What do you think you'll do? What would be a first step?

Changing health-related behaviors: Motivational interviewing (Rollnick S, Miller WR, Butler C. Motivational interviewing in health care: helping patients change behavior. New York: Guilford Press, 2008.)

ISLEEP Skills All Phases of Care (Including Health Counseling)

ISLEEP Skill	Consult/tx Plan	Treatment Visit: Preop and Postop	Treatment Visit: During Procedure (Predominant Phase)	Motivational Interviewing Skill
I. *Introduce/ Interconnect*	• names • interconnect • agenda for visit	• names • interconnect • agenda for visit	Interconnect—when a procedure has a break (i.e., waiting for anesthesia)	• names • interconnect • agenda for visit

S. *Solicit*	• Chief complaint
	• Symptoms
	• Concerns/fears
	• Needs, wants, values
	• Beliefs about condition/tx options/ previous strategies
	• How they experience the condition/tx
	• Questions
		• Questions
		• Fears/concerns
			• Comfort level (physical and emotional)
			• Details about discomfort
				• "DARN"
				  Desires
				  Ability to change what
				  Reasons to change
				  Need for the change
				• Importance of change to the patient
				• Patients' confidence in ability to change
				• Rulers—asking above questions on a scale of 1–10 then ask why not a lower number (solicits change talk)
				• Pros and cons of the behavior to the patient

L. *Listen*	• Tuning in • Expressing attention	• Tuning in • Expressing attention	Tuning in to non verbal cues about discomfort, pain, anxiety	• Reflect resistance to change • Reflect change talk • Summarize
E. *Empathize/ Validate*	• Verbal • Nonverbal (mirroring)	• Verbal • Nonverbal (mirroring)	(When patient expresses discomfort)	NOTE: Avoid scare tactics and shame

Continued

ISLEEP Skill	Consult/tx Plan	Treatment Visit: Preop and Postop	Treatment Visit: During Procedure (Predominant Phase)	Motivational Interviewing Skill
E. *Explain/ Reassure*	• Treatment options • Risks/benefits • Use visuals • Check understanding of info	• Procedure and rationale • Review risks and benefits • How will you address the fears • What patient can do to alleviate pain and anxiety • Postop—what to expect	• What sensations will be felt (especially if uncomfortable) • What the patient can do to help with pain and anxiety - Breathing techniques - Mindfulness - Distraction	• Ask what the patient already knows • Ask permission to provide info • Provide info that patient asks for • Ask for their response to the info • Talk about what others do (instead of suggesting what patient should do) • Check for understanding
P. *Power of the Patient*	• Ask permission to give info • Patient chooses tx when ready	Agree on a stop signal (esp. for pain or anxiety)	• Ask permission • Make requests • Give options • Gradual exposure	• Offer multiple choices at once (instead of one at a time) • Patient chooses next action step NOTE: Avoid suggesting what the patient should do

Source of motivational interviewing skills: Rollnick S, Miller WR, Butler C. Motivational interviewing in health care: helping patients change behavior. New York: Guilford Press, 2008.

Preprocedural Screening for Anxiety, Trauma, and Abuse

PREPROCEDURAL SCREENING

Because anxiety, trauma, and abuse are common and affect one's health and health care experiences, we ask all patients the following questions:

1. Please mark on the line your level of anxiety about your upcoming procedure.

```
0    10   20   30   40   50   60   70   80   90  100
No anxiety                              Maximum anxiety
```

2. What worries you about your upcoming procedure? _____

3. What can we do or offer you to make you more comfortable? _____

4. Is there anything else you would like us to know? _____

NOTE: The information you share is confidential and will enable us to care for you in a way that is more sensitive to your needs.

Adverse Childhood Experiences Questionnaire

The Adverse Childhood Events (ACE) Questionnaire is a simple scoring system that attributes one point for each category of adverse childhood experience. The 10 questions below each cover a different domain of trauma, and refer to experiences that occurred prior to the age of 18. Higher scores indicate increased exposure to trauma, which have been associated with a greater risk of negative consequences.

While you were growing up, during your first 18 years of life:

1. Did a parent or other adult in the household often or very often… Swear at you, insult you, put you down, or humiliate you? or Act in a way that made you afraid that you might be physically hurt?
   YES   NO   If yes, enter 1 _____

2. Did a parent or other adult in the household often or very often… Push, grab, slap, or throw something at you? or Ever hit you so hard that you had marks or were injured?
   YES   NO   If yes, enter 1 _____

3. Did an adult or person at least 5 years older than you ever… Touch or fondle you or have you touch their body in a sexual way? or Attempt or actually have oral, anal, or vaginal intercourse with you?
   YES   NO   If yes, enter 1 _____

4. Did you often or very often feel that… No one in your family loved you or thought you were important or special? or Your family didn't look out for each other, feel close to each other, or support each other?
   YES   NO   If yes, enter 1 _____

5. Did you often or very often feel that… You didn't have enough to eat, had to wear dirty clothes, and had no one to protect you? or Your parents were too drunk or high to take care of you or take you to the doctor if you needed it?
   YES   NO   If yes, enter 1 _____

6. Were your parents ever separated or divorced?
   YES   NO   If yes, enter 1 _____

7. Was your mother or stepmother: Often or very often pushed, grabbed, slapped, or had something thrown at her? or Sometimes, often, or very often kicked, bitten, hit with a fist, or hit with something hard? or Ever repeatedly hit at least a few minutes or threatened with a gun or knife?
   YES   NO   If yes, enter 1 _____

8. Did you live with anyone who was a problem drinker or alcoholic or who used street drugs?
   YES   NO   If yes, enter 1 _____

9. Was a household member depressed or mentally ill, or did a household member attempt suicide?
   YES   NO   If yes, enter 1 _____

10. Did a household member go to prison?
    YES   NO   If yes, enter 1 _____
    Now add up your "Yes" answers: _____. This is your ACE Score.

(Source: https://www.chcs.org/media/TA-Tool-Screening-for-ACEs-and-Trauma_020619.pdf)

Identifying ISLEEP Communication Skills

Video reenactment of encounter between dentist and trauma survivor.
Verbal and non-verbal ISLEEP communication skills by timestamp.

0:00 Introduce

0:31 Solicit and listen

0:50 Reflecting back after listening

0:57 Solicit/listen/empathize

1:10 Validate

1:20 Solicit/listen/empathize

1:40 Introduce plan for the visit

2:15 Solicit/listen/empathize (non verbal)

2:50 Validate

3:30 Explain, Power (offer option if pain arises)

3:40 Solicit/listen

4:20 Empathy (non verbal) and sympathy

4:40 Validate

4:50 Compassion (empathy plus the wish to help)

Identifying ISLEEP Communication Skills and Interventions for Procedural Pain and Anxiety (IPPA)

a. Dental Patient After a Dental Restoration (Video):
"What was helpful to you during the procedure?"
  i. "Talking and informing me of what you were going to do": Explain (ISLEEP skill)
  ii. "Reminder of breathing": Diaphragmatic breathing and mindfulness of the breath (IPPA)
  iii. "Making sure that I'm OK… checking in": Solicit (ISLEEP)
  iv. "Counting": Distraction (IPPA)

b. Survivor of Childhood Abuse: "My Very Best Experience With a Doctor Before Surgery"
He looked at me in the face:
  Eye contact (nonverbal communication, IPPA)
He said, "You look afraid."
  Empathize/validate (ISLEEP)
He came over and he held my hand:
  Expressive touch (IPPA)
He talked to me in a kind voice:
  Tone of voice (nonverbal communication, IPPA)
He asked me who was my favorite person:
  Interconnect (ISLEEP)
We talked about it… until they gave me the anesthesia and then I fell asleep:
  Interconnect (ISLEEP) and distraction (IPPA)

c. Sally's Visit to the Dental Clinic (new, improved version)
Stabbing, throbbing toothache in the middle of the night, again. Sally had been having pain for months in her lower left back tooth. She couldn't afford treatment and dreaded having dental work done ever since her traumatic dental experience as a child. So, she medicated herself for months and went to the ER once, too. Finally, she couldn't take it anymore.

The dental clinic nearby was swamped on the day she had her appointment. After being greeted warmly by the receptionist, she hears her name and sees a woman smiling at her ___Nonverbal Communication___ (IPPA) from the door to the clinic.
Assistant: Hi, my name is Ashley and I am a dental assistant. ___Introduce___ (ISLEEP skill). Is this your first time to our clinic? ___Interconnect___ (ISLEEP skill).
Sally: *Nods, butterflies in her stomach.*
A: Welcome! I see you have come from a distance. How was your drive? ___Interconnect (with Solicit)___ (ISLEEP skill).
S: I got stuck in a bad traffic jam.
A: It's getting harder to drive in this area with so much traffic! ___Empathy___ (ISLEEP skill). Are you ready to follow me to our room? ___Power (with Solicit)___ (ISLEEP skill).
S: *Nods and follows the assistant down a long hall to the treatment room.*
A: What brings you here today? ___Solicit___ (ISLEEP skill).
S: Bad pain in this broken tooth. It's been going on for months. *Points to the upper left tooth.*
A: That sounds really uncomfortable! I'm sorry you've been having this problem___Empathy___ (ISLEEP skill). How has this affected you in the day to day? ___Solicit___ (ISLEEP skill).
S: I can't sleep at night, which makes it hard to deal with my kids and my job.
A: That sounds really hard. ___Empathy___ (ISLEEP skill). It would be helpful to get a picture of the tooth so we can see the parts that are under the gum. ___Explain___ (ISLEEP skill) Is that OK? ___ Power___ (ISLEEP skill).

S: *Nods in approval.*

A: I'm going to recline the chair a bit and put a heavy shield on you now.____Explain_____ (ISLEEP), okay? _____Power_____ (ISLEEP skill)

S: Actually, I have a bad neck. Do you have a pillow? It would help a lot.

A: Sure! *She tucks pillow behind Sally, who adjusts it a bit until comfortable.* Ready? _____Power_____ (ISLEEP skill) *Ashley rests her hand gently on Sally's shoulder as she lowers the chair into position.* ____ Expressive touch_____ (IPPA).

I'm going to place this x-ray device next to the tooth, and then I'll need you to hold still until you hear the beep. __Explain_____ (ISLEEP skill). Ready?_____ Power_____ (ISLEEP skill).

S: *Gagging a bit.*

A: I have a suggestion—something that helps a lot of people in this situation. Would you like to try holding your foot up for about 10 seconds? ___Distraction/Power_____ (IPPA and ISLEEP skill). Perfect, thank you!
Ashley leaves to get Dr. M.

Dr. M: Hello, Sally! Welcome to our clinic. I'm Dr. M. ___Introduce_____ (ISLEEP skill). I understand you have a painful tooth. Sorry to hear about that! ___Empathy_____ (ISLEEP skill). *He sits down making eye contact.* _____Nonverbal communication_____ (IPPA). Can you tell me what the symptoms have been? _____Solicit_____ (ISLEEP skill).

S: A lot of pain for months. I've been taking a lot of pain meds, but it doesn't always help. I wish I could get the tooth out.

Dr. M: Sounds really uncomfortable! _____Empathy_____ (ISLEEP skill). If it's ok ____ Power_____ (ISLEEP skill) I would like to look in your mouth now to see what our options are. ____Explain_____ (ISLEEP skill).

S: Okay.
Dr. M performs intraoral exam.

Dr. M: Unfortunately, it looks like the tooth is not salvageable. Our options are to do nothing, which I would not recommend since the infection will continue to grow, or to take the tooth out, which we could do today. ___Explain, Power (implied by offering options)_____ (two ISLEEP skills).

S: I think I would like to take it out now.

Dr. M: OK. What concerns or worries do you have about getting the tooth out? _____ Solicit_____ (ISLEEP skill).

S: I am terrified of needles! I had a bad experience as a child and have been terrified ever since.

Dr. M: I can imagine how hard it would be for you after a bad childhood experience. It makes sense! _____ Empathy_____ (ISLEEP skill). I will do everything possible to make it easy for you. ____ Explain_____ (ISLEEP skill). And you can stop me at any time—if you can't talk just raise your hand.____Power_____ (ISLEEP skill). Here's what I can do for you: we can numb the tooth with a gel, then the numbing medicine. After a few minutes we will test the tooth to make sure it is numb. You will feel some pressure even if you are totally numb. ____Explain_____ (ISLEEP skill). My assistant, Ashley, and I work with a lot of people who have dental anxiety, and we are here to support you. I encourage you to take a few deep breaths, filling up the belly like a balloon ___ Diaphragmatic Breathing_____ (IPPA). Would you like to try right now with me? ____Power_____ (ISLEEP skill). We know that this kind of breathing helps the body to relax. Many people tend to hold their breath when they are nervous, so I will remind you every now and then to notice and feel your breath.____Mindfulness of the breath_____ (IPPA).

A: Sally, I would like to go over the risks of the tooth extraction and then we will get your blood pressure. _____Explain_____ (ISLEEP skill). Is that okay? ____Power_____ (ISLEEP skill). *After obtaining consent and preoperative vital signs… Would you be interested in some headphones with music or nature sounds? _____ Distraction_____ (IPPA).

S: That would be great! *She scans the options.* I love the beach. I'll try this one with ocean sounds and music.

A: Enjoy! Many people find it helpful to imagine the beach with all the senses…what it smells like, feels like, sounds like. _____Mental Imagery_____ (IPPA)
Dr. M returns.

Dr. M: I'm going to put the chair back now. _____ Explain_____ (ISLEEP skill), okay? _____Power_____ (ISLEEP skill).

Here is the numbing gel. ___Explain___ (ISLEEP skill). *He gently retracts Sally's cheek as he tunes into the sensations of warmth and reconnects with an intention of care.* ___Mindful Procedural Touch___ (IPPA).

Dr. M: Now I'm going to give you the numbing medicine and you may feel a slight pinch. ___Explain___ (ISLEEP skill). If it's okay, ___Power___ (ISLEEP skill) I'm going to wiggle your cheek to make it more comfortable. ___Explain___ (ISLEEP skill). *He begins to inject local anesthesia while wiggling the cheek.* ___Non-pain Stimulus___ (IPPA). *While injecting slowly….*Check in with your breathing. See if you can notice where your belly is in the breathing cycle—going up, or down or in between. ___Mindfulness of the breath___ (IPPA). How was that? ___Solicit___ (ISLEEP skill).

S: Not bad at all! Thank you!

Dr. M: Let's wait a few minutes now for the tooth to numb and then check to make sure it is comfortable for you. ___Explain___ (ISLEEP skills).

After a few minutes:

Dr. M: Are you ready? ___Power___ (ISLEEP skill).

S: Ready as I'll ever be.

Dr. M: I'm going to apply a little pressure first. ___Explain___ (ISLEEP skill) How does this feel? ___Solicit___ (ISLEEP skill).

S: Fine.

Dr. M: Okay. I'm going to apply a little more pressure now. And now I'm going to apply pressure for a few seconds. ___Gradual Exposure___ (IPPA). Are you still doing okay? ___Solicit___ (ISLEEP skill).

Assistant: Check in with your breathing. See if you can soften your belly and let the air flow down there. ___Diaphragmatic Breathing___ (IPPA) *After a short time the tooth is out.*

Dr. M: Are you doing OK? ___Solicit___ (ISLEEP skill).

Thank you for your trust in us. You did it! Ashley will give you some instructions on how to care for yourself at home. ___Explain___ (ISLEEP skill). What questions do you have before I go? ___Solicit___ (ISLEEP skill).

S: Can I make an appointment to have all my teeth fixed here? I am so grateful for your help today. You and Ashley were great!

A few hours later Dr. M calls Sally ___Postoperative communication___ (IPPA).

Dr. M: Hello this is Dr. M from the dental clinic calling for Sally ___Introduce___ (ISLEEP skill).

S: Thank you so much for calling!

Dr. M: How is the area we worked on…feeling comfortable? ___Solicit___ (ISLEEP skill)

S: Yes, I am doing great. Thank you so much.

Dr. M: You are welcome. Glad to hear you are feeling well. You must be relieved ___Empathy___ (ISLEEP skill).

S: I am!

Dr. M: Take good care and don't hesitate to call if any questions or issues arise! ___Explain/Power with options___ (two ISLEEP skills).

CARE Measure and Corresponding ISLEEP Skill

┌───┐

CARE Patient Feedback Measure for

Please write today's date here:

☐☐ / ☐☐ / ☐☐
D D   M M   Y Y

Please rate the following statements about today's consultation.

Please mark the box like this ☑ with a ball point pen. If you change your mind just cross out your old response and make your new choice. Please answer every statement.

How good was the practitioner at...	Poor	Fair	Good	Very Good	Excellent	Does not apply
1) Making you feel at ease (introducing him/herself, explaining his/her position, being friendly and warm towards you, treating you with respect; not cold or abrupt)	☐	☐	☐	☐	☐	☐
2) Letting you tell your "story" (giving you time to fully describe your condition in your own words; not interrupting, rushing or diverting you)	☐	☐	☐	☐	☐	☐
3) Really listening (paying close attention to what you were saying; not looking at the notes or computer as you were talking)	☐	☐	☐	☐	☐	☐
4) Being interested in you as a whole person (asking/knowing relevant details about your life, your situation; not treating you as "just a number")	☐	☐	☐	☐	☐	☐
5) Fully understanding your concerns (communicating that he/she had accurately understood your concerns and anxieties; not overlooking or dismissing anything)	☐	☐	☐	☐	☐	☐
6) Showing care and compassion (seeming genuinely concerned, connecting with you on a human level; not being indifferent or "detached")	☐	☐	☐	☐	☐	☐
7) Being positive (having a positive approach and a positive attitude; being honest but not negative about your problems)	☐	☐	☐	☐	☐	☐
8) Explaining things clearly (fully answering your questions; explaining clearly, giving you adequate information; not being vague)	☐	☐	☐	☐	☐	☐
9) Helping you to take control (exploring with you what you can do to improve you health yourself; encouraging rather than "lecturing" you)	☐	☐	☐	☐	☐	☐
10) Making a plan of action with you (discussing the options, involving you in decisions as much as you want to be involved; not ignoring your views)	☐	☐	☐	☐	☐	☐

Comments: If you would like to add further comments on this consultation, please do so here.

└───┘

Find the CARE measure at https://caremeasure.stir.ac.uk/CAREEng.pdf or Mercer SW, Maxwell M, Heaney D, Watt GC. The consultation and relational empathy (CARE) measure: development and preliminary validation and reliability of an empathy-based consultation process measure. *Fam Pract.* 2004;21(6):699–705.

CARE Measure Question	Corresponding ISLEEP Skill
1	Introduce, Interconnect
2	Solicit, Listen
3	Listen
4	Interconnect, Solicit
5	Empathize
6	Empathize
7	Explain, Reassure
8	Explain
9	Power (of the patient)
10	Power (of the patient)

Journal of Mindfulness Practices

Date	Practice/Technique	Duration	Emotions	Body Sensations	Thoughts

INDEX